# Financial Management for Pharmacists

## *A Decision-Making Approach*

**Third Edition**

# Financial Management for Pharmacists

## *A Decision-Making Approach*

### Third Edition

## NORMAN V. CARROLL, RPh, PhD

*Professor of Pharmacy Administration*
*School of Pharmacy*
*Virginia Commonwealth University*
*Richmond, Virginia*

Wolters Kluwer | Lippincott Williams & Wilkins
Health

Philadelphia · Baltimore · New York · London
Buenos Aires · Hong Kong · Sydney · Tokyo

*Acquisitions Editor:* David Troy
*Managing Editor:* Meredith L. Brittain
*Marketing Manager:* Marisa O'Brien
*Production Editor:* Bridget Meyer
*Project Manager:* Julie Montalbano
*Design Coordinator:* Doug Smock
*Artist:* Bob Galindo
*Compositor:* International Typesetting and Composition
*Printer:* Strategic Content Imaging

**Library of Congress Cataloging-in-Publication Data**

Carroll, Norman V.
    Financial management for pharmacists: a decision-making approach
  / Norman V. Carroll—3rd ed.
        p. ; cm.
    Includes bibliographical references and index.
    ISBN-13: 978-0-7817-6239-7 (alk. paper)
    1. Pharmacy—Practice—Finance.   I. Title.
    [DNLM:   1. Economics, Pharmaceutical.   2. Financial Management—methods.     QV 736 C319f 2008]
  RS100. C28 2008
    362.1'7820681—dc22

2006024850

13  14  15  16  17
    6   7  8  9  10

*To Charlotte, who else?*

# Preface

F *inancial Management for Pharmacists,* 3$^{rd}$ edition, was developed to meet the need for a pharmacy text that would cover the basics of financial accounting, managerial accounting, and finance.

## ORGANIZATIONAL PHILOSOPHY

The book begins with a basic introduction to financial accounting. This includes chapters on reading and interpreting financial statements, preparation of financial statements, and a discussion of accounting for inventories and cost of goods sold (Chapters 1 through 4). The material on interpretation of financial statements (Chapter 2) is a prerequisite for most of the remaining chapters. The chapters on preparing financial statements and accounting for inventory and cost of goods sold (Chapters 3 and 4) are not. These chapters can be skipped in courses that do not have sufficient time (or interest) to cover the mechanics of financial accounting.

The remaining chapters deal with those managerial accounting and finance topics of greatest relevance to pharmacy managers. Besides explaining and demonstrating the necessary calculations, the chapters in this section demonstrate the use of financial management techniques to address common managerial problems. This is done through use of detailed examples and problems. For example, the chapter on break-even analysis (Chapter 8) demonstrates use of the technique in pricing and advertising decisions, and the chapter on pricing (Chapter 9) explains how to calculate the cost of providing an asthma counseling service. The fundamentals of financial management are as applicable and necessary in HMO, hospital, and long-term care pharmacies as in traditional independent pharmacies. I have attempted to demonstrate this by including examples from a wide variety of practice sites.

The book concludes with an appendix that contains answers to the questions and problems posed throughout the text.

## WHAT IS NEW IN THIS EDITION

In addition to updating examples and problems, several significant changes have been made for this third edition. The pricing chapter (Chapter 9) has been revised to provide additional consideration to demand and especially to the interaction of unit costs, volume, demand, and price. Furthermore, a section has been added to address the common situation of pricing when the price is set by a third-party payer. Finally, the section on ingredient cost has been expanded to include MAC and WAC.

A new chapter on decision analysis (Chapter 16) has been added to the text, for two reasons. First, it presents and explains decision analysis as a technique that can be used to assist and inform decision making. Second, it augments the material on pharmacoeconomics (Chapter 15). This makes the text more useful for courses that include a pharmacoeconomics module. As with most of the other chapters, this chapter assumes that pharmacists not only need to be familiar with the techniques of financial management, they need to know how to perform the calculations and apply them to pharmacy-related problems. I believe this material will become increasingly important as pharmacists are called upon to incorporate cost-effectiveness into formulary decisions.

## SUPPLEMENTAL WEB PAGE

This edition is accompanied by a web page (connection.lww.com/carroll) to support faculty who use the text. This page, which will be available to instructors who adopt the text, will feature additional problem sets, financial management cases and exercises, slide sets, and sample examinations. In addition to the material that I post, interested faculty will be encouraged to share their own materials.

# Reviewers

**Karl D. Fiebelkorn, BS Pharm, MBA**

Assistant Dean for Student Affairs
  and Professional Relation
University at Buffalo
School of Pharmacy and Pharmaceutical
  Sciences
Amherst, New York

**Laurence Kennedy, PhD**

College of Pharmacy and Health Sciences
Butler University
Indianapolis, Indiana

**Warren Richards, PhD**

Assistant Dean and Department Chair
Palm Beach Atlantic University
West Palm Beach, Florida

**Albert Wertheimer, PhD, MBA**

Director, Center for Pharmaceutical Health
  Services Research
Department of Pharmacy Practice
Temple University School of Pharmacy
Philadelphia, Pennsylvania

# Acknowledgments

I am grateful to the Office of Instructional Development at the University of Georgia for funding the development of the first edition of this text through the Lily Teaching Fellows Program, to the students and colleagues who have provided comments and feedback about previous editions, and to the anonymous reviewers who provided suggestions and comments for the revisions.

# Contents

CHAPTER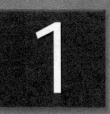

# Introduction to Financial Management

After completing this chapter, the student should be able to:

1. Discuss the importance of financial management to pharmacists,
2. Explain the goals of financial management and why they are relevant for pharmacies,
3. List and briefly describe the four most common financial statements, and
4. Discuss the limitations of financial management.

Pharmacy practice has changed dramatically over the last several years. Pharmacists are more likely to be employees than owners; to work for large organizations, such as hospitals, chain pharmacies, and managed-care pharmacies, than in small, independently owned pharmacies; and to have clinically oriented, patient care responsibilities rather than purely distributive duties. Although these changes have been associated with a dramatic decline in the number of pharmacists who own their pharmacies, they have not affected the number who are managers. In fact, the need for pharmacy managers has increased. This has occurred because large organizations, such as major hospital pharmacies, managed-care pharmacies, and chain pharmacies, need pharmacist managers for coordination and direction.

The need for pharmacist managers has also increased as technicians and automation have assumed more dispensing functions. Pharmacist managers are needed to supervise technicians and to manage the increased use of dispensing technology. Pharmacists have also found ownership and management opportunities in a variety of new settings. Contemporary pharmacists hold management and ownership positions in home health care and home IV infusion businesses, long-term care consulting organizations, disease management companies, pharmacy benefit managers (PBMs), insurance companies, and pharmaceutical care training companies.

Managers are responsible for planning, organizing, and controlling resources so that the organizations in which they are employed meet their goals. Many contemporary pharmacists meet this definition of a manager. Owners of independent pharmacies continue to function as managers, as do directors of hospital pharmacies. Chain pharmacies employ pharmacists as pharmacy and store managers, district managers, and directors of professional operations. Large hospitals and managed-care organizations employ pharmacists as clinical coordinators and formulary managers.

The essence of the manager's job is making decisions. Many of these decisions have important financial implications. The purpose of this text is to help pharmacists develop the skills they need to make more effective financial decisions.

Financial management focuses on making wise decisions about obtaining and using financial resources. These resources include both funds that the owners of an organization have invested in it and funds that the organization has borrowed. Pharmacist managers face many such decisions: how much inventory to carry, which sources of supply to use, how to set prices, which third-party prescription plans to participate in, which drugs to include on a formulary, whether a new disease management service will be profitable, whether the hospital should open a pharmacist-managed hypertension clinic. Being familiar with the tools and techniques of financial management will help pharmacists make better decisions when faced with such questions.

## GOALS OF FINANCIAL MANAGEMENT

The principal goal of financial management is to increase the value of the organization. A major part of achieving this goal is making efficient use of financial resources. Pharmacies, for example, carry inventories of prescription and nonprescription drugs. They must invest cash, a scarce financial resource, to buy inventories. Pharmacies make the most efficient use of cash that is invested in inventories when they carry the smallest amount of inventory necessary to meet consumer demand. Carrying larger inventories is inefficient because it takes cash away from other, more productive uses.

Making the most efficient use of financial resources is more important than ever before in pharmacy practice. Pharmacies of all types face substantial competition and economic challenges. The community pharmacy market has become increasingly competitive. Ambulatory consumers can obtain their prescription medicines from a number of outlets including pharmacies in supermarkets and mass merchandising stores (such as K-Mart and Wal-Mart), mail-order pharmacies, ambulatory care clinics, and physicians' offices, as well as traditional chain and independent community pharmacies. All of these face financial pressures from the reimbursement policies of government, managed-care, and other third-party prescription programs intent on controlling prescription drug costs. These policies have dramatically decreased the prices and gross margins that pharmacies receive for prescriptions. In the new competitive environment, pharmacies must use financial resources efficiently if they are to survive and grow.

Hospital pharmacies face similar financial pressures. Insurance companies, managed-care organizations, and federal and state governments have instituted a number of programs to control the increases in hospital costs. The federal Prospective Pricing System, for example, mandates that hospitals be paid no more than a fixed and predetermined amount for each inpatient with a given diagnosis. If the hospital spends more than this amount to treat the patient, it must pay for the excess. The federal government has also implemented prospective pricing programs for ambulatory care services provided in hospitals and for long-term care facilities (nursing homes).

Private insurers and managed-care organizations have implemented similar programs. As a result, hospitals and long-term care facilities must manage resources efficiently or face bankruptcy. The pressure that cost containment efforts have placed on these facilities is passed down to each department—including the pharmacy. To prosper in this environment, pharmacy managers must understand and be able to communicate the financial implications of decisions they make and programs they plan.

Pharmacies of other types—those in health maintenance organizations (HMOs), those providing home IV infusion services, and those providing consulting services to long-term care facilities—face similar pressures to control their costs. To survive and thrive in the cost-conscious health care environment, pharmacist managers must have a thorough understanding of the principles of financial management.

As these examples illustrate, financial management is as necessary and appropriate for nonprofit organizations, such as hospital pharmacies, as for profit-making firms. Both have limited resources and both are under considerable competitive pressures to make the best use of them. Using resources efficiently maximizes the value and effectiveness of both types of organizations. Even in nonprofit organizations, there is no excuse for using funds inefficiently.

## ACCOUNTING AND FINANCIAL MANAGEMENT

A proper understanding of the tools and techniques of financial management requires a basic working knowledge of accounting. Accounting is a specialized language used to communicate financial information. This information is communicated via *financial statements*.

Accounting data, and the financial statements developed from them, are maintained because they aid decision making. Financial statements facilitate decision making in three areas. First, financial statements provide information to decision makers. With this information, decision makers can better assess the financial implications of various decisions they must make. For example, bankers are decision makers. Before making loans, they will carefully evaluate the financial statements submitted by applicants to decide whether they can repay the loans. Managers are also decision makers. They use financial statements, for example, to make pricing decisions, to help decide whether to hire additional personnel, to decide whether to buy new equipment, and to decide which services to offer.

Second, financial statements aid decision makers by reporting the results of past decisions. The prudence of a banker's past lending decisions will be reflected in his or her current financial statements. Likewise, a manager who makes poor service and pricing decisions will notice, on financial statements, a decrease in profits.

Finally, financial statements keep track of a range of financial items such as cash, debts, and assets. Decision makers need this information to efficiently and effectively manage their organizations.

Financial statements provide decision makers with the following types of information:

1. Present financial status of the business. The balance sheet, or statement of financial position, indicates what a business owns and what it owes at one point in time.
2. Past profit performance of the business. The income statement, also called the profit and loss statement, indicates whether the business made a profit or suffered a loss over some period of time.

3.  Where the business is getting its *cash* and how it is spending it. This is found on the statement of changes in financial position or the cash flow statement.
4.  How the owners' investment in the business has changed over some period of time. This information is found in the statement of capital or the statement of retained earnings.

The income statement, balance sheet, and capital statement are presented and discussed in the next chapter. The cash flow statement is introduced in the next chapter and discussed in more depth in a later chapter.

## LIMITATIONS OF FINANCIAL MANAGEMENT

Financial management is a tool that managers can use to better assess the financial implications of decisions they face. Its use should be limited to deciding among potential courses of action that will help the pharmacy to reach its goals. In most cases, it should not be used to decide what those goals are, nor should most decisions be based solely on financial criteria. For example, a hospital pharmacy could decrease its expenses, and maintain its revenues, by switching from unit-dose to multiple-dose drug distribution and by cutting out all clinical and educational services. If the pharmacy's decisions were based solely on financial criteria, a financial analysis might show the advisability of this course of action. But a hospital pharmacy has a higher and more basic mission than to operate as cheaply and profitably as possible. Its primary mission is to provide pharmaceutical services that improve patient care. Unit-dose distribution and clinical and educational services substantially improve patient care. Consequently, the decision of whether to offer them should not be made solely on the basis of financial criteria. On the other hand, given that a pharmacy has limited financial resources, the decision as to which particular clinical and educational services to offer would benefit from a financial analysis.

Financial statements do not contain all the information, or in many cases even the most important information, about the factors that affect the finances of a pharmacy. Such necessary data as the state of the national and local economy, the demand for the organization's product or service, the extent and nature of the competition, and the health and loyalty of key employees are not found in financial statements. This is because financial statements deal only with those events and factors that can be readily expressed in monetary terms. In using and interpreting financial statements properly, managers must keep these limitations in mind.

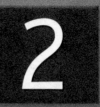

# Financial Statements

After reading this chapter, the student should be able to:

1. List and describe the primary financial statements used by pharmacies,
2. List and describe the major sections and types of information found in each of the major financial statements,
3. Explain the differences between accrual-based revenues and expenses and cash flow,
4. Compare and contrast the cash and accrual methods of accounting,
5. Define depreciation expense and accumulated depreciation,
6. Compare and contrast three major methods of calculating depreciation expense, and
7. Calculate the annual depreciation expense for a fixed asset given its acquisition cost, useful life, and residual value.

This chapter presents and discusses four financial statements used by pharmacies: the income statement, balance sheet, capital statement, and sources and uses statement. This is followed by a brief explanation of a concept that is fundamental to understanding financial statements—the accrual method of accounting. Finally, the chapter presents the concept and methods of depreciation.

## BALANCE SHEET

The balance sheet, which may also be called the statement of financial position, reports the financial status of the business. It tells what a business owns (its assets), what it owes (its liabilities), and how much is left over (owner equity), at a *specific point in time*.

The fundamental balance sheet equation is:

$$\text{ASSETS} = \text{LIABILITIES} + \text{OWNERS' EQUITY}$$

This equation states that assets must always equal the sum of liabilities plus owners' equity. If assets decrease, there must be a corresponding decrease in either liabilities or owners' equity (or their sum). If liabilities increase, either assets must increase or owners' equity must decrease.

## Components of the Balance Sheet

An example of a balance sheet is shown in Figure 2-1. The balance sheet consists of three major sections: assets, liabilities, and owners' equity.

## Assets

*Assets* are defined as valuable resources that are owned or controlled by the business and were acquired at a measurable cost. Examples include cash, accounts receivable, delivery cars, and computers.

Assets are categorized as either current or noncurrent. *Current assets* are those that will be sold, consumed, or converted to cash within the current operating cycle of the business (which is usually 1 year). Current assets are listed on the balance sheet in order of their *liquidity*, or the ease with which they are converted to cash. The current assets commonly appearing on the balance sheets of pharmacies include cash, accounts receivable, inventories, prepaid expenses, and short-term investments.

*Cash* refers to coin, currency, and other items, such as personal checks, charge card receipts, and travelers' checks, which banks will accept for deposit. Cash is the most liquid asset.

*Accounts receivable* are amounts owed to the pharmacy by its customers as a result of the ordinary extension of credit. In other words, accounts receivable are customers' promises to pay for merchandise that they have purchased on credit from the pharmacy. Conceptually, accounts receivable may be divided into those arising from credit sales and those arising from third-party sales. Credit sales are charge sales made to customers who themselves pay for the merchandise they have purchased on credit. This is the normal situation of a customer charging merchandise and then paying for it once he or she has been billed. Third-party sales are charge sales made to a customer of the pharmacy but paid for by a third party—usually an insurance company, a managed-care organization, or Medicaid. In a pharmacy, most third-party sales are for prescriptions.

Two different types of *inventories* may appear on the balance sheet: merchandise inventories and supplies inventories. The merchandise inventory is, by far, the largest and most important. In many cases, the balance sheet of a pharmacy will have only one entry labeled "Inventory." When this occurs, the notation refers to merchandise inventory. Merchandise inventory consists of goods that the pharmacy has purchased for resale. Examples of merchandise inventory in a pharmacy include over-the-counter (OTC) and prescription drugs, cosmetics, and first aid supplies.

Supplies inventory consists of goods that were purchased for use in the business rather than for resale. Supplies have low unit value and will be consumed within the year. Examples of supplies include bags, pens, and prescription labels and vials.

**Bulldog Pharmacy**
**Balance Sheet**
**12-31-20X1**

### Assets

Current assets

| | | |
|---|---|---|
| Cash | $ 71,600 | |
| Accounts receivable | 92,400 | |
| Inventory | 191,600 | |
| Total current assets | 355,600 | |

Noncurrent assets

| | | |
|---|---|---|
| Fixtures & equipment | 80,000 | |
| Less accumulated depreciation | 35,600 | |
| Net fixtures & equipment | 44,400 | |
| Total assets | | 400,000 |

### Liabilities

Current liabilities

| | | |
|---|---|---|
| Accounts payable | 64,800 | |
| Notes payable (current) | 12,000 | |
| Accrued tax payable | 23,600 | |
| Total current liabilities | 100,400 | |

Noncurrent liabilities

| | | |
|---|---|---|
| Mortgage | 52,800 | |
| Total liabilities | | 153,200 |

### Owners' equity

| | | |
|---|---|---|
| Capital stock | 25,000 | |
| Retained earnings | 221,800 | |
| Total owners' equity | | 246,800 |
| Total liabilities and owners' equity | | 400,000 |

**FIGURE 2–1** Balance sheet.

At certain times during the year, a pharmacy may have more cash than it needs to conduct its business. Rather than simply leaving the cash in a checking account, which draws little or no interest, the pharmacy may invest its excess cash in money market accounts, stocks, bonds, or certificates of deposit, which earn higher rates of interest. When management intends to sell these investments within the current operating cycle of the business (because the business will need cash), the investments are called *short-term investments,* temporary investments, or marketable securities.

*Prepaid expenses* arise from payments made for a good or service in an accounting period prior to the one during which the good or service is actually used. For example, a pharmacy may be required to prepay its rent. This would mean that January's rent would have to be paid in December. The amount of January's rent would be listed on a balance sheet prepared in December as an asset called "prepaid rent."

*Noncurrent assets* are those that under normal conditions are not sold, consumed, or converted to cash within the normal operating cycle of the business, or 1 year. They are assets that have been purchased for use in the business, which usually have high unit costs, and which are expected to last for several years. Examples include land, buildings, fixtures, cars, and computers. Noncurrent assets are also referred to as *fixed assets* or as *fixtures and equipment*.

Note that in the balance sheet shown in Figure 2-1, noncurrent assets are described in three separate lines. The first line states the acquisition cost of noncurrent assets. This is what the business paid for the assets when they were initially purchased. The second line states the amount of *accumulated depreciation*. This is an accountant's estimate of the amount of the assets' value that has been lost, or used up, as of the date on the balance sheet. The third line gives the net value of noncurrent assets. This is calculated as the acquisition cost less accumulated depreciation. (The net value of noncurrent assets is only a rough estimate of their market value, or the amount for which they could be sold.) Frequently a balance sheet will show only the net value of noncurrent assets.

## Liabilities

Liabilities are the business's debts. They arise from purchasing goods or services on credit or from borrowing money to finance the business's operations. As with assets, they are classified as either current or noncurrent.

*Current liabilities* consist of those debts that will come due during the current operating cycle of the business. For a pharmacy, the most commonly occurring current liabilities include accounts payable, short-term notes, accrued expenses, and the current portion of long-term debt.

*Accounts payable* are debts that arise from purchase of goods or services on credit. For example, purchase of accounting or janitorial services on credit would lead to an account payable. For a pharmacy, the vast majority of accounts payable come from purchase of merchandise inventory. Accounts payable that arise from purchase of inventory may also be called "trade payables."

*Current* or *short-term notes payable* are debts evidenced by formal, signed agreements called promissory notes. Notes payable arise when the pharmacy borrows money. When it does so, it must sign a written agreement that specifies when repayment must be made and at what rate of interest.

When a pharmacy orders inventory from a wholesaler, no formal signed agreement is necessary. Thus, the resulting payable is an account payable. However, when the pharmacy gets a short-term loan from a bank, a promissory note is signed, and consequently, this is a note payable. The two are also different in that interest must be paid on a note payable but, assuming payment is made on time, no interest is paid on an account payable.

*Accrued expenses* are amounts owed for goods or services that have been used during the accounting period but for which payment has not been made. For example, as of the end of the accounting period, the pharmacy may owe its employees for salaries that will not be paid until sometime in the next accounting period. This might occur if the end of the accounting period fell in the middle of a 2-week pay period. In this situation, the balance sheet for the period would show an accrued expense called accrued salaries payable to recognize that the pharmacy owed salaries as of the end of the period.

On many long-term debts, such as a 5-year car loan or a 20-year mortgage, some portion may be due in the current year. The portion of long-term debt that is due the current year is, consequently, a current liability and is called the *current portion of long-term debt.* As an example, the amount of a pharmacy's mortgage that must be paid in the current accounting period may be listed as a current liability. (The amount due in later periods would be listed as a noncurrent liability.)

*Noncurrent liabilities* are debts that will come due after the current operating cycle of the business. Examples include car loans that are paid off over 5 years and mortgages that are paid off over 20 years. Noncurrent liabilities may also be recorded as note payable (long term), mortgage, or long-term debt.

## Owners' Equity

Owners' equity is the amount left over after liabilities are subtracted from assets. Owners' equity may also be called net worth, stockholders' equity, or capital. It arises from two sources—invested capital and retained earnings.

*Invested capital* consists of cash invested into the business by its owners. For a corporation, it is called *common or capital stock.* Accountants make a strict distinction between the finances of the business and the finances of the *owners* of the business. They consider them two separate and distinct entities. This is true even when the business is a sole proprietorship (a business owned by one person). Hence, a transfer of cash from the owner's personal account to the business account is considered an investment in the business.

Owners may also withdraw cash from the business. For a sole proprietorship or partnership, such withdrawals are referred to as *owner withdrawals.* For a corporation, they are called *dividends paid.* Dividends paid or owner withdrawals decrease invested capital and, consequently, owner equity.

*Retained earnings* are profits (or losses) that the business has made during its years of operation and that have been left in the business. Profits increase retained earnings, while losses decrease them.

For a corporation, the owners' equity section of the balance sheet has separate entries for both invested capital and retained earnings. A proprietorship has only one entry that includes both. This entry is written as "owner's name, Capital." For example, if I owned a business, my owners' equity section would be entitled "N. Carroll, Capital."

## INCOME STATEMENT

The income statement, which is also called the profit and loss statement, reports the *net income* of a business for a *specific period of time.* This period may be a month, a quarter, or a year. A pharmacy will have an income statement made at least once per year. Many pharmacies generate income statements monthly to allow them to more closely monitor sales and expenses.

The basic income statement equation is:

$$\text{Revenues} - \text{Expenses} = \text{Net Income}$$

*Revenues* are sales of merchandise normally sold by the business. For a pharmacy, all sales of prescription and OTC drugs, health and beauty aids, and sundries would be considered revenues. However, sale of a delivery car would not be a revenue. This is because the pharmacy does not, as a normal part of its business, sell delivery cars. Nor would cash invested in the business by its owners be considered a revenue. Again, it is because the money coming in is not a result of the normal operation of the business. For most pharmacies revenues *include both cash and credit sales.*

*Expenses* are costs that the business incurs to make sales or earn revenues. Expenses include all costs of operating the business. Examples are the cost of merchandise sold, salaries, utilities, and interest payments. Repayment of the principal amount of a loan would not be an expense, nor would owner withdrawals from the business. One expense requires special note. The *depreciation expense* is an estimate of the amount of noncurrent assets' value that has been used up during the current operating cycle. Unlike other expenses, no direct cash payments are made for the depreciation expense. Depreciation will be discussed in greater detail later in the chapter.

*Net income* is defined as the difference between revenues and expenses for a specific period of time. Net income is also called *net profit or earnings.*

## Income Statement for a Service Firm

A service firm is one that sells a service rather than a product. Examples include physicians' and dentists' practices, architectural firms, plumbers and exterminators, and consultants. These firms may call revenues "Billings" or "Fees for Service." A sample income statement for a service firm, Erwin Consultant Pharmacy Services, is shown in Figure 2-2. This business is a service firm because it provides pharmaceutical consulting services, but not products, to patients in nursing homes.

The income statement for a service firm contains sections for revenues, operating expenses, and income tax. As shown in Figure 2-2, Erwin Consulting Service had revenues of $155,000 for the year. It had operating expenses of $137,000. This included all costs of generating the $155,000 in revenue. In this particular case, the only

| **Erwin Consultant Pharmacy Services**<br>**Income Statement**<br>**For Year Ended 12-31-20X1** | | |
|---|---:|---:|
| Revenues | | $155,000 |
| Operating expenses | | |
| Salaries | $115,000 | |
| Rent | 15,000 | |
| Utilities | 7,000 | |
| Total operating expenses | | 137,000 |
| Operating income | | 18,000 |
| Income tax | | 6,000 |
| Net income | | $ 12,000 |

**FIGURE 2-2**   Income statement for a service firm.

operating expenses were salaries, rent on the office, and utilities. The difference between revenues and operating expenses was $18,000. This amount is referred to as operating income or as net income before taxes. On this amount, the business paid income tax of $6,000. This left a net income after taxes of $12,000.

## Income Statement for a Merchandising Firm

A merchandising firm is one that sells a tangible product. Examples include super-markets, hardware stores, automobile dealerships, and pharmacies. An income state-ment for a merchandising firm is shown in Figure 2-3. The major difference between

**Bulldog Pharmacy**
**Income Statement**
**For Year Ended 12-31-20X1**

| | | |
|---|---:|---:|
| Total sales | | $2,000,000 |
| Cost of goods sold | | |
| Beginning inventory | 258,200 | |
| Purchases | 1,540,120 | |
| Cost of goods available for sale | 1,798,320 | |
| Less ending inventory | 268,320 | |
| Cost of goods sold | | 1,530,000 |
| Gross margin | | 470,000 |
| Operating expenses | | |
| Salaries | 242,000 | |
| Advertising | 10,000 | |
| Insurance | 12,000 | |
| Store supplies | 10,000 | |
| Delivery service | 6,000 | |
| Computer expense | 6,000 | |
| Rent | 22,000 | |
| Utilities | 10,000 | |
| Depreciation expense | 8,000 | |
| Other operating expenses | 54,000 | |
| Total operating expenses | | 380,000 |
| Net income before taxes | | 90,000 |
| Income taxes | | 31,500 |
| Net income after taxes | | $   58,500 |

FIGURE 2–3  Income statement for a merchandising firm.

the income statements of service and merchandising firms is the *cost of goods sold* section. Because a merchandising firm generates revenues through sales of a tangible product, the cost to the firm of the products that it sells must be included on the income statement as an expense. This expense is referred to as the *cost of goods sold*. Cost of goods sold is not the same as merchandise inventory. Inventory consists of all goods that the pharmacy holds for resale in the normal course of its business. Inventory is an asset. When a pharmacy purchases inventory, it does not incur an expense. It simply exchanges assets—cash for inventory. The expense is incurred when the inventory is sold to a customer. When it is sold, the pharmacy incurs an expense. This expense is called *cost of goods sold*. So, when merchandise is purchased, it is an asset called inventory; when merchandise is sold, it becomes an expense called cost of goods sold.

As shown in Figure 2-3, the cost of goods sold (COGS) may be determined in the following manner. The amount of inventory that the pharmacy has at the beginning of the year is referred to as beginning inventory (BI). To the beginning inventory is added all purchases (P) that the pharmacy made during the year. Purchases consist of all merchandise that the pharmacy bought for resale to its customers. The sum of BI and P is known as cost of goods available for sale (COGAS). This is the total amount of merchandise that the pharmacy had available to sell over the entire year. The ending inventory (EI) is the amount of merchandise inventory on hand at the end of the year. Cost of goods sold is calculated by subtracting ending inventory from cost of goods available for sale. So, to summarize, COGS = BI + P − EI.

## STATEMENT OF RETAINED EARNINGS

The statement of retained earnings (Fig. 2-4) reports how the business's retained earnings have changed over some period. The statement lists the amount of retained earnings at the beginning of the period and major changes to retained earnings over the period. These include dividend payments or net losses, which decrease retained earnings, and net income and additional owner investment, which increase retained earnings.

---

**Bulldog Pharmacy**
**Statement of Retained Earnings**
**For Year Ended 12-31-20X1**

| | |
|---|---|
| Beginning balance | |
| Retained earnings, January 1, 20X1 | $183,300 |
| Add net income for 20X1 | 58,500 |
| Less dividends paid in 20X1 | 20,000 |
| | |
| Ending balance | |
| Retained earnings, December 31, 20X1 | $221,800 |

---

**FIGURE 2-4**    Statement of retained earnings.

**Bulldog Pharmacy**
**Capital Statement**
**For Year Ended 12-31-20X1**

| | |
|---|---:|
| Beginning balance | |
| Owner equity, January 1, 20X1 | $208,300 |
| Add net income for 20X1 | 58,500 |
| Add owner investment for 20X1 | 0 |
| Less dividends paid in 20X1 | 20,000 |
| Ending balance | |
| Owner equity, December 31, 20X1 | $246,800 |

**FIGURE 2–5**  Capital statement.

For sole proprietorships and partnerships, a comparable statement is the capital statement (Fig. 2-5). It shows how owners' equity (which is also called capital) has changed over some period. Net income and owner investment increase owner equity (or capital), whereas net losses and owner withdrawals decrease it.

## SOURCES AND USES STATEMENT

A pharmacy's revenues and expenses for a period of time are not the same as the amounts of cash taken in and paid out during that period. For this reason, the pharmacy needs one financial statement to report its revenues and expenses and another to report its cash flows. The income statement reports revenues and expenses for the year (or operating period). The *sources and uses statement* shows how a pharmacy obtained cash during the year (or operating period) and how it used that cash. The sources and uses statement may also be called a *cash flow statement* or *a statement of changes in financial position*. An example of a sources and uses statement is presented in Figure 2-6. It shows that Bulldog Pharmacy's largest sources of cash for 20X1 were profitable operation of the pharmacy (net income plus depreciation) and an increase in accounts payable. The largest uses included purchase of noncurrent assets and dividends paid. A more in-depth discussion of the sources and uses statement is presented in Chapter 12.

## CASH VERSUS ACCRUAL ACCOUNTING

Accountants must divide the life of the business into discrete accounting periods. For a pharmacy, an accounting period is usually 1 year. One of the major problems that accountants face is that of recording and matching revenues and expenses in the proper accounting periods. If revenues and expenses are not recognized in the proper accounting periods, then net income will be measured incorrectly. There are two common methods of determining the time period in which a revenue or expense should be recorded. These are the *cash* and the *accrual methods* of accounting.

| Bulldog Pharmacy<br>Sources and Uses Statement<br>For Year Ended 12-31-20X1 | |
| --- | --- |
| Sources of cash | |
| Net income | $58,500 |
| Add depreciation | 5,000 |
| Decrease in cash account | 4,000 |
| Increase in accounts payable | 8,000 |
| Increase in other current liabilities | 3,000 |
| Total sources of cash | $78,500 |
| Uses of cash | |
| Dividends paid | 20,000 |
| Purchase of noncurrent asset | 25,000 |
| Increase in accounts receivables | 4,000 |
| Increase in inventory | 15,000 |
| Decrease in notes payable | 6,000 |
| Decrease in mortgage | 8,500 |
| Total uses of cash | $78,500 |

**FIGURE 2–6**    Sources and uses statement.

In the cash method, revenues are recognized (that is, recorded as revenues) in the period during which cash is received and expenses are recognized in the period during which cash is paid out. For example, assume that Bulldog Pharmacy dispenses a prescription to Mrs. Jones in December of 20X5. If she pays for the prescription when she receives it, Bulldog Pharmacy will recognize a revenue for the 20X5 period. If she charges it and does not pay until January 20X6, the revenue will be recognized in the 20X6 accounting period. The cash method, while simple to understand and use, is not commonly used by pharmacies.

The accrual method is more commonly used. In the accrual system, revenues are recognized in the period during which *goods are delivered or services rendered*. This is not necessarily the same period that cash is received. To continue the example used earlier, under the accrual system, Bulldog Pharmacy would recognize a revenue in the period during which the prescription was delivered to Mrs. Jones—20X5—regardless of when payment was made. Thus, in the accrual system, both cash and credit sales are recognized as revenues at the time the sale is made, not necessarily when payment is received.

There are two ways of determining when expenses are recognized in the accrual system. First, expenses are recognized in the same accounting period as the associated revenue. Thus, all the costs of making sales in 20X5 are recognized as expenses in 20X5, regardless of when payment was made. For example, property taxes for 20X5 are considered expenses of 20X5 even though they may not be paid until 20X6 or even though they may have been paid in 20X4. Why? Because the property on which the taxes are due was used to generate revenues in 20X5.

A second way of defining expense recognition in the accrual system is that expenses are recognized in the period when the associated good or service is used. Thus, all utilities used in 20X5 are recognized as expenses in 20X5 even if the bill for December's utilities is not paid until January 20X6. Or, the cost of merchandise that a pharmacy sells is not recognized as an expense until the merchandise is actually sold. So, if a bottle of Maalox is purchased and paid for in December of 19X4 and sold in January of 19X5, its cost would be recognized as an expense in 19X5, the year in which it was sold. (When merchandise is purchased it is a current asset inventory. It only becomes an expense—cost of goods sold—when it has been sold.)

Pharmacies use the accrual system because it allows for the accurate matching of the revenues of an accounting period with the expenses required to generate those revenues. In other words, they use this method because it allows for the accurate measurement of net income.

## DEPRECIATION

Noncurrent assets are assets that are purchased for use in the operation of the pharmacy and that are expected to last longer than 1 year. Noncurrent assets are also known as fixed assets, operating assets, plant and equipment, and fixtures and equipment. Examples of fixed assets include delivery cars, computers, unit dose carts, buildings, and fixtures. Pharmacies purchase noncurrent assets because they need them to generate revenues. Pharmacies purchase computers, for example, to process prescription orders and store prescription records. These functions are necessary parts of the process of generating revenues from sale of prescriptions.

Over the period of its useful life, a noncurrent asset is used up, is worn out, or otherwise loses its value in the process of generating revenues. Because it is used to generate revenues, its cost must be recognized as an expense. And, because it is used to generate revenues over several years, its total cost cannot be recognized as an expense in the year during which it was purchased. Rather, part of its total cost must be recognized as an expense in each of the years of its useful life. This expense is called the *depreciation expense. Depreciation* is the process of systematically and rationally determining how much of a noncurrent asset's initial cost is recognized as an expense in each year of its life. (Land is an exception. Land may be used to generate revenues, but it is not worn out or used up in the process. Because it does not lose value, land is not depreciated.)

### Calculating Depreciation Data

Three amounts must be known or estimated before the annual depreciation expense can be calculated.

First, the asset's *acquisition cost* must be determined. This is the amount the pharmacy paid for the asset. In addition, acquisition cost includes any reasonable costs that the pharmacy incurred in acquiring the asset and putting it into operation. Thus, transportation, taxes, and set-up costs are recorded as part of the acquisition cost of a fixed asset.

Any costs of renovating or overhauling the asset that are incurred before putting it into use are also considered part of the acquisition cost. For example, if a pharmacy purchased a building and had it renovated before using it, both the purchase price and the cost of the renovation would be included in the acquisition cost.

Next, the asset's *useful life* must be estimated. This is the length of time that the pharmacy intends to use the asset. A pharmacy might, for example, estimate the useful life of its computer at 5 years and the useful life of its building at 30 years.

Finally, the asset's estimated *residual* or *salvage value* must be estimated. This is an estimate of what the asset will be worth at the end of its useful life. In making this estimate, the pharmacy must consider what the asset could be sold for, less any costs of disposing of the asset.

The estimated useful life and residual value of a fixed asset vary depending on the pharmacy's policies. For example, Bulldog Pharmacy may replace delivery cars every 3 years, whereas Tiger Pharmacy replaces them every 5 years. The annual depreciation expense for each pharmacy will be similar, despite the difference in useful lives, because the residual value of Bulldog Pharmacy's cars will be substantially higher than that of Tiger Pharmacy's cars.

Once these quantities are determined, the pharmacy must select a depreciation method.

## Methods of Depreciation

Pharmacies may select either of three methods for calculating the annual depreciation expense. In this section, each method will be discussed and illustrated with an example. The data for the example are given in Figure 2-7.

### Straight Line Method

The straight line method of depreciation is the simplest and most straightforward of the three methods. It assumes that noncurrent assets wear out or are used up at a constant rate. As a result, the depreciation expense is the same in each year of the asset's life. The annual depreciation expense is calculated by multiplying the asset's acquisition cost less residual value by the straight line rate of depreciation. The straight line

---

Piedmont Pharmacy purchased a computer for $35,000. The manager estimates that the computer will last 5 years and have a residual value of $5,000. For this problem, the following symbols will be used:

| | |
|---|---|
| Acquisition cost | C |
| Useful life | N |
| Residual value | R |
| Depreciation expense | D |
| Depreciation rate | r |

**FIGURE 2-7**   Sample depreciation problem data.

| Year | C-R | r | D |
|------|------|------|------|
| 1 | 30,000 | 1/5 | 6,000 |
| 2 | 30,000 | 1/5 | 6,000 |
| 3 | 30,000 | 1/5 | 6,000 |
| 4 | 30,000 | 1/5 | 6,000 |
| 5 | 30,000 | 1/5 | 6,000 |
| Total | | | 30,000 |

**FIGURE 2-8**    Calculation of annual depreciation expense using the straight line method.

rate of depreciation is equal to 1 divided by the asset's useful life. Using the symbols in Figure 2-7:

$$D = (C - R) \times 1/N$$

The calculation of straight line depreciation for the sample data is illustrated in Figure 2-8. As shown, in each year, the annual depreciation expense is calculated as cost minus residual value—$30,000—multiplied by the straight line rate of 1/5. Thus, the depreciation expense is $6,000 in each of the years of the computer's useful life.

## Accelerated Methods

The other two methods are called *accelerated methods* because they take off proportionally more of an asset's value in the early years of its life and proportionally less in later years. These methods are based on the assumption that the asset is more efficient or that it loses more of its value in the early years of its life. This is a reasonable assumption for many types of noncurrent assets. Cars, for example, lose much more of their value in the first year after their purchase than in later years. The two accelerated methods most commonly used are the *sum of years digits* and the *double declining balance* methods.

### Sum of Years Digits

To calculate the annual depreciation expense by the sum of years digits method, the asset's cost minus its residual value is multiplied by a fraction that decreases each year. The numerator of the fraction is the number of years of life the asset had remaining at the beginning of the current year. The denominator is the sum of years digits.

The calculation of depreciation by this method is shown in Figure 2-9. At the beginning of the first year during which the pharmacy used the computer, it had 5 years of useful life remaining. The sum of years digits is 5 + 4 + 3 + 2 + 1 = 15. The depreciation expense for the first year is calculated as cost minus residual value—$30,000—multiplied by 5/15. This yields a first-year depreciation expense of $10,000. The annual depreciation expense declines each year. At the beginning of the fifth year, only 1 year of useful life remains. The sum of years digits remains 15, and cost

| | Year | C-R | r | D |
|---|---|---|---|---|
| | 1 | 30,000 | 5/15 | 10,000 |
| | 2 | 30,000 | 4/15 | 8,000 |
| | 3 | 30,000 | 3/15 | 6,000 |
| | 4 | 30,000 | 2/15 | 4,000 |
| | 5 | 30,000 | 1/15 | 2,000 |
| Sum of years digits | 15 | | | |
| Total depreciation | | | | 30,000 |

**FIGURE 2-9**   Calculation of the annual depreciation expense using the sum of years digits method.

minus residual value remains $30,000. Thus, the depreciation expense for the last year of the computer's life is $30,000 \times 1/15 = $2,000.

## Double Declining Balance Method

The annual depreciation expense is calculated in the double declining balance method by multiplying the *book value* of the asset by twice (or double) the straight line rate of depreciation. The book value of an asset is its acquisition cost less accumulated depreciation. Note two things about this method. First, book value, the amount that is depreciated, declines each year. Second, the total amount of depreciation recognized over the life of the asset cannot exceed the asset's acquisition cost less its residual value.

Figure 2-10 shows calculation of the annual depreciation expense using this method. In the first year of the computer's use at the pharmacy, no depreciation has accumulated. Thus, the computer's book value is the same as its cost: $35,000. This amount is multiplied by double the straight line rate—or 2/5—to give the first year depreciation expense of $14,000. In the second year of the computer's life,

| Year | Book Value | r | D | Accumulated Depreciation |
|---|---|---|---|---|
| 1 | 35,000 | 2/5 | 14,000 | 14,000 |
| 2 | 21,000 | 2/5 | 8,400 | 22,400 |
| 3 | 12,600 | 2/5 | 5,040 | 27,440 |
| 4 | 7,560 | 2/5 | 2,560 | 30,000* |
| 5 | 5,000 | — | 0 | 30,000 |

*The calculated figure for depreciation is $3,024. This amount would depreciate the asset below its residual value. The amount actually charged—$2,560—is the amount needed to reduce the asset's book value to its residual value.

**FIGURE 2-10**   Calculation of the annual depreciation expense using the double declining balance method.

| Year | Straight Line Method | Sum of Years Digits | Double Declining Balance |
|---|---|---|---|
| 1 | 6,000 | 10,000 | 14,000 |
| 2 | 6,000 | 8,000 | 8,400 |
| 3 | 6,000 | 6,000 | 5,040 |
| 4 | 6,000 | 4,000 | 2,560 |
| 5 | 6,000 | 2,000 | 0 |
| Total amount depreciated | 30,000 | 30,000 | 30,000 |

**FIGURE 2–11**  Comparison of depreciation methods.

$14,000 of depreciation has been accumulated. Thus, book value for the second year is $35,000 − $14,000 = $21,000. This amount is multiplied by 2/5 to yield the second-year depreciation expense of $8,400.

This process is continued each year. However, in the fourth year, the calculated amount of depreciation would depreciate the asset below its residual value. Because this is not allowable, the amount of depreciation expense actually recognized in this year is the amount necessary to reduce the asset's book value to its residual value. There is no depreciation expense in the fifth year of the asset's life because the full amount of allowable depreciation has been recognized in the first 4 years.

## Comparison of Depreciation Methods

The data in Figure 2-11 compare the annual depreciation expenses for the sample problem as calculated by each method. This figure illustrates that accelerated methods do, in fact, recognize more of the asset's value as an expense in the early years of its life and less in the later years. However, the total amount of depreciation expense recognized over the life of the asset is the same for all methods.

## FINANCIAL VERSUS TAX ACCOUNTING

The methods presented in this chapter are ones that a pharmacy would use for its *financial* accounting. Financial accounting differs from *tax* accounting. The purpose of financial accounting is to develop financial statements that report the performance of the pharmacy to managers, owners, and potential investors. Financial accounting is governed by a set of rules called *Generally Accepted Accounting Principles*. These rules are developed and agreed upon by accountants.

The purpose of tax accounting is to determine the amount of income tax that the pharmacy must pay. Tax accounting is governed by rules and procedures developed by the Internal Revenue Service (IRS) and the tax courts. These rules frequently differ from Generally Accepted Accounting Principles.

Because of these differences, pharmacies may legally and legitimately account for depreciation using one method for financial purposes—that is, to report the pharmacy's performance to its owners, managers, and investors—and a different method for tax purposes. Pharmacies have commonly used the straight line method for financial reporting and an accelerated method for tax purposes. It is advantageous to use accelerated methods for tax purposes because they lower income taxes in the early years of an asset's life, and thus, defer tax payments until later years. The methods that the IRS will allow a pharmacy to use for depreciation are similar to the ones presented in this chapter. Readers interested in the precise calculation of depreciation for tax purposes should consult the IRS or a tax accountant.

### Suggested Readings

Anthony RN, Breitner LK. Essentials of Accounting. 8th Ed. Upper Saddle River, NJ: Prentice Hall, 2003.
Warren CS, Reeve JM, Fess PE. Accounting. 21st Ed. Mason, OH: Thomson South-Western, 2005.
Warren CS, Reeve JM, Fess PE. Financial Accounting. 9th Ed. Mason, OH: Thomson South-Western, 2005.

## QUESTIONS

1. Identify each of the following as either an asset, liability, owner equity, revenue, or expense.
   a. Rent
   b. Salaries
   c. Accounts payable
   d. Cash
   e. Accounts receivable
   f. Depreciation charge
   g. Mortgage
   h. Retained earnings
   i. Credit sales
2. On which financial statement would a manager find each of the following?
   a. Amount the business owed
   b. Amount of cash the business had
   c. Amount of cash the owners had invested in the business
   d. Amount of cash the owners had withdrawn from the business in the past year
   e. Business's profit for the past year
   f. Business's net worth
3. Indicate whether each of the following would increase, decrease, or have no effect on owner equity.
   a. Owner withdrew $550 from the business for personal use.
   b. Business paid dividends of $1,000.
   c. Business had a net loss of $4,000 for the year.
   d. Business purchased inventory on credit.
4. Calculate the missing amount for each of the following.
   a. Assets = $50,000, liabilities = $45,000, and owner equity = ?
   b. Owner equity = $10,000, liabilities = $240,000, and assets = ?
   c. Revenues = $500,000, expenses = $480,000, and net income = ?
   d. Revenues = $400,000, expenses = $410,000, and net income = ?

e. Owner equity at the beginning of the year was $50,000, net income for the year was $5,000, no additional owner investment or withdrawal was made during the year. Owner equity at the end of the year was ?

f. Owner equity at the beginning of the year was $50,000, net income for the year was $5,000, owner equity at the end of the year was $52,000, and owner withdrawal was ?

5. Which of the following would NOT be depreciated?
   a. Building
   b. Delivery car
   c. Bottle of Maalox
   d. All of the above

6. Fiddler Pharmacy has a delivery car. The car cost $5,000 when purchased. There is presently $3,500 worth of accumulated depreciation on the car. What is the book value of the car?
   a. $5,000
   b. $3,500
   c. $1,500
   d. $8,500

7. Assuming you could use either of the three available methods of depreciation for *income tax purposes*, which would be most advantageous?
   a. Straight line method because it maximizes net income in the early years of the asset's life
   b. Double declining balance method because it minimizes income taxes
   c. Double declining balance method because it defers income taxes to the later years of the asset's life

8. Which method of depreciation gives a greater depreciation expense over the entire life of the asset?
   a. Double declining balance
   b. Straight line
   c. Both give the same depreciation expense over the entire life of the asset.

# PROBLEMS

1. Boomer Pharmacy purchased a new computer for $10,000. The computer is expected to last for 3 years. At the end of 3 years, it is expected to be worth $1,000. Calculate the annual depreciation expense for each year of the computer's estimated useful life and the accumulated depreciation at the end of each year. Use the straight line and double declining balance methods of depreciation.

2. Piggly Wiggly Pharmacy bought a new car for $5,000. They expected it to last for 5 years. At the end of 5 years it was estimated to have no value. Calculate the annual depreciation expense for each year of the car's estimated useful life and the accumulated depreciation at the end of each year. Use the sum of years digits and double declining balance methods of depreciation.

3. On January 1, 1980, Bozo Drugs bought a computer for $25,000. It had an estimated useful life of 4 years and an estimated residual value of $5,000. Calculate the annual depreciation expense for each year of the computer's estimated useful life and the accumulated depreciation at the end of each year. Use the sum of years digits and straight line methods of depreciation.

# Preparing Financial Statements

After reading this chapter, the student should be able to:

1. Describe the general process by which financial statements are prepared,
2. Define general journal, account, ledger of accounts, posting, transactions, debit and credit, trial balance, and adjusting entries, and
3. Prepare financial statements from a list of transactions.

F inancial management is based on proper use and interpretation of financial statements. This chapter will present a brief overview of the accounting involved in preparing financial statements. Students interested in a more comprehensive coverage should refer to one of the financial accounting texts listed at the end of the chapter.

The preparation of financial statements begins with analysis of transactions. Transactions are broadly defined as events that have an economic impact on the business. Examples include sale of merchandise, purchase of inventory, and paying of salaries and utilities. Because a typical business will experience thousands of transactions in a year, a system is needed to track them. The system most commonly used consists of a *general journal* and a *ledger of accounts*.

The basic component of this system is the *account*. There is a separate account for every asset, liability, owner equity, revenue, and expense that appears on the financial statements. For example, there are cash accounts, accounts payable accounts, retained earnings accounts, cash sales accounts, credit sales accounts, rent expense accounts, and salary expense accounts. The account is simply a central place used to collect relevant information about all transactions that affect a particular item on the financial statements. For example, all transactions that affect cash would be recorded in the cash account. Accounts may be kept in several physical forms. Early on, they were kept as pages in a loose-leaf folder or notebook. More recently, accounts have been kept as computer files.

Accounts are kept in a *ledger of accounts*. They appear in the ledger in the same order that they appear on the financial statements, as follows—current assets, noncurrent assets, current liabilities, noncurrent liabilities, owners' equity, revenues, and expenses.

The *general journal* is a chronologic listing of transactions. As transactions occur, they are *journalized*, or recorded in the journal. Later, they are *posted* to the proper accounts in the ledger.

In recording transactions, businesses need a system that ensures that assets always equal the sum of liabilities and owners' equity and that can be used to detect and minimize errors. The system used is called the system of *debits and credits*.

## DEBITS AND CREDITS

Every account has two sides: left and right. The left side (or column) is referred to as the *debit* side and the right side (or column) as the *credit* side. (For purposes of instruction, we will use "T-accounts" such as shown in Figure 3-1. Businesses typically use "balance column accounts" such as shown in Figure 3-2. Both are used in the same manner—only the physical appearance of the account is different.)

The following rules govern the recording of transactions in the debit and credit system:

- An increase in an asset is a debit and is recorded on the left side of the asset account.
- An increase in a liability or owners' equity is a credit and is recorded on the right side of the liability or owners' equity account.
- A decrease in an asset is a credit and is recorded on the right side of the asset account.
- A decrease in a liability or owners' equity is a debit and is recorded on the left side of the liability or owners' equity account.
- Because an expense decreases owners' equity, it is a debit and is recorded on the left side of the expense account.
- Because a revenue increases owners' equity, it is a credit and is recorded on the right side of the revenue account.

Four basic rules govern the recording of transactions:

1. Each transaction must be recorded separately.
2. The transaction must be recorded so that ASSETS = LIABILITIES + OWNERS' EQUITY. For example, if the transaction includes an increase in an asset, it must

|  | Accounts Receivable |  |
|---|---|---|
|  | 425 | 250 |
|  | 150 | 125 |
|  | 200 |  |

 **FIGURE 3-1**    T-account.

### Accounts Receivable

| Date | Debit | Credit | Balance |
|------|-------|--------|---------|
| 3-22 | 425 |  | 425 |
| 3-25 | 150 |  | 575 |
| 3-27 |  | 250 | 325 |
| 3-28 |  | 125 | 200 |

**FIGURE 3-2**   Balance column account.

also include a corresponding decrease in some other asset or a corresponding increase in a liability or owners' equity.

3. Each transaction will affect at least two accounts. Because of this, the system is referred to as dual-entry accounting. The transaction may affect more than two accounts, but it must always affect at least two.

4. Every transaction must be recorded such that debits equal credits.

The following example shows how the system of debits and credits is used to record transactions in the journal and ledger.

## SAMPLE PROBLEM: PHIL DILL CONSULTING SERVICE

Phil Dill is a pharmacist who provides consultant pharmacy services to long-term care facilities (nursing homes). He provides no drug products to the facilities. Rather, he reads patients' charts and makes suggestions as to the adequacy of their drug therapy and how it might be improved. This example presents the sequence of transactions that occurs as Phil Dill establishes his business, PD Consulting Service, and operates it for several weeks. Remember that even though Phil Dill is the owner and sole employee of the business, accountants consider him and his business as separate entities.

On June 1, 20X0, Phil Dill begins a pharmacy consulting service by investing $1,000 in a business, which he names PD Consulting Service.

To record this transaction, we must determine which accounts were affected and how they were affected. The transaction increased cash by $1,000 and owner's equity by $1,000. The increase in cash is a debit and the increase in owner's equity is a credit. Thus, as must always be true, debits equal credits and assets equal liabilities plus owner's equity.

The transaction is first entered in the journal, or journalized:

### Journal
### PD Consulting Service

| Date | Account Title and Explanation | Dr. | Cr. |
|------|-------------------------------|-----|-----|
| 6-1-X0 | Cash | 1,000 |  |
|  | P. Dill, Capital |  | 1,000 |
|  | Record owner investment in business |  |  |

Note the following practices that are used in journalizing entries:

1. Each entry is dated.
2. The debit is entered first.
3. Credits are entered last and are indented.
4. There is a short note explaining the transaction.

During the month he provides consulting services to Glow Years Retirement Home. He bills the home for $500. On June 23, Glow Years pays $300 cash and agrees to pay the remaining $200 in 30 days.

| 6-23-X0 | Cash | 300 | |
| | Accounts receivable | 200 | |
| | Revenues | | 500 |
| | Record revenues from services provided | | |
| | to Glow Years Retirement Home | | |

All $500 is recorded as a revenue on the date that services were provided. This is true in the accrual system, even though full payment has not yet been received. In this particular transaction, more than two accounts are affected. On June 28, Dill withdraws $100 in cash from the business for personal use.

| 6-28-X0 | P. Dill, Withdrawals | 100 | |
| | Cash | | 100 |
| | Record owner withdrawal of $100 | | |

On June 29, the rent of $100 is paid.

| 6-29-X0 | Rent expense | 100 | |
| | Cash | | 100 |
| | Record payment of June rent | | |

On June 30, a $25 phone bill is received. The bill will not be paid until July 15.

| 6-30-X0 | Phone expense | 25 | |
| | Accounts payable | | 25 |
| | Record phone expense for June | | |

At this point, all transactions for the month have been journalized. The journal page, as it would appear at the end of the month, is shown in Figure 3-3. The next step is to post the transactions to the ledger of accounts.

## Journal

### P. Dill, Consultant Pharmacist Services

| Date | Account Title and Explanation | Dr. | Cr. |
|------|-------------------------------|-----|-----|
| 6-1-X0 | Cash | 1,000 | |
| | P. Dill, Capital | | 1,000 |
| | Record owner investment in business | | |
| 6-23-X0 | Cash | 300 | |
| | Accounts receivable | 200 | |
| | Revenues | | 500 |
| | Record revenues from services provided to Glow Years Retirement Home | | |
| 6-28-X0 | P. Dill, Withdrawals | 100 | |
| | Cash | | 100 |
| | Record owner withdrawal of $100 | | |
| 6-29-X0 | Rent expense | 100 | |
| | Cash | | 100 |
| | Record payment of June rent | | |
| 6-30-X0 | Phone expense | 25 | |
| | Accounts payable | | 25 |
| | Record phone expense for june | | |

**FIGURE 3-3** Journal for PD Consulting Service.

## POSTING TO THE LEDGER OF ACCOUNTS

Transactions are typically journalized soon after they occur. They are posted after some longer period of time. For example, they may be journalized daily and posted weekly or monthly. This section explains how the transactions for PD Consulting Service for the month of June would be posted to the ledger.

The first transaction (June 1) involves $1,000 increases in cash and capital. Thus, the cash account would be debited $1,000. The entry is recorded as $1,000 on the left side of the cash account. Next, the $1,000 increase in capital is recorded on the right side of the P. Dill, Capital account. These entries are shown below:

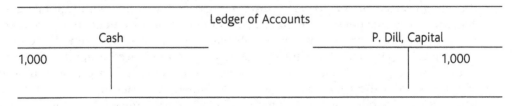

The remaining entries are posted in a similar manner. The ledger of accounts for PD Consulting Service after posting is shown in Figure 3-4.

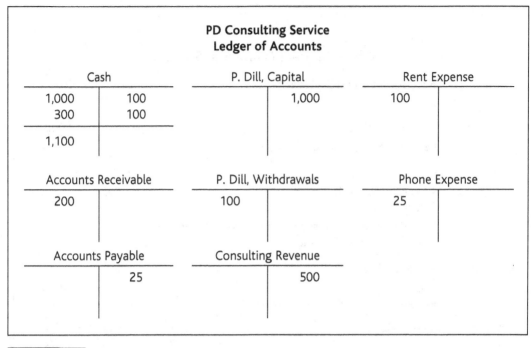

**FIGURE 3-4**   Ledger of accounts for PD Consulting Service.

## TRIAL BALANCE

At the end of the accounting period, after all journal entries have been posted to the ledger of accounts, a *trial balance* is prepared. This is a list of all accounts, in the order in which they appear in the ledger, and their debit or credit balances. The trial balance is prepared to check for errors and to place data in a convenient form for making financial statements. A trial balance for PD Consulting Service is shown in Figure 3-5.

To check for errors, the debit and credit columns of the trial balance are totaled. If the sums are not equal, an error has been made. On the other hand, if they are equal, this is not conclusive proof that no errors have been made. For example, if the accountant had mistakenly recorded a $1,000 increase in cash as a credit and the corresponding $1,000 increase in capital as a debit, the debit and credit columns would be equal, but the balances in the cash and capital accounts would be incorrect.

Financial statements can be prepared from the trial balance. Figures 3-6 through 3-8 show financial statements for PD Consulting Service for its first month of operation. The revenue and expense amounts shown on the income statement are taken directly from the trial balance. Net income is calculated as the difference between revenues and expenses (Fig. 3-6). The capital statement is then prepared using the amount of net income shown on the income statement and the amounts for capital and owner withdrawal from the trial balance (Fig. 3-7). Finally, the balance sheet is prepared using asset and liability amounts from the trial balance and the ending capital amount calculated on the capital statement (Fig. 3-8).

**PD Consulting Service**
**Trial Balance**
**June 30, 20X0**

| Account Name | Debit | Credit |
|---|---|---|
| Cash | $1,100 | |
| Accounts receivable | 200 | |
| Accounts payable | | 25 |
| P. Dill, capital | | 1,000 |
| P. Dill, withdrawal | 100 | |
| Consulting revenue | | 500 |
| Rent expense | 100 | |
| Phone expense | 25 | |
| Totals | $1,525 | $1,525 |

FIGURE 3–5   Trial balance for PD Consulting Service.

**PD Consulting Service**
**Income Statement**
**For the Month Ended June 30, 20X0**

| | | |
|---|---|---|
| Consulting revenue | | $500 |
| Expenses | | |
| Rent | $100 | |
| Phone | 25 | |
| Totals expenses | | 125 |
| Net income | | $375 |

FIGURE 3–6   Income statement for PD Consulting Service.

**PD Consulting Service**
**Statement of Capital**
**For the Month Ended June 30, 20X0**

| | |
|---|---|
| Capital, P. Dill, June 1, 20X0 | $1,000 |
| Add: Net income | 375 |
| Less: P. Dill, withdrawal | 100 |
| Capital, P. Dill, June 30, 20X0 | $1,275 |

FIGURE 3–7   Statement of capital for PD Consulting Service.

---

**PD Consulting Service**
**Balance Sheet**
**June 30, 20X0**

*Assets*

| | | |
|---|---|---|
| Cash | $1,100 | |
| Accounts receivable | 200 | |
| Total assets | | $1,300 |

*Liabilities*

| | | |
|---|---|---|
| Accounts payable | $ 25 | |
| Total liabilities | | $ 25 |

*Owner's equity*

| | |
|---|---|
| P. Dill, capital | $1,275 |
| Total liabilities plus owner's equity | $1,300 |

---

**FIGURE 3–8** Balance sheet for PD Consulting Service.

## ADJUSTING ENTRIES

Financial statements must be prepared at the end of each accounting period (which is generally the end of each fiscal year). Some transactions begin in 1 year and are not concluded until a later one. This causes problems in accurately matching expenses and revenues in the proper year. Recall that revenues are recognized in the year in which the sale is made, and that all expenses required to generate revenues are recognized in the same year as the associated revenues. If a transaction begins in 1 year and is not concluded until a later one, accountants must adjust the accounting records to indicate what portion of the transaction is a revenue or expense in each of the affected years.

For example, a pharmacy may purchase a computer and use it over a 3-year period. Because the computer is used to generate revenues in each of 3 years, part of its cost must be recognized as an expense in each of those years. To do this, the accountant must make an *adjusting entry* at the end of each year. The following journal entries record the purchase and depreciation of the computer, which was purchased for $3,000, was expected to last 3 years, and was expected to have no residual value. The first entry records the purchase of the computer. This is not an adjusting entry.

| | | | |
|---|---|---|---|
| 1-1-X0 | Computer | 3,000 | |
| | Cash | | 3,000 |
| | Record purchase of computer | | |

At the end of 20X0 an adjusting entry must be made to recognize that the computer has been used for 1 year and, consequently, that some expense for use of the computer has been incurred. The adjusting entry required is shown.

| 12-31-X0 | Depreciation expense | 1,000 | |
| | Accumulated depreciation: computer | | 1,000 |
| | Record depreciation expense on computer for 20X0 | | |

A similar entry is required at the end of each of the next 2 years.

| 12-31-X1 | Depreciation expense | 1,000 | |
| | Accumulated depreciation: computer | | 1,000 |
| | Record depreciation expense on computer for 20X1 | | |
| 12-31-X2 | Depreciation expense | 1,000 | |
| | Accumulated depreciation: computer | | 1,000 |
| | Record depreciation expense on computer for 20X2 | | |

Other common situations in which adjusting entries are used include prepaid and accrued expenses. *Prepaid expenses* occur when a pharmacy must pay for a good or service in a year prior to the one in which the good or service is used. For example, a pharmacy may have to pay rent 1 month in advance. So, as of the end of December, the pharmacy would already have paid the rent for January of the next year. The accountant would make an adjusting entry to show that rent had been paid prior to the rent expense being incurred. The prepayment would be listed on the balance sheet as an asset called *prepaid rent.*

*Accrued expenses* occur when, as of the end of the year, the pharmacy has incurred an expense but has not yet paid for it. For example, a pharmacy may have incurred an expense for property taxes but not have paid it as of the end of the year. The accountant would note this using an adjusting entry. The unpaid tax expense would appear on the balance sheet as a liability called an *accrued tax payable.*

## CLOSING ENTRIES

Balance sheet accounts accumulate transaction data over the entire life of the business. The account balances are carried from year to year such that 1 year's ending balance becomes the next year's beginning balance.

Income statement accounts, on the other hand, accumulate transaction data for a set period of time—one accounting period (which is usually 1 year). At the end of each accounting period, income statement accounts are closed. This means their balances are removed and reset to zero. Hence, the balances in the revenue and expense accounts at the beginning of each accounting period are always zero. This is necessary so that net income can be measured for each accounting period.

The closing process consists of four entries:

1. An entry to close the revenue account and transfer its balance to the income summary account (ISA). The ISA is a special temporary account used to make year-end adjusting and closing entries.

2.  An entry to close each of the expense accounts and transfer their balances to the ISA
3.  An entry to close the ISA and transfer its balance to the owners' equity account—either capital (for a sole proprietorship) or retained earnings (for a corporation)
4.  An entry to close the owner withdrawal account (of a sole proprietorship) or the dividends paid account (of a corporation) and transfer the balance to the capital account

Closing entries are dated as of the last day of the accounting period. They are journalized and then posted to the ledger. Closing entries are made after all other entries have been recorded. The closing process has two effects:

1.  It transfers net income (or net loss) to the capital account. Before it is closed, the ISA contains revenue on the credit side and expenses on the debit side. Hence, a credit balance indicates net income and a debit balance indicates net loss.
2.  It establishes zero balances in each of the income statement accounts so they are ready for use in the next accounting period.

## EXAMPLE PROBLEM: PD CONSULTING SERVICE CONTINUED

Figure 3-9 shows the year-end ledger of accounts for PD Consulting Service before closing. The balance in each account and the account name are listed to prepare the trial balance shown in Figure 3-10. The trial balance is then used to prepare the financial statements shown in Figures 3-11 through 3-13.

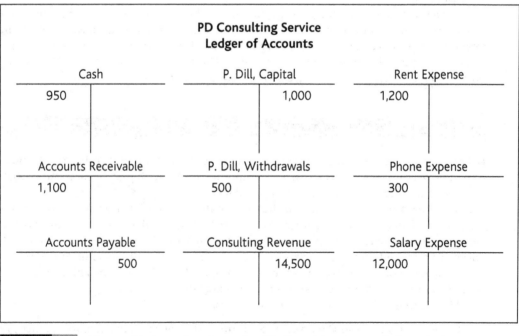

**FIGURE 3-9** Year-end ledger of accounts for PD Consulting Service before closing entries are posted.

**PD Consulting Service**
**Trial Balance**
**May 31, 20X1**

| Account Name | Debit | Credit |
|---|---|---|
| Cash | $ 950 | |
| Accounts receivable | 1,100 | |
| Accounts payable | | 550 |
| P. Dill, capital | | 1,000 |
| P. Dill, withdrawal | 500 | |
| Consulting revenue | | 14,500 |
| Rent expense | 1,200 | |
| Phone expense | 300 | |
| Salary expense | 12,000 | |
| Totals | $16,050 | 16,050 |

**FIGURE 3–10**  Trial balance for PD Consulting Service.

**PD Consulting Service**
**Income Statement**
**Year Ended May 31, 20X1**

| | | |
|---|---|---|
| Consulting revenue | | $14,500 |
| Expenses | | |
| Rent | $ 1,200 | |
| Phone | 300 | |
| Salary | 12,000 | |
| Total | | 13,500 |
| Net income | | $ 1,000 |

**FIGURE 3–11**  Income statement for PD Consulting Service.

**PD Consulting Service**
**Statement of Capital**
**For the Year Ended May 31, 20X1**

| | |
|---|---|
| Capital, P. Dill, June 1, 20X1 | $1,000 |
| Add: Net income | 1,000 |
| Less: P. Dill, withdrawal | 500 |
| Capital, P. Dill, May 31, 20X1 | $1,500 |

**FIGURE 3–12**  Statement of capital for PD Consulting Service.

**PD Consulting Service**
**Balance Sheet**
**May 31, 20X1**

### Assets

| | | |
|---|---|---|
| Cash | $ 950 | |
| Accounts receivable | 1,100 | |
| Total assets | | $2,050 |

### Liabilities

| | | |
|---|---|---|
| Accounts payable | $ 550 | |
| Total liabilities | | $ 550 |

### Owner's equity

| | | |
|---|---|---|
| P. Dill, capital | | $1,500 |
| Total liabilities plus owner's equity | | $2,050 |

**FIGURE 3–13**    Balance sheet for PD Consulting Service.

**Journal**

**PD Consulting Services**

| Date | Account Title and Explanation | Dr. | Cr. |
|---|---|---|---|
| 5-31-X1 | Consulting revenue | 14,500 | |
| | Income summary account | | 14,500 |
| | Close consulting revenue to income summary account | | |
| 5-31-X1 | Income summary account | 13,500 | |
| | Rent expense | | 1,200 |
| | Phone expense | | 300 |
| | Salary expense | | 12,000 |
| | Close expenses to income summary | | |
| 5-31-X1 | Income summary account | 1,000 | |
| | P. Dill, capital | | 1,000 |
| | Close income summary to capital | | |
| 5-31-X1 | P. Dill, capital | 500 | |
| | P. Dill, withdrawal | | 500 |
| | Close owner withdrawal to capital | | |

**FIGURE 3–14**    Closing entries for PD Consulting Service.

Figure 3-14 shows the entries necessary to close PD Consulting Service's temporary accounts. Figure 3-15 shows the balances in the income summary, capital, and withdrawal accounts after each closing entry is made. As indicated, the first closing entry closes the consulting revenue account to the ISA. As shown in Figure 3-15, this results in a $14,500 credit balance in the ISA. It also results in a zero balance in the consulting revenue account. The second closing entry closes the expense accounts and transfers their balances to ISA. In our example, this adds a $13,500 debit to the ISA and results in zero balances in each of the expense accounts. The ISA is then closed to the capital account. This is done by means of a $1,000 debit to the ISA and a $1,000 credit to the P. Dill, Capital account. At this point, the ISA has a zero balance and the P. Dill, Capital account has a $2,000 credit balance. The last entry closes the owner withdrawal account to capital. This results in a $500 debit to P. Dill, Capital and a final balance of $1,500 in the P. Dill, Capital account. This is the same figure calculated on the capital statement (Fig. 3-12) and listed on the balance sheet (Fig. 3-13).

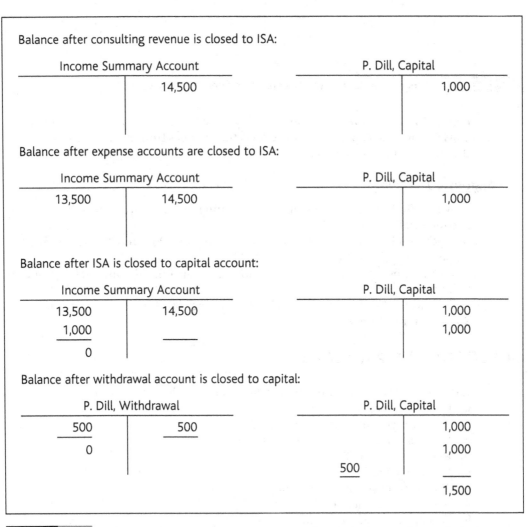

FIGURE 3–15   Balance in income summary account and capital amount after each closing entry.

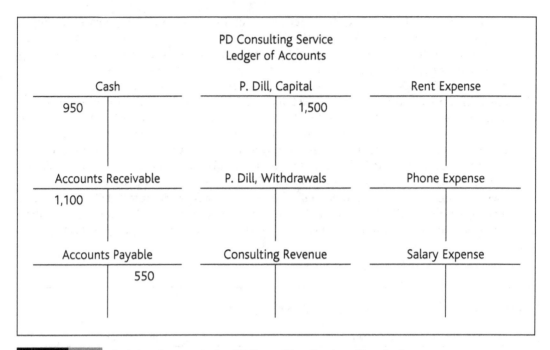

**FIGURE 3-16**  Ledger of accounts for PD Consulting Service after closing.

Figure 3-16 shows the ledger after closing. The balances for the asset and liability accounts remain, the capital account reflects the changes from net income and owner withdrawal, and the balances in the revenue and expense accounts are now set to zero.

### Suggested Readings

Anthony RN, Breitner LK. Essentials of Accounting. 8th Ed. Upper Saddle River, NJ: Prentice Hall, 2003.

Anthony RN, Breitner LK. Essentials of Accounting and Post Test Booklet 8. 8th Ed. Upper Saddle River, NJ: Prentice Hall, 2003.

Warren CS, Reeve JM, Fess PE. Accounting. 21st Ed. Mason, OH: Thomson Southwestern, 2005.

Warren CS, Reeve JM, Fess PE. Financial Accounting. 9th Ed. Mason, OH: Thomson Southwestern, 2005.

## QUESTIONS AND PROBLEMS

1. Indicate whether each of the following would be a debit or a credit.
   a. Cash increases by $1,000
   b. Accounts payable increase by $1,000
   c. Owners' equity increases by $500
   d. Rent expense of $850
   e. Revenue of $250
   f. Accounts receivable decrease by $400
   g. Notes payable increase by $5,000
   h. Owner withdrawal of $100
   i. Fixed assets increase by $5,000
   j. Inventory increases by $500

2. Record the following transactions.
   a. On January 1, 20X1, Jones Pharmacy has cash sales of $5,000.
   b. On January 5, 20X1, Jones Pharmacy pays its rent expense of $500.
   c. On March 10, 20X1, Jones Pharmacy buys a computer for $9,000 cash.
   d. On April 1, 20X1, Jones Pharmacy pays salaries of $5,000.
   e. On May 30, 20X1, Jones Pharmacy pays its utility bill for $200.
   f. On June 1, 20X1, Jones Pharmacy sells $500 worth of merchandise on credit.
   g. On July 3, 20X1, Jones Pharmacy purchases $200 of supplies on credit.
   h. On December 27, 20X1, Jones Pharmacy purchases $500 of supplies and pays cash for them.
3. Shown is a year-end ledger of accounts for Big Bill's Consulting Service. Using the ledger, make a trial balance, financial statements, and necessary closing entries.

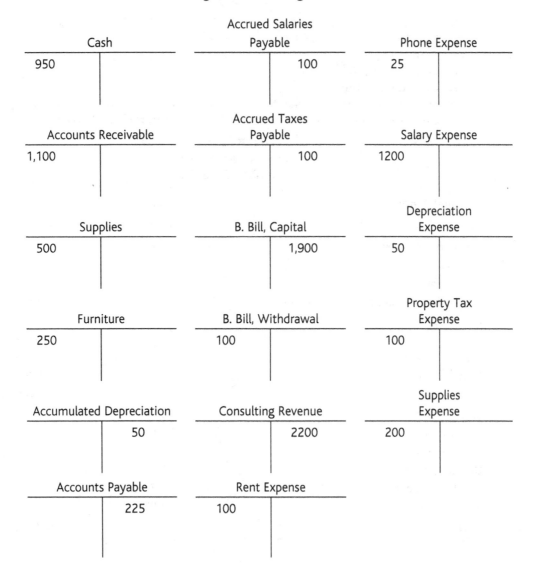

**Ledger of Accounts**
**Big Bill's Consulting Service**

| Cash | | Accrued Salaries Payable | | Phone Expense | |
|---|---|---|---|---|---|
| 950 | | | 100 | 25 | |

| Accounts Receivable | | Accrued Taxes Payable | | Salary Expense | |
|---|---|---|---|---|---|
| 1,100 | | | 100 | 1200 | |

| Supplies | | B. Bill, Capital | | Depreciation Expense | |
|---|---|---|---|---|---|
| 500 | | | 1,900 | 50 | |

| Furniture | | B. Bill, Withdrawal | | Property Tax Expense | |
|---|---|---|---|---|---|
| 250 | | 100 | | 100 | |

| Accumulated Depreciation | | Consulting Revenue | | Supplies Expense | |
|---|---|---|---|---|---|
| | 50 | | 2200 | 200 | |

| Accounts Payable | | Rent Expense | |
|---|---|---|---|
| | 225 | 100 | |

4. Assume Piedmont Pharmacy's fiscal year ends on December 31. Which of the following would require adjusting entries? Explain your answers.
   a. Rent for November was paid the following December.
   b. Rent for December was paid the following January.
   c. Salary expense of $5,000 was incurred and paid in December.
   d. Salary expense of $2,500 was incurred, but not paid, during the last 2 weeks of December. Salaries will be paid on January 14.
   e. Credit sales of $1,000 are made during the last week of December. Payment for these sales will be made during the following January.
   f. A car is purchased and paid for, in cash, on March 31.
   g. A computer with an estimated life of 5 years is purchased on April 30. The money used to buy the computer was borrowed from a bank on a 5-year loan. Both principal and interest are due in 5 years.
5. For what period of time is transaction data collected in an income statement account? In a balance sheet account?
6. Which of the following accounts must be closed at the end of an accounting period?
   a. Cash
   b. Accounts receivable
   c. Sales
   d. Rent expense
   e. Owner withdrawal
   f. Consulting revenues
7. A year-end trial balance for New Service Company is shown. From this balance, prepare financial statements and necessary closing entries for New Service Company.

## Trial Balance
## New Service Company
## December 31, 20X2

| Account Name | Debit | Credit |
| --- | --- | --- |
| Cash | 4,000 | |
| Accounts receivable | 17,000 | |
| Supplies | 3,000 | |
| Equipment | 40,000 | |
| Accumulated depreciation: equipment | | 4,000 |
| Accounts payable | | 9,000 |
| Note payable | | 10,000 |
| Accrued interest payable | | 375 |
| J. Smith, Capital | | 39,000 |
| Consulting revenue | | 60,000 |
| Salary expense | 46,200 | |
| Utility expense | 1,800 | |
| Misc. expense | 1,000 | |
| Depreciation expense | 4,000 | |
| Supplies expense | 5,000 | |
| Interest expense | 375 | |
| Totals | 122,375 | 122,375 |

8. On August 1, 20X5, Linda Smith established a nursing home pharmacy consulting business named Long-Term Care Consultants. The business had the following transactions during the month:
   a. On August 1, Smith invested $1,000 in the business.
   b. On August 3, she purchased $100 of supplies with cash.
   c. On August 5, she purchased $500 of office furniture on account.
   d. On August 7, she provided services to the Golden Agers Home. She billed them for $250, which they agreed to pay in 30 days.
   e. On August 10, she provided services to the Old Sailors Home. She billed them for $400, which they paid.
   f. On August 18, she paid rent of $250 with cash.
   g. On August 25, she withdrew $100 cash for personal use.
   h. On August 28, she received and paid a utilities bill for $50.
   i. On August 30, she paid $100 on account for the previously purchased furniture.

Smith's accountant has set up the following accounts for use by the business:

| | |
|---|---|
| Cash | L. Smith, Withdrawals |
| Accounts receivable | Consulting Fees |
| Supplies | Rent expense |
| Furniture | Utilities expense |
| Accounts payable | L. Smith, Capital |

Record these transactions, post them to the ledger of accounts, and prepare a trial balance, income statement, balance sheet, and a statement of capital for August.

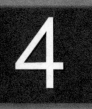
# Accounting for Inventory and Cost of Goods Sold

## OBJECTIVES

After completing this chapter, the student should be able to:

1. Compare and contrast the two systems used to measure inventory and cost of goods sold,
2. Describe the method used for accounting for purchases,
3. Compare and contrast three methods of valuing inventory,
4. Describe the effects of each method of valuing inventory on cost of goods sold, net income, income tax payments, and cash flow during periods of inflation, and
5. Use a pharmacy's gross margin percent and its sales to estimate its inventory level.

The typical pharmacy has a greater investment in merchandise inventory than in any other asset. The *NARD—Pfizer Digest* indicates that inventory accounts for about 44% of an independent community pharmacy's total assets. During this same time period, no other asset has accounted for more than 22% of total investment. Cost of goods sold, which is closely related to inventory, accounts for about 75% of the typical independent community pharmacy's operating expense.[1] An examination of the financial statements of the larger chain pharmacies shows similar figures for inventory and cost of good sold.[2]

Inventory holds a comparable importance in the financial structure of hospital pharmacies. According to a national survey conducted by the American Society of Health System Pharmacists (ASHP), the inpatient pharmacy inventory value for a majority of hospital pharmacies ranged between $100,000 and $499,999. For hospitals with 400 or more beds, average inventory values ranged from $500,000 to over $1 million.[3] An earlier ASHP survey indicated that the typical hospital's pharmacy purchases averaged $3,848,000 in 2000.[4]

Because inventory and cost of goods sold are such major factors in the financial operations of pharmacies, accounting for them accurately is important. Two major issues affect accounting for inventory and cost of goods sold. The first is the system used to measure inventory and cost of goods sold. The second is the method of calculating these two values when prices change over the accounting period.

As discussed in the chapter on financial statements, it is important to remember that inventory and cost of goods sold are not the same. Inventory consists of all goods that the pharmacy holds for resale. It is an *asset*. Cost of goods sold refers to the cost of the merchandise that the pharmacy sold during the year. Cost of goods sold is an *expense*.

## MEASUREMENT OF INVENTORY AND COST OF GOODS SOLD

Inventory and cost of goods sold may be measured using either of two systems. The *perpetual system* is the more useful and logical of the two. Use of the perpetual system, however, requires a great deal of record keeping. The *periodic system* requires much less record keeping and, consequently, has historically been the one used by pharmacies.

### The Perpetual System

The perpetual system of measurement maintains current and accurate accounts for inventory and cost of goods sold. This is accomplished by constantly (or perpetually) updating the balances in these accounts. When the pharmacy purchases merchandise, the balance in the inventory account is increased by the amount of the purchase. When it sells merchandise, the amount in the inventory account is decreased and the balance in the cost of goods sold account is increased by the cost (to the pharmacy) of the items sold. Thus, the perpetual system maintains constant, accurate, and up-to-date records of the pharmacy's cost of goods sold and inventory.

The perpetual system also requires that separate inventory accounts be kept for each stock keeping unit (SKU). An SKU is a unique size, strength, and type of item. For example, Valium is available in 2-, 5-, and 10-mg strengths and in 100- and 500-tablet package sizes. A pharmacy that stocked both sizes of all three strengths would stock six different Valium SKUs. If it used the perpetual system, the pharmacy would, consequently, maintain six different inventory accounts for Valium. For each SKU, the account shows the beginning inventory, all purchases, and all sales of the item. Each time a sale or purchase of the SKU is made its inventory account must be updated. As a result, the perpetual system provides a complete sales history for each SKU.

As should be obvious, the perpetual system requires a great deal of record keeping. Historically, firms such as pharmacies, supermarkets, and hardware stores—which sell thousands of different SKUs—have not been able to use the perpetual system because of the extensive record keeping required. As a result of computerization, many such businesses, including pharmacies, can and now do use the perpetual system. This is a direct result of the computer's ability to quickly and accurately process and store large amounts of data, such as individual inventory accounts for thousands of SKUs.

### The Periodic System

The periodic system has historically been used by businesses—such as pharmacies, hardware stores, and supermarkets—that sell many different items, each of which has relatively low unit cost. It is a simpler system to use than the perpetual system.

The periodic system requires accounts for sales, purchases, and inventory. There are no accounts for cost of goods sold or for individual SKUs. Merchandise purchases are recorded in the purchases account. No adjustment is made to the inventory account for either sales or purchases. Consequently, the inventory account usually does *not* reflect the actual amount of inventory the firm holds.

Cost of goods sold (COGS) is determined in the periodic system in the following manner. The balance in the inventory account at any time during the year shows the value of inventory at the beginning of the year. This is called beginning inventory (BI). The balance in the purchases account shows the amount of purchases (P) made for the year. At the end of the year, a physical inventory is taken. A physical inventory consists of counting the numbers of each SKU in stock, multiplying the number of each SKU by its cost to determine the dollar value of the inventory of that SKU, and then adding the dollar values of all SKUs to determine the total dollar value of the pharmacy's inventory. The year-end physical inventory indicates the value of ending inventory (EI). Cost of goods sold is then calculated by the following formula: COGS = BI + P − EI. The sum of beginning inventory and purchases is cost of goods available for sale (COGAS). This is the total value of merchandise that the pharmacy had available for sale for the year. The amount the pharmacy did not sell (ending inventory) is subtracted from the cost of goods available for sale to determine the value of goods actually sold—or the cost of goods sold. The ending inventory for the present year is then recorded in the inventory account. It will be the beginning inventory for the next year.

When the periodic system is used, cost of goods sold may only be accurately and reliably determined after a physical inventory has been taken. As a result, generating accurate financial statements requires first taking a physical inventory. Because physical inventories are expensive, time consuming, and frequently disruptive, they are generally taken only once a year. Consequently, firms that use the periodic system usually generate accurate financial statements only once a year.

## Comparison of the Two Systems

The perpetual system is more useful for managers. It offers the following advantages:

1. It provides the cost of goods sold without a physical inventory. Consequently, financial statements can be generated easily and inexpensively at any time during the year.
2. It provides information that managers can use to control inventory levels. Individual inventory accounts show frequency of sales for each SKU. Managers can use this to determine optimal purchase quantities and maximum and minimum inventory levels for SKUs.
3. It provides a basis for measuring *shrinkage*. Shrinkage refers to the amount of inventory that is lost, broken, or stolen. Shrinkage is estimated by comparing the inventory level recorded in the inventory account with that found by a physical inventory. The difference between these two levels represents shrinkage.

As mentioned earlier, the perpetual system has one major disadvantage: it requires much record keeping. Because of this, noncomputerized pharmacies continue to use the periodic system.

## ACCOUNTING FOR PURCHASES

Purchases refer to merchandise a pharmacy buys for resale to its customers. In most cases, the pharmacy makes purchases on credit, then pays for the merchandise several days or weeks after it is received. Manufacturers frequently offer cash discounts to encourage pharmacies to pay early. For example, a frequently offered discount is 2/10, net 30. This means that payment for the merchandise is due within 30 days of the date of sale (the date on the invoice), but that the firm can take a 2% discount if it pays within 10 days of the date of sale. If a pharmacy bought $100 worth of merchandise and was offered terms of 2/10, net 30, it could pay either $100 within 30 days or $98 within 10 days. Firms almost always take such discounts. Not taking the discount amounts to losing 2% in order to delay payment for 20 days. This has the same effect as paying 2% interest to borrow money for 20 days. Two percent for 20 days works out to be an annual rate of 36.5%. A pharmacy can almost always borrow money for less than 36.5%; consequently, pharmacies almost always take their cash discounts. Because pharmacies generally take these discounts, purchases should be recorded at their *discounted price*. Then, if the pharmacy fails to take the discount, the amount of the lost discount is recorded as an interest expense, not as a part of the purchase price or of cost of goods sold.

Besides purchase discounts, two other factors affect the final value of purchases and, consequently, cost of goods sold. Most suppliers allow customers to return unsatisfactory merchandise. When a pharmacy returns merchandise to the supplier, the pharmacy records the return in a "purchase returns and allowances" account.

The cost of shipping merchandise to the pharmacy from the supplier must also be considered. Shipping costs that are paid by the pharmacy are considered part of purchase costs. The account used to record shipping costs is frequently called the "freight-in" account.

On the income statement the purchases amount used to calculate cost of goods sold is calculated by adding gross purchases—at the discounted price—and freight-in and subtracting purchase returns and allowances. Any purchase discounts *not* taken would be considered as an interest expense and not part of purchases.

## ACCOUNTING FOR CHANGES IN PRICES

The basic equation for calculating cost of goods sold in the periodic system is:

$$BI + P - EI = COGS,$$

where BI = Beginning Inventory,
    P = Purchases, and
    EI = Ending Inventory

The calculation is straightforward as long as the prices of goods remain the same over the year; however, problems occur if prices change during the year. The problem is one of determining whether the higher costs are assigned to the items sold or to the items remaining in stock. This decision has a significant impact on the values of ending inventory and cost of goods sold and, consequently, on income tax payments, net income, and cash flow.

For example, assume Bulldog Pharmacy had 20 bottles of Valium in stock at the beginning of the year, that it bought 10 in January, 15 in June, and 10 in December, and had 15 left at year end. If all bottles cost $65 (or any other price) each, then there is no problem. There is a problem if the 20 bottles in beginning inventory cost $60 each and the ones purchased in January, June, and December cost more. The problem, as stated earlier, arises in determining if the 15 bottles in ending inventory will be valued at $60 or at the higher cost.

## Physical Flow of Goods

In almost all cases pharmacies sell first the merchandise that they purchased first. This is referred to as the physical flow of goods. The assignment of costs to inventory does *not* have to match the physical flow of goods. If it did, there would be no problem; ending inventory would always be valued at the cost of the most recently purchased merchandise. But the valuation of inventory does *not* have to match the physical flow of goods. Consequently, pharmacies must decide how they wish to assign costs to inventory.

## Inventory Valuation Methods

Pharmacies may use either of three methods of assigning costs to inventory. These methods are weighted average cost; first-in, first-out; and last-in, first-out. Each method will be explained and illustrated using the data presented in Figure 4-1.

### Weighted Average Cost Method

The weighted average cost method yields a cost that is representative of the cost of the product over the entire accounting period. The weighted average cost of a unit of inventory (such as a bottle of Valium) is determined and all units are assigned this cost. The average cost is weighted by the number of units purchased at each cost.

As shown in Figure 4-1, the sample pharmacy had 55 bottles of Valium available for sale during the year. The cost of goods available for sale was $3,700. The weighted average cost (WAC) per bottle is calculated as:

$$WAC = COGAS/No.\ bottles\ available\ for\ sale$$
$$= \$3,700/55$$
$$= \$67.27\ per\ bottle$$

| | No. Bottles | Unit Cost | Total Cost |
|---|---|---|---|
| Beginning inventory | 20 | $60 | $ 1,200 |
| January purchases | 10 | $65 | $ 650 |
| June purchases | 15 | $70 | $ 1,050 |
| December purchases | 10 | $80 | $ 800 |
| Goods available for sale | 55 | | $ 3,700 |
| Ending inventory | 15 | | ? |
| Goods sold | 40 | | ? |

**FIGURE 4-1** Sample data for inventory valuation example (using the periodic system).

Fifteen bottles remained in ending inventory. Therefore, 55 − 15, or 40, bottles were sold. From this we calculate:

$$\text{Ending inventory} = 15 \text{ bottles} \times \$67.27 \text{ per bottle}$$
$$= \$1,009 \text{ and}$$
$$\text{COGS} = 40 \text{ bottles} \times \$67.27 \text{ per bottle}$$
$$= \$2,691$$

## First-in, First-out

An alternate method is called FIFO, or first-in, first-out. The FIFO method is based on the assumption that the first units bought are the first sold. In the example, the FIFO method would assume that the 20 bottles of Valium in beginning inventory are sold first, the 10 purchased in January next, the 15 in June next, etc. This method is simple, is rational, and is not subject to manipulation.

Using the data in Figure 4.1, FIFO assumes that the 40 bottles sold were the *first* 40 available. Thus, the cost of goods sold is the cost of the first 40 bottles available. This is calculated as:

$$\text{COGS} = (20 \text{ bottles} \times \$60 \text{ per bottle}) + (10 \text{ bottles} \times \$65 \text{ per bottle})$$
$$+ (10 \text{ bottles} \times \$70 \text{ per bottle})$$
$$= \$2,550$$

A total of 15 bottles remained in ending inventory. FIFO assumes that these were the last 15 purchased. Ending inventory is calculated as:

$$\text{EI} = (5 \text{ bottles} \times \$70 \text{ per bottle}) + (10 \text{ bottles} \times \$80 \text{ per bottle})$$
$$= \$1,150$$

## Last-in, First-out

The final method that could be used by a pharmacy is known as LIFO, or last-in, first-out. This method is based on the assumption that the *last* units bought are the first ones sold, and that the first bought are the last sold. This does not accurately reflect the physical flow of goods, but it is an acceptable assumption to make for purposes of valuing inventory.

Continuing the example, LIFO assumes that the 40 units sold were the *last* 40 purchased. Therefore, the cost of goods sold is calculated as:

$$\text{COGS} = (10 \text{ bottles} \times \$80 \text{ per bottle}) + (15 \text{ bottles} \times \$70 \text{ per bottle})$$
$$+ (10 \text{ bottles} \times \$65 \text{ per bottle}) + (5 \text{ bottles} \times \$60 \text{ per bottle})$$
$$= \$2,800$$

LIFO assumes that the 15 bottles in ending inventory are the first 15 available. Ending inventory is calculated as:

$$\text{EI} = (15 \text{ bottles} \times \$60 \text{ per bottle})$$
$$= \$900$$

The LIFO method of assigning costs to inventory can be manipulated. Cost of goods sold can be artificially changed by buying extra units of a good at the end of the accounting period. If prices are increasing, this will artificially inflate the cost of goods sold for the period.

## Comparison of Methods

The data in Figure 4-2 compare the cost of goods sold and ending inventory values calculated by each of the methods. In this example prices were increasing over time. Because of this, FIFO gave the lowest cost of goods sold and LIFO gave the highest. All methods would have given the same cost of goods sold if prices had not changed over the year. FIFO would have yielded the highest cost of goods sold and LIFO the lowest if prices had decreased.

Over the last several years the costs of pharmaceuticals have been increasing. Thus, LIFO would give most pharmacies the highest cost of goods sold. Because of this, LIFO would yield the lowest pretax net income and, consequently, the lowest tax payments. This would maximize the pharmacy's cash flow and its actual cash income. LIFO would also produce the lowest net income (both before and after income taxes). This is, for most pharmacies, a less important consideration than the improved cash flow.

To understand why this is true, note that the inventory valuation technique selected does not actually affect what the pharmacy paid for the merchandise it sold during the year. This amount is the same regardless of the valuation method selected. The valuation methods also have no effect on the pharmacy's revenues or operating expenses. The valuation method selected will, however, affect the amount of cash paid out for income taxes. In a period of inflation, LIFO will minimize tax payments and, consequently, maximize cash flow.

Over the entire life of the pharmacy all methods will give the same total income tax expense. LIFO may still be preferred in inflationary times because it defers income taxes until later years.

## Consistency

A pharmacy must choose one of the methods and use it consistently. It cannot change methods from year to year. A pharmacy may change methods, but before doing so it must secure the approval of the Internal Revenue Service and, because of the effect of a change on net income and inventory value, it must report the change in the notes accompanying its financial statements.

## Periodic versus Perpetual

The explanation and examples given in this chapter have assumed that the pharmacy uses the periodic system of inventory measurement. The same principles apply to the

| Method | COGS | EI | Total |
|---|---|---|---|
| Weighted average | 2,691 | 1,009 | 3,700 |
| First-in, first-out | 2,550 | 1,150 | 3,700 |
| Last-in, first-out | 2,800 | 900 | 3,700 |

FIGURE 4-2   Comparison of three methods of inventory valuation.

perpetual system. However, because cost of goods sold is calculated continually during the year in the perpetual system, rather than once at the end of the year as in the periodic system, there is not as great a difference between the cost of goods sold produced by the FIFO and LIFO methods. (An explanation and examples of calculations in the perpetual system can be found in the references listed in the Suggested Reading at the end of this chapter.)

## Lower of Cost or Market

Inventory valuation is complicated by an additional factor; items in inventory must be valued at the *lower* of cost or market value. *Cost* refers to the amount the pharmacy paid for the item when it bought it. *Market value* refers to the replacement value of the item. This is the amount the pharmacy would have to pay to buy the item at current prices. For most items, cost is lower than market value. However, if market value is lower, the item should be valued at its market or replacement cost. When this occurs, the value of ending inventory declines. The difference between the calculated value of ending inventory and the value after the adjustment represents a loss on inventory for the pharmacy. This amount is recorded and recognized as an expense called "loss on write down of inventory."

For example, assume a pharmacy had 10 bottles of penicillin on hand at the end of the year. The pharmacy had paid $25 per bottle for the penicillin. If, at year end, penicillin prices had declined to $20 per bottle, the pharmacy would have to value its penicillin at the lower market (or replacement) price of $20 per bottle. It would also recognize an expense for the year of $50 (10 bottles multiplied by the price decrease of $5 per bottle) for the drop in the cost of the penicillin.

## ESTIMATING INVENTORY LEVELS

Taking a physical inventory is a time-consuming and expensive task. Consequently, most pharmacies take a physical inventory only once a year. As noted previously, this means that pharmacies using the *periodic system* of inventory measurement can generate accurate financial statements only once a year. A pharmacy may want to generate financial statements more often than this. This can be done, without taking a physical inventory, by estimating the current level of inventory. (The current inventory level would be used as the ending inventory in all calculations.) This is done using the *gross margin method*.

At any point during the year, current levels of sales, purchases, and beginning inventory can be found in the pharmacy's accounting records. The cost of goods sold and ending inventory can be *estimated* by assuming that the pharmacy's current gross margin percent is the same as the gross margin percent the pharmacy has earned in the past. The estimation procedure can be illustrated using the following data. Assume that a pharmacy's beginning inventory is $30,000, purchases for the year are $100,000, sales for the year are $112,500, and the pharmacy's gross margin percent has averaged about 30% over the past few years.

By definition, the dollar amount of cost of goods sold for a pharmacy is equal to the product of sales and the cost of goods sold percent. The cost of goods sold percent is equal to 1 minus the gross margin percent. Thus, for the sample data the cost of goods sold percent is estimated as:

$$COGS\% = 1 - GM\%$$
$$= 1 - 30\%$$
$$= 70\% \text{ or } 0.70$$

The dollar amount of cost of goods sold can then be estimated as:

$$COGS = Sales \times COGS\%$$
$$= \$112,500 \times 0.70$$
$$= \$78,750$$

Once the cost of goods sold is determined, the ending inventory can be estimated as:

$$COGS = BI + Purchases - EI$$
$$\$78,750 = \$30,000 + \$100,000 - EI$$
$$EI = \$30,000 + \$100,000 - \$78,750$$
$$EI = \$51,250$$

With estimates of the cost of goods sold and ending inventory, the pharmacy can generate financial statements.

### References

1. West DS, ed. 2004 NARD—Pfizer Digest. Alexandria, VA: National Community Pharmacists Association and Pfizer Inc., 2004.
2. Financial statements for Walgreens, CVS, and Rite Aid were accessed through the EDGAR database, www.sec.gov/edgar.shtml. Accessed April 7, 2005. The EDGAR database is a government-maintained database of the financial statements of corporations listed with the Securities and Exchange Commission.
3. Peterson CA, Schneider PJ, Scheckelhoff DJ. ASHP national survey of pharmacy practice in hospital settings: dispensing and administration—2002. Am J Health Syst Pharm 2003;60:52.
4. Peterson CA, Schneider PJ, Santell JP. ASHP national survey of pharmacy practice in hospital settings: prescribing and transcribing—2001. Am J Health Syst Pharm 2001;58:2251.

### Suggested Readings

Horngren CT, Sundem GL, Elliott JA. Introduction to Financial Accounting. 7th Ed. Englewood Cliffs, NJ: Prentice-Hall, 1998.
Kieso DE, Weygandt JJ, Warfield TD. Intermediate Accounting. 10th Ed. New York: John Wiley & Sons, Inc., 2001.

## QUESTIONS

1. Cost of goods sold refers to which of the following?
   a. The amount the pharmacy paid for the merchandise it sold during the year
   b. The amount the pharmacy paid for the merchandise it purchased during the year
   c. The amount the pharmacy received for merchandise it sold during the year

2. When merchandise is purchased by a firm, it is considered as part of <u>B</u>, when it is sold it is part of <u>C</u>.
   a. B is inventory and C is cost of goods sold.
   b. B is cost of goods sold and C is inventory.
3. Which system of inventory measurement:
   a. allows measurement of merchandise lost due to theft and breakage?
   b. is simpler to use?
   c. allows better inventory control?
   d. allows a pharmacy to generate monthly financial statements without taking a monthly physical inventory?
   e. requires a cost of goods sold account?
   f. requires a purchases account?
   g. requires more record keeping?
4. A pharmacy buys $1,500 worth of merchandise and is offered credit terms of 3/10, net 30. If the firm pays within 10 days of the date on the invoice, what amount is due?
   a. $1,500
   b. $1,470
   c. $1,455
5. If the pharmacy in question did <u>not</u> take the discount, at what price would the purchase be recorded (assuming normal accounting convention is followed)?
   a. $1,500
   b. $1,470
   c. $1,455
6. The discount not taken in question 5 is considered as:
   a. a part of purchases
   b. a part of cost of goods sold
   c. an interest expense

# PROBLEMS

1. Jack's Pharmacy has an inventory of 25 bottles of Maalox at the beginning of the year. These are valued at $1.00 each. The pharmacy purchases 50 more in January for $1.10 each, 100 in March for $1.15 each, and 400 in July for $1.20 each. At year end, 50 bottles remain.

   Assume Jack's Pharmacy uses the periodic system of inventory control. What would Jack's Pharmacy's ending inventory and cost of goods sold be for Maalox using each of the three inventory valuation methods?

2. Jack's Pharmacy also has an inventory of five bottles of amoxicillin 250 mg at the beginning of the year. These are valued at $20 each. The pharmacy purchases 100 more in March for $18 each and 250 more in October for $15 each. At year end 20 bottles remain.

   Assume Jack's Pharmacy uses the periodic system of inventory control. What would Jack's Pharmacy's ending inventory and cost of goods sold be for amoxicillin 250 mg using each of the three inventory valuation methods?

3. Halfway through the year Jack, the owner of Jack's Pharmacy, decides he would like to know how the pharmacy is doing financially and, consequently, that he

needs financial statements for the first 6 months of the year. From the ledger of accounts, he determines that:

$$\text{Sales} = \$500,000$$
$$\text{Beginning inventory} = \$75,000$$
$$\text{Purchases} = \$300,000$$

Historically, Jack's gross margin has been 35%.

What is Jack's estimated ending inventory and gross margin at this point during the year?

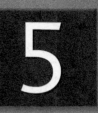
# Financial Statement Analysis

## OBJECTIVES

After completing this chapter, the student should be able to:

1. List and described the five basic management questions that ratio analysis addresses,
2. Evaluate the financial performance of a pharmacy using ratio analysis, common size statements, and the DuPont Model of Profitability. Based on this analysis, suggest ways to improve the pharmacy's financial performance,
3. Explain the differences between solvency and liquidity and between profitability and return on equity, and
4. Define, calculate, and interpret the performance ratios used by managed care organizations.

Financial statements provide decision makers with information that they can use to make better decisions. This chapter will discuss two commonly used techniques for analyzing financial statements: ratio analysis and common size statements. In addition, it will present the DuPont Model of Profitability as a related method of analyzing financial performance.

## RATIO ANALYSIS

Ratio analysis is a method of using income statement and balance sheet data to detect trends and problems in the business. For example, it can be used to identify inventory and credit management problems, poor pricing policies, or declining sales and profitability. A ratio analysis can provide insight into five basic questions of interest to decision makers. The five basic questions are:

1. Does the business earn adequate profits? That is, does it earn as much as other firms in the same type of business and having the same financial resources? These are *tests of profitability*.
2. Are funds available to the business and its management being used wisely? In this context, funds include both debt and equity. Debt consists of funds borrowed by the business. Equity consists of funds that the owners have invested in the business. Ratios used to answer this question are referred to as *tests of overall performance*.
3. Can the firm pay its short-term debts as they come due? This is referred to as *liquidity*. A firm that can pay short-term debts on time is said to have adequate liquidity.
4. Can the firm pay its long-term debt on a continuing basis? This is referred to as *solvency*.
5. How efficiently are the firm's assets being managed? An efficiently run pharmacy will minimize the assets, such as inventory and accounts receivable, which it needs to generate a given level of sales and income.

The next several sections discuss the ratios that address each of these questions and illustrate how they are calculated. Data used to calculate the ratios are found in Figures 5-1 and 5-2, the balance sheet and income statement for Geri-care Pharmacy.

Ratios that measure overall performance, liquidity, and solvency are usually not used by pharmacies that are part of larger outlets. These pharmacies include those found in health care institutions (such as hospitals, long-term care facilities, or health maintenance organization [HMOs]), mass merchandisers (such as Wal-Mart and K-Mart), and supermarkets. This is because the larger outlet (e.g., hospital or supermarket) does not typically account for the amount of debt or equity specific to the pharmacy. These larger outlets do, however, account for many of the assets used by the pharmacy and for the pharmacy's expenses and level of activity (e.g., medication orders dispensed, sales, consults provided). Consequently, tests of efficiency and profitability can be used to assess the performance of these pharmacies.

## TESTS OF PROFITABILITY

Tests of profitability indicate the pharmacy's ability to cover its expenses plus some excess to reward its owners (profit). Two ratios measure profitability: the gross margin percent and the net income percent.

### Gross Margin Percent

The gross margin percent (GM%) is a measure of the profitability of the pharmacy before operating expenses are considered. It tells the percent of every dollar of sales that is available to cover operating expenses and profit. It is calculated as:

$$GM\% = (\text{Sales} - \text{COGS}) \times 100\%/\text{Sales},$$

where COGS = cost of goods sold

| | Geri-care Pharmacy | | | | | | Typical LTC Pharmacy | |
| | 20X4 | | 20X5 | | 20X6 | | 20X6 | |
| | $000 | % | $000 | % | $000 | % | $000 | % |
|---|---|---|---|---|---|---|---|---|
| **Assets** | | | | | | | | |
| Cash | 45 | 0.1 | 35 | 0.1 | 25 | 0.1 | 830 | 3.0 |
| Accounts receivables | 4,100 | 11.6 | 4,950 | 13.5 | 5,800 | 15.6 | 5,420 | 19.5 |
| Inventory | 1,400 | 3.9 | 900 | 2.5 | 1,400 | 3.8 | 1,980 | 7.1 |
| Prepaid expenses | 400 | 1.1 | 75 | 0.2 | 50 | 0.1 | 1,610 | 5.8 |
| Total current assets | 5,945 | 16.8 | 5,960 | 16.3 | 7,275 | 19.5 | 9,840 | 35.5 |
| Property & equipment | 9,320 | | 9,300 | | 12,380 | | | |
| Less accumulated depreciation | (1,220) | | (1,300) | | (1,380) | | | |
| Net property & equipment | 8,100 | 22.8 | 8,000 | 21.9 | 11,000 | 29.5 | 13,910 | 50.2 |
| Total assets | 14,045 | 39.6 | 13,960 | 38.1 | 18,275 | 49.1 | 23,750 | 85.6 |
| **Liabilities and equity** | | | | | | | | |
| Accounts payable | 830 | 2.3 | 735 | 2.0 | 700 | 1.9 | 1,810 | 6.5 |
| Accrued expenses payable | 300 | 0.8 | 625 | 1.7 | 600 | 1.6 | 1,020 | 3.7 |
| Note payable—current | 315 | 0.9 | 300 | 0.8 | 175 | 0.5 | 150 | 0.5 |
| Total current liabilities | 1,445 | 4.1 | 1,660 | 4.5 | 1,475 | 4.0 | 2,980 | 10.7 |
| Total long-term debt | 2,700 | 7.6 | 2,500 | 6.8 | 2,300 | 6.2 | 9,160 | 33.0 |
| Total liabilities | 4,145 | 11.7 | 4,160 | 11.4 | 3,775 | 10.1 | 12,140 | 43.8 |
| Common stock | 7,000 | 19.7 | 7,000 | 19.1 | 7,000 | 18.8 | | |
| Retained earnings | 2,900 | 8.2 | 2,800 | 7.7 | 7,500 | 20.1 | | |
| Total owner equity | 9,900 | 27.9 | 9,800 | 26.8 | 14,500 | 38.9 | 11,610 | 41.9 |
| Total liabilities & equity | 14,045 | 39.6 | 13,960 | 38.1 | 18,275 | 49.1 | 23,750 | 85.6 |

**FIGURE 5–1** Balance sheets for Geri-care Pharmacy and the "typical" long-term care pharmacy.

| | Geri-care Pharmacy | | | | | | Typical LTC Pharmacy | |
| | 20X4 | | 20X5 | | 20X6 | | 20X6 | |
| | $000 | % | $000 | % | $000 | % | $000 | % |
|---|---|---|---|---|---|---|---|---|
| **Net sales** | | | | | | | | |
| Pharmacy | 34,000 | 95.9 | 35,000 | 95.6 | 36,000 | 96.6 | 36,000 | |
| Consulting | 460 | 1.3 | 500 | 1.4 | 250 | 0.7 | 250 | |
| Other | 1,000 | 2.8 | 1,100 | 3.0 | 1,000 | 2.7 | 1,000 | |
| Total | 35,460 | 100.0 | 36,600 | 100.0 | 37,250 | 100.0 | 27,730 | 100.0 |
| **Cost of goods sold** | | | | | | | | |
| Pharmacy | 23,000 | 64.9 | 24,000 | 65.6 | 26,000 | 69.8 | 26,000 | |
| Consulting | — | 0.0 | — | 0.0 | — | 0.0 | — | |
| Other | 700 | 2.0 | 800 | 2.2 | 800 | 2.1 | 800 | |
| Total | 23,700 | 66.8 | 24,800 | 67.8 | 26,800 | 71.9 | 21,040 | 75.9 |
| **Gross margin** | | | | | | | | |
| Pharmacy | 11,000 | 31.0 | 11,000 | 30.1 | 10,000 | 26.8 | 10,000 | |
| Consulting | 460 | 1.3 | 500 | 1.4 | 250 | 0.7 | 250 | |
| Other | 300 | 0.8 | 300 | 0.8 | 200 | 0.5 | 200 | |
| Total | 11,760 | 33.2 | 11,800 | 32.2 | 10,450 | 28.1 | 6,690 | 24.1 |
| **Operating expenses** | | | | | | | | |
| Rent | 600 | 1.7 | 625 | 1.7 | 640 | 1.7 | | |
| Utilities | 175 | 0.5 | 185 | 0.5 | 190 | 0.5 | | |
| Salaries and benefits | 4,500 | 12.7 | 4,200 | 11.5 | 4,300 | 11.5 | | |
| Depreciation | 120 | 0.3 | 80 | 0.2 | 80 | 0.2 | | |
| Delivery | 570 | 1.6 | 495 | 1.4 | 500 | 1.3 | | |
| Bad debt | 370 | 1.0 | 240 | 0.7 | 350 | 0.9 | | |
| Misc. | 710 | 2.0 | 785 | 2.1 | 705 | 1.9 | | |
| Total | 7,045 | 19.9 | 6,610 | 18.1 | 6,765 | 18.2 | 4,510 | 16.3 |
| Net income before income taxes | 4,715 | 13.3 | 5,190 | 14.2 | 3,685 | 9.9 | 2,180 | 7.9 |
| Income tax | 1,792 | 5.1 | 1,972 | 5.4 | 1,400 | 3.8 | 790 | 2.8 |
| Net income after taxes | 2,923 | 8.2 | 3,218 | 8.8 | 2,285 | 6.1 | 1,390 | 5.0 |

**FIGURE 5-2** Income statements for Geri-care Pharmacy and the "typical" long-term care pharmacy.

For Geri-care Pharmacy, the gross margin percent for 20X6 is:

$$GM\% = (37,250 - 26,800)/37,250 \times 100\% = 28.1\%$$

Pharmacies earn higher gross margins when they charge higher prices or buy merchandise less expensively. Lower gross margins might result from any of the following:

1. Low prices
2. Improper purchasing—the cost of goods sold could be too high due to not taking cash discounts or not purchasing from the least expensive suppliers
3. Shoplifting or other theft
4. Owner or employees not ringing up sales

Different types of pharmacies typically have different gross margins. Gross margins of independently owned community pharmacies have averaged around 23% to 24% over the past few years.[1] HMO pharmacies, mail-order pharmacies, and hospital pharmacies typically have higher gross margins. This is because they are able to negotiate larger discounts and rebates from drug manufacturers.

## Net Income Percent

A second measure of profitability is the net income percent (NI%). The NI% is also referred to as the net profit margin. It is a measure of profitability after expenses are considered.

The net income percent is calculated as:

$$NI\% = \text{Net income} \times 100\%/\text{Sales}$$

For Geri-care Pharmacy:

$$NI\% = 2,285 \times 100\%/37,250 = 6.1\%$$

The net income percent may be increased by increasing the gross margin percent, which would require raising prices or purchasing goods at lower cost, or by decreasing expenses.

In comparing the computed net income percentage with those reported for other pharmacies, a manager must make sure that he or she has calculated net income the same way the source of comparison did. For example, some sources use net income after taxes, some use net income before taxes, and some use net income before taxes and before interest payments. In our example we have used net income after taxes.

## TESTS OF OVERALL PERFORMANCE

Tests of overall performance indicate how effectively funds available to the manager have been used.

## Return on Equity

The first test of overall performance is referred to as return on equity (ROE). This measure of performance is also known as return on investment (ROI) and return on net worth (RONW). ROE measures how effectively funds invested in the firm by its owners or stockholders have been used. This measure is oriented toward investors. It indicates the rate of return they would, or did, earn by investing in the business. The ROE is calculated as:

$$\text{ROE} = \text{Net income} \times 100\% / \text{Owners' equity}$$

For Geri-care Pharmacy, ROE for 20X6 would be calculated as:

$$\text{ROE} = 2{,}285 \times 100\% / 14{,}500 = 15.8\%$$

As with net income percent, ROE can be calculated with net income before taxes or net income after taxes. We have used net income after taxes. For consistency, in the remainder of the text, unless otherwise specified we will use net income after taxes whenever net income is specified.

An examination of the calculation of ROE indicates that it can be improved in two ways. First, ROE can be improved by increasing the pharmacy's net income. If the unit volume of sales can be maintained, then net income can be increased by raising prices or by lowering expenses.

Second, ROE can be improved by decreasing owners' equity. This may be accomplished by operating the business with more debt and less owner investment. That is, the owner can borrow more of the funds needed to run the business and use less capital. This is known as *financial leverage*. Pharmacies that have high financial leverage operate with much debt and little owner investment. This will produce higher levels of ROE for a given net income, but it is also risky. If a financial crisis occurs, such as losing a major source of revenue or having to pay a large and unanticipated bill, the pharmacy is at greater financial risk because it must continue to make loan payments.

Owners' equity can also be decreased by decreasing assets. If the manager is able to operate the pharmacy using less cash, accounts receivable, inventory, or fixed assets, then less owner investment is needed. For most pharmacies, the most reasonable way to increase ROE is to carry less inventory or accounts receivable.

## Return on Assets

Another ratio that assesses overall performance is return on assets (ROA). This ratio measures how effectively all funds available to the manager, both debt and equity, have been used. ROA is a better indicator of a manager's performance than ROE because it considers all funds at the manager's disposal, not just invested funds. ROA is calculated as:

$$\text{ROA} = \text{Net income} \times 100\% / \text{Total assets}$$

For Geri-care Pharmacy:

$$\text{ROA} = 2{,}285 \times 100\% / 18{,}275 = 12.5\%$$

ROA may be improved by increasing net income or by decreasing total assets. Increasing borrowing will have no effect. As with ROE, the most likely method by which pharmacies can improve ROE is to decrease investment in assets by proper management of accounts receivable and inventory.

ROE and ROA are regarded as the best measures of the overall performance of a firm. This is because they consider not only the firm's profits, but also the amount of investment needed to generate those profits.

## TESTS OF LIQUIDITY

Tests of liquidity measure the firm's ability to pay its current debt as it comes due.

## Current Ratio

The current ratio (CR) compares a pharmacy's current assets, which supply the cash to pay current debt, with its current debt. Creditors, such as bankers or wholesalers (who supply the pharmacy with merchandise on credit), are interested in this ratio because it measures the pharmacy's ability to repay them on time. The current ratio is calculated as:

$$CR = \text{Current assets/Current liabilities}$$

For Geri-care Pharmacy:

$$CR = 7,275/1,475 = 4.9$$

Creditors prefer high current ratios, that is, a high proportion of current assets to current debt. A rule of thumb suggests that the current ratio should be between 2 and 3.8. A lower ratio indicates that the pharmacy may have problems paying current debts on time. A ratio greater than 3.8 suggests that the pharmacy has too much invested in current assets. (For pharmacies, if the CR is too high, the pharmacy probably has too much invested in accounts receivable or inventory.) As discussed earlier, having more assets than the pharmacy needs to operate efficiently has a negative effect on return on equity and assets.

## Quick Ratio

The quick ratio (QR; or acid test) is similar to the current ratio but is a more stringent test of the firm's liquidity. It is calculated as:

$$QR = (\text{Current assets} - \text{inventory})/\text{Current liabilities}$$

For Geri-care Pharmacy:

$$QR = (7,275 - 1,400)/1,475 = 4.0$$

The quick ratio measures the excess of very liquid current assets—cash and accounts receivable—to current liabilities. The ratio takes the perspective of whether the firm could pay its current debts if it were not able to sell its inventory. The rule of thumb indicates that the quick ratio should be between 1.1 and 2. Pharmacies can operate with lower quick ratios than other businesses because their inventories are composed of merchandise that sells quickly (and is, therefore, readily converted to cash) as compared with, say, cars or appliances.

## Accounts Payable Period

The accounts payable period (APP) indicates how long it takes the pharmacy to pay for its credit purchases. It is the average number of days between when a pharmacy makes a purchase on credit and when it pays for the purchase. The accounts payable period is calculated as:

$$APP = Accounts\ payable/Purchases\ per\ day$$

The amount of annual purchases is frequently not shown on the income statement or balance sheet. However, it can be calculated from the available information using the following formula,

$$COGS = BI + P - EI,$$

where COGS = cost goods sold
     BI = beginning inventory
      P = purchases
     EI = ending inventory

In using this formula, remember that the inventory shown on the balance sheet is the inventory as of the last day of the fiscal year. Therefore, this number is the ending inventory for that year. The inventory shown on the balance sheet for the previous year is this year's beginning inventory. So, the ending inventory for 20X6 is 1,400 and the beginning inventory for 20X6 is 900.

So, for Geri-care Pharmacy,

$$COGS = BI + P - EI$$
$$26,800 = 900 + P - 1,400$$
$$P = 26,800 - 900 + 1,400 = 27,300$$

We can now calculate the accounts payable.

$$APP = 700/(27,300/365) = 9.4\ days$$

## SOLVENCY TESTS

Solvency ratios measure a business's ability to meet its long-term debt payments. They are also called debt-to-equity ratios because they compare the amount the pharmacy has borrowed to the amount its owners have invested.

*Debt* refers to funds that have been lent to the business. Debt must be repaid according to a set schedule. Regardless of whether the firm is profitable, it is legally obligated to pay its debts on time. Consequently, debt is a risky method of raising funds to finance a business. On the other hand, debt confers no ownership of the business to the lender. If the business does well, the owner is required only to repay the debt and interest.

*Equity* refers to funds that have been invested in the business. It does not have to be repaid. However, it gives the investor ownership of part of the business.

The solvency ratios are calculated as:

Current liabilities to owner's equity = Current liabilities × 100%/Owners' equity
Long-term debt to owner's equity = Long-term debt × 100%/Owners' equity
Total debt to owner equity = Total debt × 100%/Owners' equity
Financial leverage = (Total liabilities + Owners' equity)/Owners' equity

For Geri-care Pharmacy:

$$CL/OE = 1,475/14,500 \times 100\% = 10\%$$
$$LTD/OE = 2,300/14,500 \times 100\% = 16\%$$
$$TD/OE = 3,775/14,500 \times 100\% = 26\%$$
$$\text{Financial leverage} = 18,275/14,500 = 1.3$$

Lenders, such as bankers, prefer that pharmacies have low debt-to-equity ratios. This indicates that the owners have more invested in the business than does the lender, so the owners should have a strong incentive to do well.

A rule of thumb suggests that total debt to owner equity should be 80% or less. This rule must be interpreted loosely because of the relationship between a pharmacy's age and its debt level. New pharmacies typically have higher solvency ratios than older ones because of the debt associated with starting a business. Over time, a successful pharmacy will make profits that it can use to repay debt or increase owners' equity. This reduces the solvency ratios.

## TESTS OF EFFICIENCY

These ratios measure how efficiently the pharmacy's assets are used. Efficient use involves generating a given level of activity—such as sales, medication orders dispensed, or consults—with the smallest possible investment in assets. Efficient use can also be thought of as making the maximum use of available assets.

## Accounts Receivable Collection Period

The accounts receivable collection period (ARCP) is an estimate of the average number of days it takes the pharmacy to collect an account receivable. Or, it estimates the average number of days between when a charge sale is made and when payment for the sale is collected.

The accounts receivable collection period is calculated as:

$$ARCP = \text{Accounts receivable/Net credit sales per day}$$

For Geri-care Pharmacy:

$$ARCP = 5,800/(37,250/365) = 56.8 \text{ days}$$

In this example, net credit sales were the same as net sales. That was true in this example because long-term care pharmacies typically send out bills to all customers at the end of each month. Because they do not have direct contact with most of their patients, they do not deal in cash sales. Consequently, all sales are credit sales. The situation is different for community pharmacies. Most prescription sales in community pharmacies are paid for by third parties such as insurance companies, HMOs, or state Medicaid agencies and are therefore credit sales. However, most community pharmacies have a substantial amount of cash prescription sales and most find that much of their nonprescription sales are paid for by cash.

The rule of thumb states that the ARCP should be no greater than 1.5 times the firm's credit terms (the length of time customers are given to pay their bills after the bills are sent). Longer periods indicate poor credit management. They also suggest that many of the pharmacy's customers are not paying on time.

## Inventory Turnover

Inventory turnover (ITO) measures the rate of movement of inventory. That is, it indicates how quickly inventory is purchased, sold, and replaced.

Inventory turnover is calculated as:

$$ITO = COGS/\text{Average inventory at cost}$$

For Geri-care Pharmacy:

$$ITO = 26,800/((900 + 1,400)/2) = 23.3 \text{ times}$$

(Average inventory is calculated using inventory levels at the beginning and end of the year.)

A high turnover is desirable. It indicates that the pharmacy is being run with a minimum investment in inventory. Because inventory is frequently the pharmacy's largest asset, this is very important. If inventory can be minimized, then ROA and ROE will be maximized. However, if inventory turnover is too high, the pharmacy may frequently find itself out of stock. Inventory turnover may be increased by either increasing sales without increasing inventory or by decreasing inventory and maintaining the same volume of sales.

## Asset Turnover

Asset turnover (ATO) measures how efficiently the pharmacy's total assets are used. ATO is calculated by dividing the pharmacy's sales for the year by its total assets. ATO for Geri-care Pharmacy is calculated as:

$$ATO = \text{Sales/Total assets}$$
$$\text{ATO for Geri-care Pharmacy} = 37,250/18,275 = 2.0 \text{ times}$$

As with ITO, a high ATO is desirable. It indicates that the pharmacy is being operated with a minimum investment in assets. For a given net income, this will result in higher rates of ROE and ROA. ATO can be improved by increasing sales while holding asset investment constant or by decreasing asset investment while increasing or maintaining sales.

## Tests of Efficiency for Institutional Pharmacies

As mentioned earlier, ratios measuring overall performance, liquidity, and solvency are not applicable to most institutional pharmacies. Tests of efficiency, however, are frequently used to assess the performance of these pharmacies.

An institutional pharmacy's largest expense items are purchases and payroll. These two items account for the great majority of a hospital pharmacy's direct expenses.[2] Thus, if an institutional pharmacy is to operate efficiently, it must make the best possible use of inventory and personnel. (While personnel is not an asset in the normal financial sense, that is, it does not appear on a balance sheet, it is a resource that must be managed efficiently.)

The inventory turnover ratio (discussed earlier in the chapter) is as important for an institutional pharmacy as for a community pharmacy. Other efficiency ratios compare usage of inventory or personnel to some basic measure of workload such as prescriptions dispensed or patient days. Wilson stated that as institutional pharmacy has moved away from dispensing to more clinical functions, the number of prescriptions dispensed has become a less meaningful measure of pharmacy workload[2]. Therefore, he recommends using measures like patient days or acuity-adjusted patient days. Acuity-adjusted patient days adjusts the number of patient days for the intensity of services required to treat different patients. The idea behind the adjustment is that patients who require more care will use more drugs and manpower. Examples of some commonly used efficiency ratios for institutional pharmacies follow.

## Personnel Expense per Patient Day

The efficiency with which personnel are utilized is measured by the personnel expense per patient day ratio. The ratio is calculated as:

$$\text{Personnel expense per patient day} = \text{Total annual pharmacy payroll/Annual patient days}$$

(Annual patient days is a measure of workload based on the number of patients treated and their average length of stay in the hospital. A patient in the hospital for 1 day would equal 1 patient day. Ten patients in the hospital for 5 days each would equal 50 patient days.)

## Drug Expense per Patient Day

The efficiency with which pharmaceutical expenditures are managed is measured by the drug expense per patient day ratio. The ratio is calculated as:

$$\text{Drug expense per patient day} = \text{Total annual drug expense/Annual patient days}$$

## Example of Efficiency Ratios for an Institutional Pharmacy

The Comera Community Hospital is a 250-bed community hospital. For the most recent year, the hospital's pharmacy had an average inventory of $400,000, drug acquisition costs (which are the same as cost of goods sold) of $5,500,000, and an annual payroll expense of $1,900,000. The hospital provided 60,000 patient days of service during the year. Assume that the typical hospital pharmacy in a hospital this size has a drug expense per patient day of $96.50, a personnel expense per patient day of $33.21, and an inventory turnover of 10.

Inventory turnover for the pharmacy was:

$$\text{ITO} = \text{Cost of goods sold/Average inventory at cost}$$
$$\text{ITO} = \$5,500,000/400,000 = 13.8$$

The personnel expense per patient day (PEPPD) for the pharmacy was:

PEPPD = Total annual pharmacy payroll/Annual patient days
PEPPD = $1,900,000/60,000 = $31.67

The drug expense per patient day (DEPPD) for the pharmacy was:

DEPPD = Total annual drug expense/Annual patient days
DEPPD = $5,500,000/60,000 = $91.67

Compared to the typical pharmacy, Comera Community Hospital's pharmacy has a higher inventory turnover and a lower drug expense per patient day. This indicates that the pharmacy's efficiency in controlling drug expense is better than average. Comera Community Hospital's pharmacy has a lower personnel expense per patient day, indicating that it uses personnel more efficiently than the typical hospital pharmacy.

## Managed-Care Pharmacy Ratios

Managed-care organizations (MCOs) also use ratios to evaluate performance. Although these ratios are not based on the financial statements, they are used in a similar manner to financial ratios. Managed-care organizations use these ratios to evaluate the performance of their own pharmacies and of the community pharmacies with which they contract.

The most commonly used ratio is probably the per member per month (PMPM) drug expense. This ratio is used to measure and track the amount the managed-care organization spends on prescriptions. It is calculated as follows:

$$\text{PMPM drug expense} = \frac{\text{Total drug expense for the month}}{\text{Total number of MCO members for the month}}$$

The ratio indicates the average drug expenditure per MCO member for a month. (The ratio may also be calculated on a per year basis.) A ratio that increases over time indicates that the MCO's drug expenses are increasing over time and suggests that the MCO may be doing a poor job of controlling drug costs. Pharmacy managers who work for MCOs are frequently evaluated based on how well they can control the PMPM drug expense over time. The average PMPM drug expense for an HMO in 2003 was $28.02.[3]

The generic fill ratio measures the extent to which generic drugs, rather than brand-name products, are dispensed. The ratio is calculated as:

$$\text{GFR} = \frac{\text{Number of prescriptions dispensed with the generic product}}{\text{Total number of prescriptions dispensed}}$$

Because generic drugs are almost always much less expensive than their brand-name counterparts, increasing the use of generic drugs results in a decrease in drug expenses. Consequently, MCOs want pharmacies to have high generic fill ratios. In some situations, they may provide bonuses to pharmacies that meet or exceed a target generic fill ratio. Because generic equivalents are not available for all prescription products, the maximum generic fill ratio is less than 100%; it is closer to 50%. The generic fill ratio for pharmacies serving patients in HMOs was about 46% in 2003.[3]

## INTERPRETING RATIOS

Ratios are meaningful only when compared to some standard. There are two commonly used standards. The first is the pharmacy's ratios for past years. Comparison of the present year's ratios with those for past years identifies trends. This indicates whether the pharmacy's financial performance is improving or deteriorating. The second standard is the ratios of other pharmacies of the same type (e.g., chain community, in-house HMO, long-term care) and with similar financial resources. Comparing this year's performance to performance in past years is called internal benchmarking. Comparing this year's performance to that of other, similar pharmacies is called external benchmarking.

Many professional organizations provide financial information and ratios through periodic surveys of their membership. Ratios for independently owned community pharmacies may be found in the *NCPA Digest*.[1] Pharmacies that are members of chains can compare their ratios with those of other pharmacies in the chain. Many types of pharmacies are part of chains. Examples include the Walgreens and Revco chains of community pharmacies, Humana and Columbia hospital chains, and Prudential and Kaiser Permanente HMOs. Comparisons with other pharmacies must be done cautiously. Problems arise when pharmacies differ in their accounting for inventories, methods of depreciation, or the age of their fixed assets.

## CAUTIONS

Ratio analysis is best viewed as a diagnostic technique. A thorough ratio analysis will identify a pharmacy's problems and their probable causes but may give little information about how to solve the problems. A ratio analysis yields suggestive, rather than definitive, results. The results of a ratio analysis guide the manager in asking appropriate questions and in identifying areas in need of further investigation. The analysis seldom yields final, definitive answers. Consequently, managers must use caution in interpreting the results of a ratio analysis. A proper and correct interpretation requires use of other data, such as particular policies, peculiarities, and practices of the pharmacy.

Ratios are based on balance sheet and income statement data. Consequently, they suffer from many of the limitations of these statements. For example, on the balance sheet, fixed assets are valued at their historical, rather than replacement, costs. Thus, two pharmacies owning land and buildings with similar market or replacement costs may value the assets at vastly different amounts if one bought its land and building recently and one bought its several years ago.

## DuPONT MODEL OF PROFITABILITY

The DuPont Model of Profitability provides another way of assessing a pharmacy's financial performance. Although it uses the same information and many of the same calculations as a ratio analysis, it has the advantage of showing how the various ratios and their components interact to determine the pharmacy's overall performance. The DuPont Model assumes that the best measure of performance for a business is ROE.

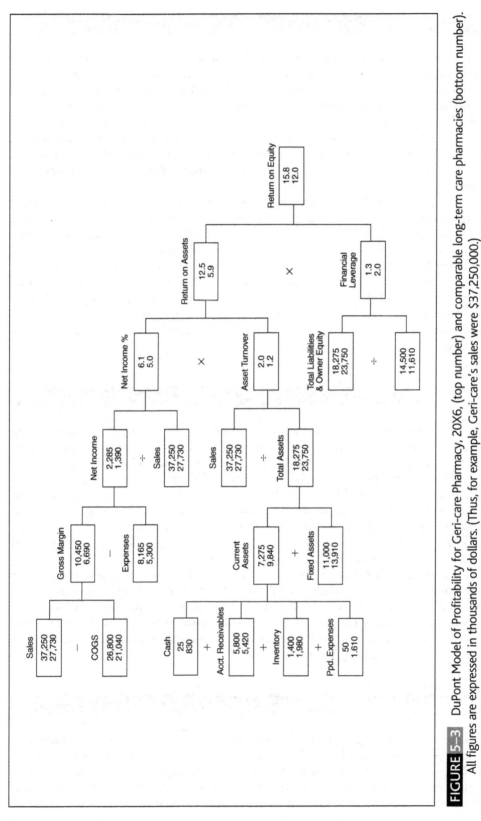

**FIGURE 5-3** DuPont Model of Profitability for Geri-care Pharmacy, 20X6, (top number) and comparable long-term care pharmacies (bottom number). All figures are expressed in thousands of dollars. (Thus, for example, Geri-care's sales were $37,250,000.)

In the DuPont Model, ROE is calculated as the product of net income percent, asset turnover, and financial leverage, as shown below:

$$ROE = NI\% \times ATO \times \text{Financial leverage}$$
$$= \frac{NI}{\text{Sales}} \times \frac{\text{Sales}}{\text{Total Assets}} \times \frac{TL + OE}{OE}$$

The complete DuPont Model is shown in Figure 5-3. It shows the three components of profitability—net profitability, asset turnover, and financial leverage—the financial variables that determine each component, and the interrelationships among the variables and components.

The DuPont Model is useful because it helps the manager identify trouble spots and plan for increased profits. For example, a manager might determine that his or her pharmacy had a poor ROE. Considering the three components of ROE would allow him or her to more precisely identify the source of the problem by determining whether the problem resulted from low profit margin, inefficient use of assets, or low financial leverage. Once that was determined, the manager could work back through the model to more precisely identify the source of the profitability, asset turnover, or leverage problem. Knowing the source of the problem helps the manager determine the most effective actions for solving it. In addition, the model shows that improving any of the components—either net profitability, asset turnover, or financial leverage—will lead to an improvement in ROE.

## COMMON SIZE STATEMENTS

Managers can obtain additional useful information about their pharmacies' performance by comparing current financial statements with those of similar pharmacies or with past years' statements. The comparisons are simplified by restating each item on the income statement and balance sheet as a percent of sales. After making these changes, statements for pharmacies with different sales volumes, assets, and liabilities can be more easily and directly compared. Such financial statements are called *common size statements*. Common size income statements are used to compare expenses and profits. Common size balance sheets are used to compare levels of current and fixed assets and sources of financing. Common size statements for Geri-care Pharmacy are shown in the last columns of Figures 5-1 and 5-2.

## FINANCIAL STATEMENT ANALYSIS EXAMPLE

In this section, a more complete financial statement analysis for Geri-care Pharmacy will be presented. The analysis will demonstrate the use of ratio analysis, common size statement analysis, and the DuPont Model. Figures 5-1 and 5-2 show financial and common size statements for Geri-care Pharmacy for the years 20X4 to 20X6 and for the "typical" long-term care (LTC) pharmacy for 20X6. Figure 5-4 shows calculated ratios for Geri-care Pharmacy and the typical LTC pharmacy.

### Comparison with Similar Pharmacies

The first step in the analysis is to compare Geri-care Pharmacy's 20X6 ratios with those of the typical LTC pharmacy. The comparison indicates that Geri-care Pharmacy's financial performance is considerably better than that of the typical LTC pharmacy.

| | Geri-care Pharmacy | | | Typical LTC Pharmacy |
| | 20X4 | 20X5 | 20X6 | 20X6 |
| --- | --- | --- | --- | --- |
| Net income percent | 8.2 | 8.8 | 6.1 | 5.0 |
| Gross margin percent | 33.2 | 32.2 | 28.1 | 24.1 |
| Return on equity | 29.5 | 32.8 | 15.8 | 12.0 |
| Return on assets | 20.8 | 23.1 | 12.5 | 5.9 |
| Current ratio | 4.1 | 3.6 | 4.9 | 3.3 |
| Accounts payables period | 12.5 | 11.0 | 9.4 | 31.4 |
| Total debt to owner equity | 0.42 | 0.42 | 0.26 | 1.0 |
| Financial leverage | 1.4 | 1.4 | 1.3 | 2.0 |
| Inventory turnover | 20.6 | 21.6 | 23.3 | 10.6 |
| Accounts receivables collection period | 42.2 | 49.4 | 56.8 | 71.3 |
| Asset turnover | 2.5 | 2.6 | 2.0 | 1.2 |

**FIGURE 5–4** Calculated financial ratios for Geri-care Pharmacy and the "typical" long-term care pharmacy (assume that inventory for 20X3 was $900).

Geri-care Pharmacy's ROE and ROA were considerably better than those of the typical LTC pharmacy. Profitability is a major determinant of both ROA and ROE. Geri-care Pharmacy's gross margin percent and net income percent were higher than those of the typical pharmacy. The common size statements indicate that Geri-care Pharmacy had about the same owner investment (as a percentage of sales) as the typical pharmacy. Therefore, Geri-care Pharmacy's higher ROE resulted primarily from its higher profitability. The common size statements also indicate that Geri-care Pharmacy had fewer assets (as a percentage of sales) than the typical pharmacy. Higher profitability and lower asset investment both contributed to Geri-care Pharmacy's higher ROA.

Geri-care Pharmacy's gross margin percentage was 4.0 percentage points greater than that of the typical LTC pharmacy (28.1% versus 24.1%). The net income percent was only 1.1 percentage point higher than the typical pharmacy's (6.1% versus 5.0%). Because the only difference between the gross margin and net income percents is expenses, this suggests that Geri-care Pharmacy does not control expenses as well as the typical pharmacy. Common size statements bear this out. The typical pharmacy had operating expenses equal to 16.3% of sales and income taxes equal to 2.8% of sales. By comparison, the figures for Geri-care Pharmacy were 18.2% and 3.8%, respectively.

Geri-care Pharmacy's liquidity was much better than that of the typical pharmacy. It had a current ratio of 4.9 and an accounts payable period of 9.4 days. Figures for the typical pharmacy were 3.3 and 29.3 days, respectively. Geri-care's current ratio of 4.9 suggests that the pharmacy may have more current assets than it needs to operate efficiently. However, common size statements indicate that Geri-care had considerably lower amount of current assets than did the typical pharmacy (19.5% versus 35.5%). Apparently, Geri-care Pharmacy's high current ratio is a result of low current liabilities. Common size statements indicate that Geri-care's current liabilities were less than those of the typical pharmacy (4.0% compared with 10.7%).

Geri-care Pharmacy's total debt to owner equity and financial leverage ratios were also lower than those of the typical LTC pharmacy. (While this is preferable to the alternative, it is not a convincing indicator of Geri-care's solvency. The typical long-term care pharmacy had more debt than equity.) Geri-care pharmacy had much lower levels of debt than the typical pharmacy. Common size statements show that Geri-care's total debt was equal to 10.1% of sales compared with 43.8% for the typical pharmacy.

Finally, Geri-care used its assets more efficiently than the typical LTC pharmacy. Both inventory turnover and asset turnover were higher and the accounts receivables collection period was shorter than those of the typical pharmacy. Common size statements show a similar pattern. Geri-care Pharmacy's inventory and total assets were equal to 3.8% and 49.1% of sales, respectively. Comparable figures for the typical pharmacy were 7.1% and 85.6%, respectively.

## Trend Analysis

A comparison with the typical LTC pharmacy indicates that Geri-care Pharmacy had much better than average financial performance in 20X6. Trend analysis, however, suggests potential problems with profitability and efficiency. (To calculate the ratios for Geri-care Pharmacy for 20X4, note that inventory for 20X3 was $900.)

The gross margin percentage fell considerably from 20X4 to 20X6. As discussed earlier, declining gross profitability could result from falling prices, improper purchasing, increased theft, or failure to record sales. Unfortunately, we do not have sufficient information to determine the correct reason. However, the manager should investigate the situation further.

Geri-care's net income percent increased between 20X4 and 20X5, then decreased in 20X6. We might have expected decreases in both years given the decreases in the gross margin percent. The fact that the net income percent increased 1 year and decreased less than the decrease in the gross margin percent the next year indicates that Geri-care Pharmacy is doing a better job of controlling its expenses. Further, this indicates that the problem with profitability is caused more by the declining gross margin percent than by failure to control operating expenses.

Both ROE and ROA increased in 20X5, then decreased in 20X6. This is the same pattern we saw with the net income percent and is most likely to be a result of the changes in the net income percent. Common size statements indicate that both total assets and owner equity increased (as a percentage of sales) in 20X6. These changes also contributed to the decreases in ROA and ROE.

The current ratio declined from 20X4 to 20X5, then increased in 20X6. Common size statements indicate that this was primarily due to changes in the level of current assets, primarily accounts receivables. The accounts payable period declined in both 20X5 and 20X6. Common size statements showed that accounts payable as a percent of sales also declined in both years.

The trend analysis showed no problems with solvency. Both total debt to owner equity and financial leverage remained the same in 20X5 and declined in 20X6.

Inventory turnover improved from 20X4 to 20X6. The accounts receivables collection period increased over this period. Common size statements indicated that accounts receivables (as a percent of sales) increased over the period. Both measures indicate a growing problem with collection of accounts receivables. Asset turnover improved from 20X4 to 20X5, then declined in 20X6. This was due to increases in accounts receivables and fixed assets. This is another indication that accounts receivables may be a problem.

## DuPont Model

A financial analysis using the DuPont Model provides similar results. An advantage of using the DuPont Model is that it provides a structure for analyzing Geri-care Pharmacy's financial performance and for identifying problems. Using this structure consists of beginning the analysis at the far right-hand side of the model; Geri-care's ROE is compared with that of the typical LTC pharmacies to determine how well Geri-care performed. If Geri-care's ROE is below average, then working backwards (or to the left) through the model will identify the source of the problem. The DuPont Model for Geri-care Pharmacy for 20X6 is shown in Figure 5-3. The number on top in each box is the figure for Geri-care; the number on the bottom is the figure for a group of comparison pharmacies.

The figure shows that Geri-care Pharmacy's ROE was greater than that of the typical pharmacy (15.8% versus 12.0%). To determine why, the primary determinants of ROE are examined. These are net income percent, asset turnover, and financial leverage.

Geri-care was more profitable than the typical LTC pharmacy. It had a net income percent of 6.1%. The net income percent of the typical pharmacy was 5.0%. This is a primary reason for higher ROE. The DuPont Model shows that net income is a function of the pharmacy's gross margin and its total expenses. Comparison of common size income statements indicates that Geri-care's gross margin percent was substantially higher than average, and thus a primary reason for its higher profitability. Total expenses (as a percentage of sales) were also higher than average. Higher expenses lead to lower profit. Individual expense figures (such as salaries, depreciation, and bad debt) were not available for the typical pharmacy, so it is not possible to determine which expenses were out of line.

Geri-care Pharmacy's asset turnover was also higher than that of the typical pharmacy (2.0 versus 1.2). This is another reason for higher than average ROE. The model shows that asset turnover is calculated as sales divided by total assets. Common size statements indicate that Geri-care had a much lower investment in total assets (as a percent of sales) than did the typical pharmacy. Consequently, it had higher asset turnover and ROE. Tracing back through the model and comparing common size statements reveals that Geri-care's lower investment in total assets resulted, in great part, from lower net property and equipment. However, Geri-care's investment in all types of assets was lower than that of the typical pharmacy.

Geri-care's financial leverage was lower than average. Lower financial leverage leads to lower ROE, so this would not be a reason for Geri-care's higher than average ROE. The lower financial leverage also indicates that Geri-care is at lower financial risk than similar pharmacies. Common size balance sheets indicate that Geri-care had lower financial leverage because it had substantially less debt (as a percent of sales) than the typical LTC pharmacy.

## Summary of Financial Analysis

A complete financial statement analysis using ratio analysis, common size statements, and the DuPont Model indicates that Geri-care Pharmacy has considerably better financial performance than the typical LTC pharmacy. Profitability, overall performance, and solvency are all better, as is inventory turnover.

The analyses suggest that Geri-care may have problems in three areas: expense control, declining gross margin, and control of accounts receivables. Despite higher than average operating expenses and declining gross margin percentages, Geri-care Pharmacy has better than average profitability. Nevertheless, the manager should investigate these areas further to determine the causes of less than average performance. Over time, declining gross margins and poor expense control could result in declining profitability, ROE, and ROA.

Geri-care's investment in accounts receivables and its accounts receivables collection period are both better than those of the typical pharmacy. However, both have been increasing over time. This could indicate a growing problem with management of accounts receivables. Over time these problems could result in cash flow problems.

### References

1. NCPA—Pfizer Digest 2004. Alexandria, VA: National Community Pharmacists Association, 2004.
2. Wilson AL. Financial management and cost control. In: Handbook of Institutional Pharmacy Practice. 4th Ed. Bethesda, MD: American Society of Health-System Pharmacists, 2005.
3. Anon. Managed Care Digest Series 2004: HMO-PPO/Medicare-Medicaid Digest. Bridgewater, NJ: Aventis Pharmaceuticals, 2004.

### Suggested Reading

Besley S, Brigham EF. Essentials of managerial finance. 13th Ed. Mason, OH: Thomson South-Western, 2005.

Higgins RC. Analysis for financial management. 6th Ed. Boston: Irwin McGraw-Hill, 2001.

Keown AJ, Petty JW, Martin JD, et al. Foundations of finance: the logic and practice of finance management. 5th Ed. Upper Saddle River, NJ: Prentice Hall, 2006.

## PROBLEMS

1. Shown are financial statements for Apple Blossom Pharmacy, a long-term care pharmacy. Also shown are financial statements for the "typical" long-term care pharmacy. Perform a financial statement analysis for Apple Blossom Pharmacy. Your analysis should include a ratio analysis, common size statement analysis, and DuPont Model of Profitability analysis. Use the results of your analysis to discuss Apple Blossom Pharmacy's liquidity, solvency, efficiency, profitability, and overall performance. Because beginning inventories are not given, assume that beginning inventory is equal to ending inventory.

| | Apple Blossom Pharmacy | | Typical Long-Term Care Pharmacy | |
|---|---|---|---|---|
| | $ | % | $ | % Sales |
| Sales* | 1,325,000 | 100.0 | 2,004,163 | 100.0 |
| Cost of goods sold | 900,000 | 67.9 | 1,146,248 | 57.2 |
| Gross margin | 425,000 | 32.1 | 857,915 | 42.8 |
| Operating expenses | | | | |
|  Salaries and benefits | 280,000 | 21.1 | 453,454 | 22.6 |
|  Rent | 12,000 | 0.9 | 27,222 | 1.4 |
|  Utilities | 10,000 | 0.8 | 15,986 | 0.8 |
|  Professional fees | 9,000 | 0.7 | 26,658 | 1.3 |
|  Taxes and licenses | 2,500 | 0.2 | 3,110 | 0.2 |
|  Insurance | 10,500 | 0.8 | 8,739 | 0.4 |
|  Interest | 11,000 | 0.8 | 9,855 | 0.5 |
|  Computer expenses | 9,500 | 0.7 | 13,515 | 0.7 |
|  Depreciation | 19,000 | 1.4 | 32,116 | 1.6 |
|  Marketing | 1,000 | 0.1 | 4,166 | 0.2 |
|  Miscellaneous | 42,000 | 3.2 | 85,513 | 4.3 |
| Total expenses | 406,500 | 30.7 | 680,334 | 33.9 |
| Net income before taxes | 18,500 | 1.4 | 177,581 | 8.9 |
| Assets | | | | |
|  Cash | 39,000 | 2.9 | 129,733 | 6.5 |
|  Accounts receivables | 185,000 | 14.0 | 316,558 | 15.8 |
|  Inventory | 125,000 | 9.4 | 156,111 | 7.8 |
|  Prepaid expenses | 41,000 | 3.1 | 71,724 | 3.6 |
|  Total current assets | 390,000 | 29.4 | 674,126 | 33.6 |
| Net fixed assets | 90,000 | 6.8 | 92,283 | 4.6 |
| Total assets | 480,000 | 36.2 | 766,409 | 38.2 |
| Liabilities | | | | |
|  Accounts payable | 176,000 | 13.3 | 105,099 | 5.2 |
|  Note payable | 6,000 | 0.5 | 24,012 | 1.2 |
|  Accruals | 31,000 | 2.3 | 84,323 | 4.2 |

| | | | | |
|---|---|---|---|---|
| Total current liabilities | 213,000 | 16.1 | 213,434 | 10.7 |
| Total long-term debt | 190,000 | 14.3 | 128,780 | 6.4 |
| Total liabilities | 403,000 | 30.4 | 342,214 | 17.1 |
| Owner equity | 77,000 | 5.8 | 424,195 | 21.2 |
| Total liabilities and owner equity | 480,000 | 36.2 | 766,409 | 38.2 |

*All sales are credit sales.

2. Shown are 2 years of financial statements for Tarboro Pharmacy, an independently owned community pharmacy. Perform a financial statement analysis for Tarboro Pharmacy. Your analysis should include a ratio analysis, common size statement analysis, and DuPont Model of Profitability evaluation. Use the results of your analysis to discuss Tarboro Pharmacy's liquidity, solvency, profitability, efficiency, and overall performance. Financial statements for a comparable group of independent pharmacies are also provided.

| | Tarboro Pharmacy | | | | Typical Pharmacy | |
|---|---|---|---|---|---|---|
| | Year Ended 12/31/20X1 | | Year ended 12/31/20X2 | | Year ended 12/31/20X2 | |
| | $ | % | $ | % | $ | % |
| *Sales* | | | | | | |
| Cash | 339,180 | | 317,085 | | 519,480 | |
| Credit | 791,420 | | 739,865 | | 779,220 | |
| Total | 1,130,600 | 100.0 | 1,056,950 | 100.0 | 1,298,700 | 100.0 |
| *Cost of goods sold* | | | | | | |
| Beginning inventory | 190,000 | | 187,000 | | 159,000 | |
| Purchases | 773,500 | | 730,750 | | 946,050 | |
| COGAS | 963,500 | | 917,750 | | 1,105,050 | |
| Ending inventory | 187,000 | | 176,500 | | 160,900 | |
| Cost of goods sold | 776,500 | 68.7 | 741,250 | 70.1 | 944,150 | 72.7 |
| Gross margin | 354,100 | 31.3 | 315,700 | 29.9 | 354,550 | 27.3 |
| *Operating expenses* | | | | | | |
| Owner salary | 64,100 | 5.7 | 65,650 | 6.2 | 80,150 | 6.2 |
| Employee salaries | 121,850 | 10.8 | 110,100 | 10.4 | 107,500 | 8.3 |
| Rent | 23,300 | 2.1 | 25,300 | 2.4 | 21,350 | 1.6 |
| Utilities | 16,750 | 1.5 | 15,500 | 1.5 | 9,300 | 0.7 |
| Prescription containers | 6,050 | 0.5 | 6,400 | 0.6 | 6,050 | 0.5 |
| Computer expenses | 2,950 | 0.3 | 5,400 | 0.5 | 6,750 | 0.5 |
| Security | 7,000 | 0.6 | 9,100 | 0.9 | 7,400 | 0.6 |
| Delivery | 2,900 | 0.3 | 1,450 | 0.1 | 4,600 | 0.4 |
| Advertising | 9,950 | 0.9 | 4,400 | 0.4 | 7,600 | 0.6 |
| Miscellaneous | 36,850 | 3.3 | 31,300 | 3.0 | 56,700 | 4.4 |
| Total expenses | 291,700 | 25.8 | 274,600 | 26.0 | 307,400 | 23.7 |
| Net income before taxes | 62,400 | 5.5 | 41,100 | 3.9 | 47,150 | 3.6 |

| Assets | | | | | | |
|---|---|---|---|---|---|---|
| Cash | 5,300 | 0.5 | 900 | 0.1 | 56,600 | 4.4 |
| Accounts receivables | 54,250 | 4.8 | 51,500 | 4.9 | 73,200 | 5.6 |
| Inventory | 187,000 | 16.5 | 176,500 | 16.7 | 160,900 | 12.4 |
| Prepaid expenses | 17,100 | 1.5 | 16,100 | 1.5 | 18,200 | 1.4 |
| Total current assets | 263,650 | 23.3 | 245,000 | 23.2 | 308,900 | 23.8 |
| Net fixed assets | 25,500 | 2.3 | 19,150 | 1.8 | 37,600 | 2.9 |
| Total assets | 289,150 | 25.6 | 264,150 | 25.0 | 346,500 | 26.7 |
| Liabilities | | | | | | |
| Accounts payable | 70,200 | 6.2 | 82,400 | 7.8 | 60,650 | 4.7 |
| Note payable | 10,700 | 0.9 | 11,050 | 1.0 | 17,800 | 1.4 |
| Accruals | 2,000 | 0.2 | 2,400 | 0.2 | 17,150 | 1.3 |
| Total current liabilities | 82,900 | 7.3 | 95,850 | 9.1 | 95,600 | 7.4 |
| Total long-term debt | 9,200 | 0.8 | 42,200 | 4.0 | 42,300 | 3.3 |
| Total liabilities | 92,150 | 8.2 | 138,050 | 13.1 | 137,900 | 10.6 |
| Owner equity | 197,000 | 17.4 | 126,100 | 11.9 | 208,600 | 16.1 |
| Total liabilities and owner equity | 289,150 | 25.6 | 264,150 | 25.0 | 346,500 | 26.7 |

3. The Sawbones Medical Center is a 600-bed university teaching hospital. During the most recent year, it provided 175,000 days of patient care. During this same period of time, the hospital pharmacy had drug acquisition costs of $21,000,000 and an annual payroll of $2,000,000, and maintained an average inventory of $2,400,000. Assume that the typical hospital pharmacy of this size has an inventory turnover of 12, a drug expense per patient day of $104, and a personnel expense per day of $30.50. Evaluate the director's performance in managing inventory and personnel.

4. Shown below are financial statements for Rivbo Drugs, a large national chain of pharmacies, and comparison figures for a similar group of chain pharmacies. Perform a financial statement analysis for Rivbo Drugs for both years. Your analysis should include both a ratio analysis and an evaluation of common size statements. Use the results of your analysis to discuss Rivbo's liquidity, solvency, efficiency, profitability, and overall performance. Also do an analysis using the DuPont Model of Profitability and present suggestions for improving Rivbo's performance. Note: Credit sales are not specified, so the accounts receivables collection period cannot be calculated. Rivbo's inventory at the end of 20X2 was $475,000,000.

| | Chain Averages | Rivbo—20X4 | | Rivbo—20X3 | |
|---|---|---|---|---|---|
| | % | $ | % | $ | % |
| Income statement | | | | | |
| Sales | 100.0 | 2,504 | 100.0 | 2,242 | 100.0 |
| COGS | 71.7 | 1,742 | 69.6 | 1,568 | 69.9 |
| Gross margin | 28.3 | 762 | 30.4 | 674 | 30.1 |

| | | | | | |
|---|---|---|---|---|---|
| Operating expenses | 24.6 | 685 | 27.4 | 639 | 28.5 |
| Net income before taxes | 3.7 | 77 | 3.1 | 35 | 1.6 |
| *Balance sheet* | | | | | |
| Current assets | | | | | |
| Cash | 0.7 | 24 | 1.0 | 18 | 0.8 |
| Accounts receivables | 2.4 | 42 | 1.7 | 34 | 1.5 |
| Inventory | 17.9 | 505 | 20.2 | 488 | 21.8 |
| Prepaid expenses | 0.5 | 13 | 0.5 | 12 | 0.5 |
| Total current assets | 21.5 | 584 | 23.3 | 552 | 24.6 |
| Net fixed assets | 14.6 | 429 | 17.1 | 467 | 20.8 |
| Other assets | 2.0 | 48 | 1.9 | 26 | 1.2 |
| Total assets | 38.1 | 1,061 | 42.4 | 1,045 | 46.6 |
| *Current liabilities* | | | | | |
| Accounts payable | 5.9 | 181 | 7.2 | 154 | 6.9 |
| Accrued liabilities | 5.2 | 159 | 6.4 | 152 | 6.8 |
| Short-term notes | 0.4 | 1 | 0.0 | 24 | 1.1 |
| Total current liabilities | 11.5 | 341 | 13.6 | 330 | 14.7 |
| Long-term debt | 12.1 | 220 | 8.8 | 261 | 11.6 |
| Total liabilities | 23.6 | 561 | 22.4 | 591 | 26.4 |
| Owners' equity | 14.5 | 500 | 20.0 | 454 | 20.3 |
| Total liabilities and owner equity | 38.1 | 1,061 | 42.4 | 1,045 | 46.6 |

($ Figures in millions)

| Ratio | Chain Averages |
|---|---|
| ROE | 20.0 |
| ROA | 9.8 |
| GM% | 28.3 |
| NI% | 3.7 |
| CR | 1.9 |
| QR | 0.3 |
| APP | 30.1 |
| CL TO OE | 57.6 |
| LTD TO OE | 44.1 |
| TD TO OE | 101.8 |
| Fin. Leverage | 2.0 |
| ITO | 4.1 |
| ATO | 2.7 |

# Budgeting

After completing this chapter, the student should be able to:

1. Name and define the three types of budgets commonly prepared by pharmacies,
2. Develop simple demand forecasts for new and existing pharmacies,
3. List and discuss the steps in the planning process,
4. List and discuss the steps in developing an operating budget,
5. Use a performance report to identify and analyze budget variances,
6. Define and differentiate price, volume, and mix effects in analyzing budget variances, and
7. Define and differentiate controllable and noncontrollable expenses and their use in evaluating and motivating employees.

Planning and controlling operations of the business are two of a manager's most important functions. Budgeting is a process that assists the manager in carrying out both functions. A budget is most simply defined as a plan expressed in monetary terms. It shows what a pharmacy's goals are and the expenditures the pharmacy expects to make to meet them. Because it expresses the pharmacy's goals and plans in dollar terms, the budget provides a standard with which actual performance can be compared. This provides the manager with a means of controlling the operation of the pharmacy.

Pharmacies commonly prepare three different types of budgets. An *operating budget* shows the pharmacy's anticipated revenues and expenses for the coming 6 to 12 months. A *cash budget* is a schedule of forecasted cash receipts and payments. It shows the pharmacy's anticipated cash inflows and outflows for the next 6 to 12 months. A *capital budget* shows the pharmacy's planned investment in fixed assets. Capital budgets are more common in large organizations such as hospitals, chain pharmacy organizations, or large multisite long-term care pharmacy providers. Examples of the types of projects found in capital budgets include purchase and installation of a computer system, purchase of a robotic dispensing system, and major renovation of the pharmacy itself. This chapter will discuss operating budgets. Cash budgets will be discussed in the next chapter. Chapter 11 will discuss capital budgets.

Proper budgeting depends on two other processes: demand forecasting and planning. Each of these will be addressed before the discussion of budgeting is continued.

## FORECASTING

The initial and most crucial step in preparing both cash and operating budgets is constructing a forecast of demand. The demand forecast made in community pharmacies is typically a sales forecast. In hospital pharmacies, it is more common to forecast a measure of demand such as patient admissions or discharges or patient days.

A forecast is an estimate of demand for the next 6 to 12 months. Because developing a forecast requires predicting what will happen in the future, it is a difficult and inexact process. Most forecasting techniques fall into one of two categories: analyzing past years' data or employing expert judgment. The method suggested here utilizes both types of techniques.

### Forecasting for an Existing Pharmacy

Demand forecasts are frequently based on the *trend* of demand over the past several years. For example, if the director of a hospital pharmacy determines that patient discharges have decreased by 4% per year for the past 5 years, then his or her initial estimate of next year's discharges would be made by subtracting 4% from the current year's discharges.

As a more specific example, the data in Figure 6-1 present annual sales for a pharmacy for a 7-year period. From these data, the annual percentage increase in sales has been calculated for each year. For example, the sales increase for 20X7 is calculated by subtracting 20X6's sales from 20X7's sales and dividing this amount by 20X6's sales.

| Year | Sales | % Increase |
|------|-------|------------|
| 20X7 | $594,000 | 4.0 |
| 20X6 | 571,000 | 7.9 |
| 20X5 | 529,000 | 6.2 |
| 20X4 | 498,000 | 13.4 |
| 20X3 | 439,000 | 5.5 |
| 20X2 | 416,000 | 6.1 |
| 20X1 | 392,000 | — |
| Average | | 7.2 |

**FIGURE 6-1**    Annual pharmacy sales and percentage sales increases.

Using the numbers:

$$20X7 \text{ \% sales increase} = [(\$594,000 - 571,000)/571,000] \times 100\%$$
$$= 4.0\%$$

The average annual increase for the 7-year period was 7.2%. This represents the *expected* or *forecasted* increase in sales for 20X8. In this case, the sales forecast for 20X8 would be 20X7 sales ($594,000) plus the 7.2% increase (594,000 × 0.072). Thus, 20X8 sales would be estimated as $637,000.

Any estimate based on past years' data assumes that future conditions will be similar to past conditions. Because of changes in competition, economic conditions, government regulation, and the pharmacy's own marketing programs, this assumption is often untrue. As a result, the initial forecast based on past data must be supplemented by the manager's judgment of the effects of changing conditions.

In revising the forecast, the manager must consider both external and internal factors that may affect demand. External factors are those over which the manager has no control, such as inflation, business conditions, new government regulations, new methods of treatment, and changes in competition. Internal factors are those over which the manager has some control. They include changes in prices, promotion, service, hours of operation, and products. Because of the difficulty of developing accurate forecasts, managers often develop three forecasts. One is based on optimistic estimates, one on pessimistic estimates, and one on what the manager believes most likely to occur.

## Forecasting for a New Pharmacy

Developing a demand forecast for a new pharmacy is more difficult because no data on past demand are available. Forecasting demand for a new pharmacy first requires that the manager develop an estimate of *market potential*. Market potential refers to total demand in the pharmacy's market area of those goods and services provided by the pharmacy. For a community pharmacy that sells only prescription and over-the-counter (OTC) drugs, market potential consists of all sales of these items in the area from which the pharmacy draws its patients. For an ear, nose, and throat hospital, market potential consists of all hospital-based ear, nose, and throat procedures performed in the area from which the hospital draws its patients.

Estimates of market potential may be developed from published statistics on area demand. *Sales and Marketing Management Magazine* publishes an annual "Survey of Buying Patterns," which estimates sales of drugs and drug sundries for each county in the United States. For pharmacies with trading areas smaller than the entire county, local census records can be used to develop estimates of market potential. Census records are available in local libraries and online at the U.S. Bureau of the Census site (http://census.gov/home). *The American Fact Finder* link provides, for example, estimates of population for various sized areas such as blocks, census tracts, and cities. Census data also provide breakdowns of each of these areas by age, sex, education, and race. Statistics on prescription usage and average prescription prices can be applied to population estimates to develop estimates of market potential. Statistics describing prescription usage and prices are available from the National Center for Health Statistics, from publications of major pharmacy benefits managers (PBMs) such as the *Medco Drug Trend Report* and Express Scripts' *Drug Trend Report*, and in trade journals such as *Drug Topics* or *US Pharmacist*. The Kaiser Family Foundation website

| Age Range | Population | Rx Purchases Per Person Per Year | Total Rx Purchases Per Year | Average Rx Price Price | Total Rx Expenditures Per Year |
|---|---|---|---|---|---|
| 0 to 18 | 595 | 4.2 | 2,499 | $53.00 | $  132,897 |
| 19 to 64 | 2,135 | 13.7 | 29,250 | 53.00 | 1,555,488 |
| 65 plus | 770 | 28.7 | 22,099 | 53.00 | 1,175,225 |
| Totals | 3,500 | | 53,848 | | $ 2,863,610 |

**FIGURE 6-2**  Calculation of market potential for prescription sales.

(www.kff.org) includes statistics on prescription drug use by age and average prescription prices. Figure 6-2 illustrates the calculation of market potential for prescriptions for a community pharmacy.

The *American Journal of Health-System Pharmacy* periodically publishes information on hospital drug expenditures.[1,2] In addition, it annually publishes an article aimed at assisting managers in estimating drug expenditures for the coming year.[3]

Once market potential is estimated, the manager must attempt to determine the share, or proportion, of total area demand that the pharmacy can attract. This will depend on the pharmacy's or hospital's marketing program (its pricing and advertising, what products it carries, its hours of operation and services, for example) and its competition. For example, the manager of the pharmacy to which the data in Figure 6-2 applied may estimate that his or her pharmacy can attract 20% of sales in the pharmacy's market area. Assuming a 20% share, the pharmacy's sales forecast would be $2,863,610 × 0.20 = $572,722.

## PLANNING

All organizations need to plan. Planning makes explicit what the organization expects to accomplish and how it intends to accomplish it. Proper planning provides guidance to employees and a structure for determining how well the organization is performing.

## Planning Process

All planning should begin with a careful consideration of the organization's *mission*. This is typically defined in the organization's mission statement. The mission statement is a broad, general description of the basic societal need that the organization satisfies. Because it deals with the organization's basic function, a mission statement should guide the organization over very long periods of time. All of the organization's plans should flow directly from and be consistent with its mission statement. The mission statement for Omnicare, a large provider of pharmacy services to long-term care residents, is shown in Figure 6-3.

An organization's mission statement should answer the question, "What is the organization's business?" That is, what service does the organization provide to society? The answer to this question determines, in a very basic way, how the organization is operated.

Omnicare's mission statement indicates that it provides pharmacy services for the elderly. This both defines and limits the types of business opportunities that Omnicare

*Mission Statement:*

"Omnicare's mission is to build the nation's preeminent pharmacy services organization dedicated to enhancing the quality and cost-effectiveness of care for the elderly."

*Goals:*

- ■ "By assisting the health care facilities we serve in achieving positive, healthy outcomes for their residents in a cost-effective manner, we create value for our Customers."

- ■ "By fostering an environment where commitment to achievement and personal growth is encouraged and by recognizing each individual's contribution to the success of the whole, we create value for our Employees."

- ■ "By recognizing our obligation to achieve superior financial performance and provide a competitive return on investment, we create value for our Shareholders."

*Strategy:*

"Omnicare's vision is that a national organization dedicated to lowering costs through economies of scale and consolidation and to enhancing care through specialization can be an important force in the long-term care pharmacy industry. Our objective is to build such an organization through a two-pronged growth strategy. First, we seek to acquire quality regional providers of institutional pharmacy services in new and existing geographic markets. Second, we promote and support strong internal growth in the companies we acquire by capitalizing on opportunities for increased market penetration and expansion of the services we offer.

. . . . Our consolidation strategy allows us to lower costs significantly. We believe the Omnicare strategy puts us on course to make a significant contribution to the quality and cost-effectiveness of care for the elderly and, in turn, achieve substantial growth and improved return on investment."

*Objectives: (suggested by annual report)*

1. Acquire three strong regional long-term care pharmacies operating in the midwestern U.S. by end of year. The pharmacies must be in areas which expand our geographic reach and solidify our market position.

2. Increase the number of nursing facility residents served by 5% by year end. This will include increases brought about through acquisitions and by increasing the numbers of residents served by current facilities.

3. Develop and implement a "clinically-based drug formulary specifically tailored for the geriatric population" by the end of the third quarter.

4. Complete formation of Professional Services Committee (PSC) by the end of the first quarter. The PSC will "bring together some of the nation's highest quality pharmacy providers" to "develop and implement leading edge geriatric pharmaceutical care."

5. Consolidate purchasing for pharmacies acquired during the past year by the end of the second quarter.

6. Complete development of clinical training programs for consultant pharmacists by the end of the second quarter. Train 75% of consultant pharmacists by year end.

7. Raise $50 million to finance growth and acquisitions by the end of the third quarter by issue of convertible subordinated notes. (A convertible subordinated note is a type of debt.)

**FIGURE 6–3**    Omnicare: mission, goals, strategy, and objectives (taken from Omnicare, Inc. Annual Report 1993: Creating Value in Long-Term Care Pharmacy, Cincinnati, Omnicare, Inc., 1994).

will pursue. For example, Omnicare currently serves elderly patients who are cared for in long-term care facilities. Given this ability to serve institutionalized patients, it might make sense for Omnicare to look for opportunities in other types of institutions that need pharmaceutical services, such as prisons and mental hospitals. But, Omnicare has defined its mission as serving elderly patients. Because prisons and mental hospitals care for people of all ages, Omnicare is not likely to seek their business. On the other hand, a growing number of noninstitutionalized elderly patients need home IV infusion services. Serving these patients would be different from Omnicare's current business but consistent with its mission.

The second step in the planning process is to define the *goals* of the organization. Goals are endpoints that must be accomplished for the organization to fulfill its mission. Goals are, consequently, more specific than the mission statement. Omnicare's goals are shown in Figure 6-3. Omnicare's goals recognize that to be successful it must provide pharmaceutical services that result in positive, cost-effective outcomes in the patients it serves, a positive environment for its employees, and a competitive return for its investors.

Once goals have been decided upon, the *strategies* that will be used to reach those goals must be specified. Strategies are broad guidelines, or basic operating principles, that indicate how the organization will meet its goals. They serve as guides and constraints for more specific, functional plans. Omnicare's strategy, as described in Figure 6-3, is to decrease costs through economies of scale and consolidation and to enhance patient care by specializing in pharmaceutical treatment of geriatric patients.

The next step in the planning process is to decide upon the organization's *objectives*. Objectives are statements of specific tasks that must be accomplished in the next 1 to 5 years if the organization is to meet its goals. Each of an organization's objectives should specify, in measurable terms, what is to be accomplished, by what date it should be accomplished, and its priority relative to the organization's other objectives. Omnicare's second objective, for example, states that the company should increase the number of residents served by 5% by the end of the year (Fig. 6-3).

*Functional plans* are detailed specifications of how each objective will be met. Functional plans cover the same time periods as the objectives on which they are based. Functional plans must be evaluated continuously. This is done by comparing what was planned with what has actually been accomplished. Major discrepancies indicate either problems with which the manager needs to deal or changing conditions that require revising the plans.

## Planning and Budgeting

A budget translates the pharmacy's objectives and functional plans into monetary terms. Operating budgets forecast the costs of implementing plans and the revenues that will result from fulfilling objectives. Cash budgets forecast the impact of plans on cash inflows and outflows. Capital budgets reflect the costs of purchasing fixed assets that are required to meet the organization's objectives.

As an example, one of Omnicare's objectives is to increase the number of nursing home residents served by 5%. Omnicare's operating budget for the year would reflect the additional revenues it would earn from serving 5% more nursing home residents. Similarly, the operating budget would estimate the extra costs required to attract and serve a larger number of residents. This would involve additional sales, marketing, and administrative costs for attracting additional nursing home contracts and the higher drug, supply, and personnel costs required to serve additional patients.

## OPERATING BUDGET

The operating budget shows the pharmacy's planned revenues and expenses for some future period of time, usually 12 months. Typically, the budget will be prepared so that it also shows budgeted revenues and expenses for shorter periods of time, such as months or quarters. This is done to allow managers to compare actual and budgeted performance and to take corrective actions in a timely manner. Examples of operating budgets for a chain community and hospital pharmacy are shown in Figures 6-4 and 6-5.

| Operating Budget<br>Wellrun Pharmacy<br>For the year ended 12-31-20X8 | |
| --- | --- |
| Sales | |
| Prescription | $4,649,200 |
| Other | 2,339,230 |
| Total | 6,988,430 |
| Gross profit | |
| Prescription | 890,000 |
| Other | 812,520 |
| Total | 1,702,520 |
| Salary | |
| Pharmacists | 353,370 |
| Technicians & clerks | 339,000 |
| Management | 41,850 |
| Total salary | 734,220 |
| Other controllable expenses | |
| Repair & maintenance | 18,870 |
| Utilities | 36,670 |
| Supplies | 770 |
| Other | 129,480 |
| Total other controllable | 185,790 |
| Noncontrollable expenses | |
| Tax & license | 6,340 |
| Insurance | 67,690 |
| Depreciation | 26,200 |
| Promotion | 10,760 |
| Rent | 284,760 |
| Other | 71,790 |
| Total noncontrollable expenses | 467,540 |
| Total expenses | 1,387,550 |
| Net income | $ 314,970 |

FIGURE 6-4   Operating budget for a chain community pharmacy.

**Operating Budget**
**Goodcare Hospital Pharmacy**
**Year ended 12-31-20X9**

| | |
|---|---:|
| Prescription orders | |
| Inpatient | 4,349,292 |
| Outpatient | 481,749 |
| Revenues | |
| Inpatient | $43,492,920 |
| Outpatient | 24,087,450 |
| Total | $67,580,370 |
| Expenses | |
| Salaries—Management | 665,000 |
| Salaries—Pharmacists and technicians | 7,300,000 |
| Salaries—Support staff | 300,000 |
| Salaries—Other | 105,000 |
| Employee benefits | 2,000,000 |
| Total salaries and benefits | 10,370,000 |
| Drugs | 38,000,000 |
| Intravenous supplies | 700,000 |
| Blood and blood products | 5,500,000 |
| Medical/surgical supplies | 500,000 |
| Computer | 250,000 |
| Rent—buildings | 200,000 |
| Leased equipment | 275,000 |
| Office expense | 190,000 |
| Miscellaneous | 975,000 |
| Total nonpersonnel | 46,500,158 |
| Total operating expenses | 56,870,158 |
| Surplus | $10,710,212 |

**FIGURE 6-5**  Operating budget for a hospital pharmacy.

## Preparing an Operating Budget

The basic steps involved in preparing an operating budget are the same for all organizations. In a large organization, such as a hospital, health maintenance organization (HMO), or chain of pharmacies, the process is more complicated because many operating units and individuals are involved. We will first consider the case of preparing a budget in a small organization. This illustrates the basic steps. We then will consider the additional steps involved in budgeting in larger organizations.

### Basic Steps in Preparing the Operating Budget

In a small organization, such as an independently owned community pharmacy, the process of preparing an operating budget is relatively simple. The person responsible for the budget, usually the owner or manager, begins by considering the pharmacy's objectives for the coming year. Attaining a targeted net income is almost always a critical objective. The manager then decides what programs and activities are required to achieve the pharmacy's objectives. In terms of the planning process, the manager develops functional plans for the pharmacy.

Next, the manager develops revenue and expense budgets. These are forecasts of revenues for the coming year and of the expenses required to generate those revenues. The revenue and expense budgets are based on the initial forecast of demand. They also incorporate the expected results of any plans the manager has to increase demand or control expenses in the coming year and the expected impact of changes in external conditions (such as inflation and increased competition) that would affect sales or costs.

Once revenue and expense budgets have been prepared, the manager can determine whether projected revenues and expenses will yield the target income. If not, he or she must revise either the revenue budget, the expense budget, or both. The process of preparing revenue and expense budgets, checking them against the target net income, and revising them continues until a satisfactory budget is achieved.

## Preparing a Budget in a Larger Organization

While the basic steps involved in preparing an operating budget are the same in a large organization, the process is complicated by having more employees and operating units involved. Typically, each operating unit will prepare its own budget. (Each department in a hospital or HMO would be an operating unit.) Preparation of the unit operating budgets is done in much the same manner as discussed in the previous section. The organization's budget is then prepared by aggregating, or "rolling up," the budgets of each of the operating units.

Because the overall budget for a large organization is based on the individual operating units' budgets, someone in upper management must coordinate the budgets of the various operating units. Because many different individuals are involved, a great deal of discussion and negotiation may be required.

In a large organization, annual objectives are decided on by top management and passed down to lower levels of the organization. Along with the annual objectives, top management provides data on other factors that affect revenue and expense estimates. These may include forecasts of economic conditions and demand, allowable salary increases, and anticipated increases in operating costs and prices.

Based on this information, the head of each operating unit sets annual objectives for the unit and develops plans to meet the objectives. Each unit's objectives must be consistent with the overall goals, objectives, and mission of the organization. After formulating plans for the year, the unit head prepares an operating budget that will allow implementation of the plans.

The head of each operating unit then submits the unit budget to his or her superior. The superior reviews and coordinates the budgets of the individual operating units. The review ensures that the budgets of the operating units are consistent with the overall goals and objectives of the organization, that the roll-up budget based on the operating unit budgets meets the organization's revenue and expense goals, and that the budgets of units that are dependent on each other are coordinated. A hospital administrator, for example, would check to ensure that the department of nursing budgeted for sufficient nurses and the pharmacy budgeted for sufficient drugs to cover the volume of surgeries anticipated by the department of surgery.

If the superior uncovers problems with the unit's budget, he or she and the unit head meet to discuss and resolve the problems. This involves negotiation. The superior attempts to convince the unit head that some of the budget estimates are unreasonable. The unit head attempts to justify them. The negotiation should continue until mutually acceptable estimates are agreed upon. It is important that the superior not force the unit head to accept budget estimates that he or she believes to be unreasonable. Unit heads, and other employees, will not be motivated to work to attain levels of performance that they believe are unrealistic. The endpoint of the negotiation should be a mutually acceptable budget. The unit head's acceptance of the budget indicates that he or she agrees budgeted figures are realistic goals that the department should be able to meet. The superior's acceptance indicates agreement that if budgeted revenue and expense budgets are met, the operating unit and its head would have performed at an acceptable level. The agreement of both parties is contingent upon there being no major departures from the assumptions underlying the budget. For example, if wage rates increased much faster than anticipated, the unit head should not be held to budgeted estimates of personnel costs.

Review and negotiation continue until all operating unit budgets are acceptable. At this point, upper management approves the individual units' budgets, prepares the final roll-up budget, and distributes it throughout the organization.

## An Example of the Budget Process in a Hospital

An example may clarify the process of budget construction. We will use a small hospital as an example of a larger organization. The hospital's management consists of an administrator and several department directors. These include the directors of pharmacy, nursing, housekeeping, and central supply.

The hospital's budget process begins with the administrator identifying the hospital's objectives for the year. In conjunction with the hospital's fiscal department, the administrator then gathers relevant statistics—such as last year's patient discharges and number of surgeries—and projections, such as the projected number of admissions, patient mix, and increases in operating costs for the coming year. In addition, he or she decides on other data needed for budget preparation, such as allowable amounts for raises, promotions, and new personnel. The administrator then passes this information to the department directors.

Each director then determines the programs that the department needs to contribute to reaching the hospital's objectives. If one of the hospital's objectives was to increase its involvement in home health care, the pharmacy director might see the pharmacy's contribution as implementing a home IV therapy service. Based on the information given to the director by the administrator and the more specific objectives of the pharmacy, the director then develops revenue and expense budgets for the pharmacy. In developing these estimates, he or she should consult with staff members most knowledgeable about various pharmacy areas. For example, the director should confer with the outpatient pharmacy supervisor to determine the personnel expenses for that area and with the director of outpatient clinics to determine the volume and type of outpatient visits anticipated for the coming year. Each of the other department directors develops an operating budget in similar manner.

The department budgets are submitted to the hospital administrator for review. The review covers several areas. First, he or she ensures that departmental budgets are consistent with the hospital's objectives and plans for the year. Second, he or she coordinates the budgets of departments that work closely with each other. Finally, he or she rolls up the individual department budgets into an aggregate hospital budget. This is necessary to ensure that total revenues are adequate to cover the hospital's total expenses.

If the administrator has problems with the pharmacy budget, he or she meets with the pharmacy director to discuss them. Assume that the administrator felt the forecast for pharmaceuticals expense was too high. He or she would point this out to the director, along with his or her reasons for believing the projection was too high. The pharmacy director might justify his or her estimates based on anticipated increases in prescription volume or prices or on the high cost of new products expected to be marketed during the coming year. The negotiation should continue until mutually satisfactory estimates were agreed upon. The administrator holds similar meetings with all other department directors.

After concluding the meetings with the department directors, the administrator prepares a roll-up budget based on the revised departmental budgets. If this budget is satisfactory, the administrator approves it, publishes it, and sends it to the department heads for implementation. If it is not satisfactory, the process of negotiation and revision continues.

## Revision of the Budget during the Year

An operating budget is based on assumptions about what will happen during the coming year. The revenue budget, for example, is based on management's assumptions about business conditions, government regulations, prescriber and consumer response to changes in advertising, and competition. The expense budget is based on assumptions about costs, wages, and employee productivity. If the assumptions on which the budget are based turn out to be inaccurate, that is, if actual conditions turn out differently than expected, the budget may be unrealistic. There is much disagreement about whether the operating budget should be revised to reflect changes in operating conditions.

Many authorities believe that budgets should be revised to reflect changes in operating conditions. Not revising, they believe, results in a budget that is not realistic. Unrealistic budgets are not as useful for planning and coordinating operations or for evaluating employee performance.

Proponents of not revising the budget base their argument on the use of a budget as a standard against which performance can be measured. To be useful, a standard must be stable and reliable. A budget that is revised provides neither a stable nor a reliable standard. Thus, such a budget has little use for controlling operations or for motivating employees. Also, a policy of allowing revisions gives employees an incentive to argue that any departure from the budget is due to changes in external conditions rather than inadequate performance. Proponents of this position believe that, rather than revising the budget, managers should consider changes in conditions when deciding how to deal with departures from the budget. For example, in deciding whether some action should be taken with regard to higher than expected utility costs, a manager's superior would take into consideration that the winter was unusually cold.

## Fixed versus Flexible Budgets

A *fixed budget* is one that is based on a single level of forecasted demand. The manager develops the best possible forecast of demand and bases revenue and expense projections on this forecast. The budgets shown in Figures 6-3 and 6-4 are examples of fixed budgets.

A *flexible budget* is one that allows budgeted *variable* expenses to change in response to changes in demand. Variable expenses are those that increase or decrease in direct proportion to changes in demand. Expenses such as cost of goods sold and prescription labels and vials are examples of variable expenses. As sales or number of medication orders dispensed increase, these costs increase proportionately. Variable expenses can be differentiated from fixed expenses, such as depreciation and property taxes, which stay the same regardless of changes in demand. A flexible budget explicitly recognizes that when demand is higher (or lower) than anticipated, the budgeted figures for cost of goods sold, supplies, and other variable costs should be allowed to change proportionately. Flexible budgets are preferable for pharmacies that typically experience wide or unexpected variations in demand.

A flexible budget may be constructed by specifying several likely levels of demand and the expected revenues and expenses at each. An example of a flexible budget for a hospital pharmacy is shown in Figure 6-6.

**Operating Budget**
**Goodcare Hospital Pharmacy**
**Year ended 12-31-20X9**

| Prescription orders | | | |
|---|---|---|---|
| Inpatient | 3,000,000 | 4,000,000 | 5,000,000 |
| Outpatient | 400,000 | 450,000 | 500,000 |
| Total | 3,400,000 | 4,450,000 | 5,500,000 |
| Revenues | | | |
| Inpatient | $30,000,000 | $40,000,000 | $50,000,000 |
| Outpatient | 20,000,000 | 22,500,000 | 25,000,000 |
| Total | 50,000,000 | 62,500,000 | 75,000,000 |
| Fixed expenses | | | |
| Salaries—Management | 665,000 | 665,000 | 665,000 |
| Salaries—Support staff | 300,000 | 300,000 | 300,000 |
| Salaries—Other | 105,000 | 105,000 | 105,000 |
| Employee benefits—Fixed salaries | 256,000 | 256,000 | 256,000 |
| Computer | 250,000 | 250,000 | 250,000 |
| Rent—buildings | 200,000 | 200,000 | 200,000 |
| Leased equipment | 275,000 | 275,000 | 275,000 |
| Office expense | 190,000 | 190,000 | 190,000 |
| Total fixed expenses | 2,241,000 | 2,241,000 | 2,241,000 |
| Variable expenses | | | |
| Salaries—Pharmacists and technicians | 5,134,000 | 6,719,500 | 8,305,000 |
| Employee benefits—V | 1,227,400 | 1,606,450 | 1,985,500 |
| Drugs | 26,758,000 | 35,021,500 | 43,285,000 |
| Intravenous supplies | 493,000 | 645,250 | 797,500 |
| Blood and blood products | 3,876,000 | 5,073,000 | 6,270,000 |
| Medical/surgical supplies | 353,600 | 462,800 | 572,000 |
| Miscellaneous | 686,800 | 898,900 | 1,111,000 |
| Total variable expenses | 38,528,800 | 50,427,400 | 62,326,000 |
| Total expenses | 40,769,800 | 52,668,400 | 64,567,000 |
| Surplus | $ 9,230,200 | $ 9,831,600 | $10,433,000 |

**FIGURE 6–6**  Flexible budget for a hospital pharmacy.

## Using the Operating Budget

Operating budgets are used for short-term planning, financial control, and employee motivation and evaluation. Different organizations stress some uses more than others. Churchill points out that larger, more stable organizations depend on budgets more for financial control, while smaller, more entrepreneurial firms rely on them more for planning.[4]

Use of budgets in planning has been covered. This section will discuss using budgets for financial control and employee motivation and evaluation.

## Financial Control

A budget provides a standard against which actual performance can be compared. By comparing the pharmacy's actual and budgeted revenues and expenses on a regular basis (usually monthly or quarterly), the manager can identify emerging problems and take timely action to remedy them.

Identification of problems is facilitated through use of periodic *performance reports*. A simple performance report consists of three columns. The first column shows the pharmacy's *actual* revenues and expenses, the second shows *budgeted* revenues and expenses, and the last column shows the *difference* between actual and budgeted revenue and expenses. An example is shown in Figure 6-7.

The differences between budgeted and actual amounts are referred to as *budget variances*. When an item of revenue or expense is greater than the budgeted amount, the variance is positive; when it is less than budgeted, it is negative. Whether a variance is positive or negative denotes only its numerical difference from the budgeted amount; it does not indicate whether the variance is favorable. Whether a variance is favorable or unfavorable depends on its effect on net income. If the variance increases net income, such as a positive revenue variance or a negative expense variance, it is a favorable variance (which is abbreviated F). If the variance decreases net income, such as a negative revenue variance or a positive expense variance, the variance in unfavorable (U).

*Analysis of Budget Variances*   Performance reports are prepared on a monthly or quarterly basis to allow managers to monitor performance in a timely manner. From the performance report, the manager can determine in what areas budget variances have occurred. The manager must then analyze the variances. Two analyses must be made. First, the manager must determine which variances are large enough to merit further investigation. Second, for the significant variances, the manager must determine why the variance occurred. Once the manager has determined the cause of the variance, he or she is in a position to develop and implement plans to resolve the problem. Both positive and negative variances should be analyzed.

Several methods may be used to determine whether a variance is significant. One is size of the variance. Size may be examined in either absolute terms (e.g., $1,000 over budget), in percentage terms (e.g., 10% below the budgeted amount), or in some combination of the two. Buchanan points out that larger variances may be acceptable for items over which the manager has less control.[5] For example, he suggests that a 10% variance in revenues may be acceptable because the manager has little control over revenues. However, a 10% variance in personnel expenses would not be acceptable because the manager has a great deal of control over staffing levels. Managers should also take into account the frequency of occurrence of the variance. A variance that occurs chronically should be investigated. Finally, the manager should pay special

**Wellrun Pharmacy**
**Performance Report**
**Month ended 10-31-20X8**

| | Actual ($) | Budget ($) | Variance ($) | Variance (%) | |
|---|---|---|---|---|---|
| Sales | | | | | |
| Prescription | 464,920 | 525,000 | (60,080) | (11.44) | U |
| Other | 233,923 | 225,000 | 8,923 | 3.97 | F |
| Total | 698,843 | 750,000 | (51,157) | (6.82) | U |
| Gross profit | | | | | |
| Prescription | 89,000 | 99,750 | (10,750) | (10.78) | U |
| Other | 81,252 | 78,750 | 2,502 | 3.18 | F |
| Total | 170,252 | 178,500 | (8,248) | (4.62) | U |
| Gross profit percent | | | | | |
| Prescription | 19.1 | 19.0 | 0.1 | 0.75 | F |
| Other | 34.7 | 35.0 | (0.3) | (0.76) | U |
| Total | 24.4 | 23.8 | 0.6 | 2.36 | F |
| Salary | | | | | |
| Pharmacist | 35,337 | 30,000 | 5,337 | 17.79 | U |
| Technicians & clerks | 33,900 | 37,500 | (3,600) | (9.60) | F |
| Management | 4,185 | 4,150 | 35 | 0.84 | U |
| Total salary | 73,422 | 71,650 | 1,772 | 2.47 | U |
| Other controllable expenses | | | | | |
| Repair & maintenance | 1,887 | 1,800 | 87 | 4.83 | U |
| Utilities | 3,667 | 3,600 | 67 | 1.86 | U |
| Supplies | 77 | 50 | 27 | 54.00 | U |
| Other | 12,948 | 12,950 | (2) | (0.02) | F |
| Total other controllable | 18,579 | 18,400 | 179 | 0.97 | U |
| Noncontrollable expenses | | | | | |
| Tax & license | 634 | 625 | 9 | 1.44 | U |
| Insurance | 6,769 | 6,750 | 19 | 0.28 | U |
| Depreciation | 2,620 | 2,620 | — | — | |
| Promotion | 1,076 | 2,300 | (1,224) | (53.22) | F |
| Rent | 28,476 | 28,475 | 1 | 0.00 | U |
| Other | 7,179 | 7,200 | (21) | (0.29) | F |
| Total noncontrollable expenses | 46,754 | 47,970 | (1,216) | (2.53) | F |
| Total expenses | 138,755 | 138,020 | 735 | 0.53 | U |
| Net income | 31,497 | 40,480 | (8,983) | (22.19) | U |

**FIGURE 6-7**  Performance report for a community pharmacy.

attention to variances that may have a large impact on long-run performance. For example, a pharmacy may regularly show favorable variances on housekeeping and repair expenses. Rather than being an indication of effective expense control, this may indicate a failure of the manager to spend sufficient amounts on keeping the pharmacy clean and in good repair. Because patients do not like to shop in dirty, ill-kept pharmacies, in the long run these favorable variances may result in loss of sales and profits.

In determining why a variance occurred, the manager must consider the components that make up the variance. Variances may be caused by volume, price, or mix differences. An unfavorable salary variance could be due to employees working more hours than budgeted (volume), being paid higher than budgeted salaries (price), or using more pharmacists and fewer technicians than budgeted (mix). A favorable revenue variance for prescription sales could be caused by more than the budgeted number of prescriptions being dispensed (volume), by higher than budgeted prices (price), or by dispensing a higher than budgeted number of more expensive products (mix).

The manager must consider the components of the variance because different components suggest different causes and, thus, different solutions. For example, a hospital pharmacy's drug budget (which indicates its cost of goods sold) may show an unfavorable variance because more patients than expected were served (volume), because drug prices increased, or because a more expensive mix of drugs was used. If the cause of the variance was increased numbers of patients, then no action is warranted. If the cause was an increase in drug prices, further analysis is needed. The pharmacy's drug costs may have increased either because of manufacturers' price increases or because of improper purchasing. This might have occurred from buying improper quantities or buying from suppliers who charge higher prices. If the cause of the increase was a manufacturer's price increase, there is little the manager could do. If the cause was improper purchasing, then corrective action could be taken. If a more expensive mix of drugs was used, the manager would want to determine if less expensive, but equally effective, alternatives were available.

***An Example of Analysis of Variances***    Figure 6-7 shows a performance report for Wellrun Pharmacy. The pharmacy has a policy of examining any sales or gross margin variance that exceeds 10% of the budgeted amount and any expense variance that exceeds $1,000. In examining the performance report, the manager determined that the variances for prescription sales, prescription gross margin, pharmacist salaries, technician and clerk salaries, and promotion needed further investigation.

Prescription sales had a negative, unfavorable variance. Actual sales were about 11% lower than budgeted. This could have been due to a smaller number of prescriptions dispensed, lower prices charged, or a greater proportion of less expensive drugs dispensed. Budgeted and actual prescription gross margin percents indicated that the unfavorable variance was not due to lower prices or less expensive drugs. The budgeted gross margin percent was just one tenth of 1% lower than the actual. Because little of the variance was due to price and mix changes, most of it must have been due to lower prescription volume. This was verified by comparing actual and budgeted numbers of prescriptions dispensed. (This comparison is not shown.) The manager's next step was to determine the cause of the lower volume so action could be taken to increase it.

Pharmacists' salaries were higher than budgeted. This could have been due to pharmacists working more hours or being paid at a higher rate than budgeted. Because prescription volume was lower than budgeted, there was no obvious reason for pharmacists to have worked more hours. The manager also noted that technician and clerk salaries were well under budget. This suggests that the salary variances were due to using a lower proportion of technicians and clerks and a higher proportion of pharmacists than budgeted. This could be corrected by more attention to scheduling in the next month.

Finally, promotion expense was lower than budgeted. This could have been due to running fewer promotions than budgeted or running less expensive ads. The manager checked the pharmacy's records and found that neither the mix nor prices of promotions was lower than planned, but that fewer promotions had been run. This problem could be easily solved by simply running more promotions in the coming months. It is possible that the negative prescription variance could be related to lower than budgeted promotion. If so, then increasing promotions should improve prescription volume.

## Motivating and Evaluating Employees

Just as the budget provides a performance standard for the organization as a whole, it provides a performance standard for individual employees, especially managers, within the organization. A comparison of actual and budgeted performance for the operating unit under the manager's control will indicate how well the manager performed for the year.

By providing a standard, the budget gives employees a goal to work toward. Reasonable, realistic goals motivate employees. To ensure that employees perceive budget goals as being reasonable, managers must involve those employees responsible for implementing the budget in setting budget goals. For example, the hospital pharmacy director should seek the input of the pharmacists who work in a hospital's outpatient pharmacy when estimating the unit's revenues and expenses for the coming year. Besides leading to greater motivation, employee involvement in budgeting usually leads to more accurate budgets because employees have first-hand, day-to-day working knowledge of the areas in which they work.

To improve the budget's usefulness for motivating and evaluating employees, large organizations may classify operating expenses as *controllable* or *noncontrollable* in operating units' budgets. Controllable expenses are those over which the head of the unit can exert a significant level of control. Noncontrollable expenses are those over which he or she can exert little control. A chain pharmacy manager, for example, could control the pharmacy's salary, housekeeping, and supplies expenses. Thus, these would be controllable expenses for him or her. The manager would have little control over lease payments or depreciation expenses. These would be, for that manager, noncontrollable.

Whether an expense is controllable depends on the manager's level in the organization; it is not an inherent characteristic of the expense itself. For the chain pharmacy manager, the depreciation expense is noncontrollable. The depreciation expense depends on the value of the pharmacy's fixed assets. The pharmacy manager does not make decisions about purchase of fixed assets. Consequently, he or she has little control over the depreciation expense. The vice president of the chain, on the other hand, does make decisions about purchases of fixed assets and, as a result, can control the depreciation expense. So, the depreciation expense is noncontrollable for the pharmacy manager but controllable for the vice president.

To improve motivation and for evaluation, employees' performance should be evaluated primarily in terms of controllable expenses. Employees should not be held accountable for those expenses over which they have no control.

## References

1. Pedersen CA, Schneider PJ, Santell JP. ASHP national survey of pharmacy practice in hospital settings: prescribing and transcribing—2001. Am J Health Syst Pharm 2005;58:2251–2266.
2. Pedersen CA, Schneider PJ, Scheckelhoff DJ. ASHP national survey of pharmacy practice in hospital settings: dispensing and administration—2002. Am J Health Syst Pharm—2003;60:52–68.
3. Hoffman JM, Shah ND, Vermeulen LC, et al. Projecting future drug expenditures—2005. Am J Health Syst Pharm—2005;62:149–167.
4. Churchill NC. Budget choice: planning versus control. Harvard Business Rev 1984;62:150.
5. Buchanan C. Budgeting and financial reporting. Topics Hosp Pharm Manage 1986;6:29.

## Suggested Reading

Warren CS, Reeve JM, Fess PE. Accounting. 21st Ed. Mason OH: Thomson South-Western, 2005.

Wilson AL. Financial management and cost control. In: Brown TR, ed. Handbook of Institutional Pharmacy Practice. Bethesda, MD: American Society of Health-System Pharmacists, 2005.

## QUESTIONS

1. The process of budgeting assists a manager in which of the following functions?
   a. Business planning
   b. Financial control of the business
   c. Business organization
   d. All of the above
   e. a and b only
2. A demand forecast is:
   a. precise measurement of past years' demand
   b. precise measurement of future demand
   c. estimate of past years' sales
   d. estimate of future sales
3. A sales forecast for a *new* community pharmacy would consider which of the following?
   a. Past years' sales for the pharmacy
   b. Potential sales in the pharmacy's market area
   c. Pharmacy's competition
   d. Pharmacy's marketing programs
   e. All of the above
   f. b, c, and d only
4. A demand forecast for an *existing* hospital pharmacy would consider which of the following?
   a. Past years' patient admissions
   b. New drug therapies
   c. New government regulation of hospital reimbursement

      **d.** Pharmacy's marketing programs
      **e.** All of the above
      **f.** b, c, and d only

  **5.** The operating budget typically covers a time period of:
      **a.** 6 to 12 months
      **b.** 12 to 24 months
      **c.** 12 to 60 months

  **6.** Preparation of operating budgets for large and small organizations differ in that:
      **a.** the larger organization requires a clearer and more precise delineation of its goals
      **b.** the larger organization will be more concerned with negotiation and coordination
      **c.** the smaller organization really does not need a budget
      **d.** All of the above
      **e.** a and b only

  **7.** The revenue budget:
      **a.** is the same as the demand forecast
      **b.** is derived from the demand forecast
      **c.** incorporates any plans management has to increase demand
      **d.** All of the above
      **e.** b and c only

  **8.** The endpoint of the budgeting process in a large organization should be:
      **a.** a budget that is acceptable to upper management
      **b.** a budget that is acceptable to unit heads
      **c.** a budget that is acceptable to both upper management and unit heads

  **9.** Budgets that are revised during the year are less useful for which of the following:
      **a.** planning
      **b.** control of financial operations
      **c.** employee motivation
      **d.** All of the above
      **e.** b and c only

**10.** A budget that allows variable expenses to vary in proportion to changes in demand is called a:
      **a.** fixed budget
      **b.** flexible budget

**11.** A pharmacy that typically experiences stable, constant demand would be most likely to use a:
      **a.** fixed budget
      **d.** flexible budget

**12.** A manager should analyze those budget variances that:
      **a.** are large in absolute terms and unfavorable
      **b.** are large in percentage terms and unfavorable
      **c.** occur frequently and are favorable
      **d.** are large in absolute terms and favorable
      **e.** All of the above
      **f.** a, b, and c only

**13.** A negative sales variance may be the result of a:
      **a.** decline in prices charged by the pharmacy
      **b.** decline in the number of units sold by the pharmacy
      **c.** change in the mix of products sold by the pharmacy

     **d.** All of the above

     **e.** a and b only

14. A negative salary variance may be the result of:
    **a.** employees working fewer hours than budgeted
    **b.** employees making lower hourly wages than budgeted
    **c.** using fewer pharmacists and more technicians than budgeted
    **d.** All of the above

15. A controllable expense:
    **a.** is the same as a variable expense
    **b.** is one over which a manager can exert complete control
    **c.** is one over which a manager can exert substantial control
    **d.** a and b
    **e.** a and c

16. A budget may be useful for motivating managers because:
    **a.** it provides specific goals for them
    **b.** it lets them know what is expected of them
    **c.** it provides flexible standards
    **d.** All of the above
    **e.** a and b only

17. A pharmacy's mission:
    **a.** is a broad, general statement of the societal role that the pharmacy should fulfill
    **b.** should be revised annually to reflect changes in external and internal factors affecting the pharmacy's sales
    **c.** should be the starting point for the pharmacy's planning
    **d.** All of the above
    **e.** a and c only

18. Strategies are:
    **a.** what the pharmacy plans to accomplish in the next 12 months
    **b.** specific plans the pharmacy has for accomplishing its annual objectives
    **c.** broad guidelines, or basic operating principles, that indicate how the pharmacy will meet its long-term goals

19. An operating budget shows the forecasted costs and revenues associated with a pharmacy's:
    **a.** mission
    **b.** long-term goals
    **c.** strategies
    **d.** functional plans

## DISCUSSION QUESTIONS

1. How does the budgeting process facilitate planning?
2. Pharmacist Small is developing a budget for the coming year for his community pharmacy. He has determined that the pharmacy's average annual sales increase for the past 5 years has been 6.5%. In addition, he has identified five major changes that might affect the coming year's sales. These factors include the recent opening of a chain pharmacy down the street, a plan to increase hours of operation during the coming year, a plan to offer a new home IV prescription service, a decrease in the amount Medicaid pays for prescriptions, and a large increase in

the elderly population of the pharmacy's trading area. Discuss how each of these factors would affect the sales forecast.

3. Briefly list the steps required in developing an operating budget for a small community pharmacy. What additional steps would be necessary if the pharmacy were a unit in a large chain?

4. Why should the endpoint of the budget negotiation process be a budget that is mutually acceptable to both unit head and his or her superior? In what ways would the organization suffer if the superior forced overly optimistic budget goals on the unit head? In what ways would it suffer if the unit head were able to negotiate lax goals?

5. Large organizations are typically concerned with maintaining control. Given this bias, would you expect large organizations to be for or against the practice of revising budgets to reflect changes in operating conditions? Why?

6. Explain several ways in which involving lower level employees (such as staff pharmacists and technicians) improves the budgeting process.

7. Why is the budgeting process for a large organization characterized by much negotiation and a need for coordination?

## PROBLEMS

1. A 5-year sales history for Steady-gro Pharmacy is shown.
   a. Based on the sales history, and assuming economic conditions remain stable, what would Steady-gro Pharmacy's estimated sales be for 20X6?
   b. What would estimated sales be for 20X6 if the manager expected a 5% increase in the inflation rate?
   c. What would estimated sales be for 20X6 if the manager expected increased advertising to increase sales between 10% and 15%?

### Sales History for Steady-gro Pharmacy

| Year | Sales |
|------|-------|
| 20X1 | $250,000 |
| 20X2 | 280,000 |
| 20X3 | 315,000 |
| 20X4 | 340,000 |
| 20X5 | 380,000 |

2. Community General Hospital anticipates admitting its first patients in the near future. The director of the hospital's pharmacy is currently developing the pharmacy budget. The hospital administrator has supplied her with the following information:

   - Anticipated patient visits to hospitals in Community Hospital's market area in the next year should total 50,000.
   - The average patient visit lasts 4 days.
   - Community Hospital anticipates gaining a 30% market share.
   - Drug and IV fluid purchases average $50 per patient day.
   - Pharmacy personnel expenses average $20 per patient day.
   - Other direct pharmacy expenses average $5 per patient day.

Given this information, please answer the following questions:
a. What is Community Hospital's *market potential* in terms of patient days? (Patient days can be calculated as number of visits multiplied by average visit length.)
b. What is the Community Hospital's *demand forecast* in patient days?
c. Develop an expense budget for the pharmacy. (Assume the pharmacy only has drug and IV purchase, personnel, and other direct expenses.)
d. Develop a flexible expense budget for the pharmacy assuming hospital market shares of 20%, 30%, and 40%. Assume that the only variable expense is purchasess and that personnel expenses will be fixed at $1,200,000 per year and other direct expenses at $300,000 per year.

3. A monthly performance report for the NoGro Pharmacy is shown. The pharmacy has a policy of analyzing sales and gross margin variances that differ from the budget by 10% or more and analyzing expense variances greater than $100.
a. Which variances would the manager analyze?
b. What is the most likely cause of the sales variance? (Hint: compare the gross margin percents for budgeted and actual performance.)
c. Are the expense variances favorable or unfavorable? If these variances occur regularly, could they be contributing to the sales variance? Explain your answer.

### Monthly Performance Report for NoGro Pharmacy

|  | Actual | Budgeted | Variance |
|---|---|---|---|
| Sales | $65,000 | $75,000 | (10,000) |
| Gross margin | 22,750 | 26,250 | (3,500) |
| Expenses |  |  |  |
| Salaries |  |  |  |
| Pharmacist | 5,250 | 6,250 | (1,000) |
| Nonpharmacist | 12,000 | 12,000 | 0 |
| Housekeeping | 0 | 200 | (200) |
| Utilities | 500 | 550 | (50) |
| Advertising | 500 | 2,000 | (1,500) |
| Depreciation | 1,500 | 1,500 | 0 |
| Net income | $ 3,000 | $ 3,750 | (750) |

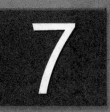

CHAPTER

# Cash Budgeting

After completing this chapter, the student should be able to:

1. Compare and contrast cash budgets and operating budgets,
2. Explain why a manager needs a cash budget,
3. Construct a cash budget, and
4. Use the cash budget to determine when a pharmacy will need to borrow cash and when it will be able to repay the cash or to invest excess cash.

A cash budget is a weekly or monthly forecast of cash inflows and outflows. It estimates, for each week or month, how much cash will come into the pharmacy and how much will be paid out. A cash budget is essential for proper planning and budgeting for the cash needs of the pharmacy.

A cash budget is needed because cash does not flow into and out of a pharmacy at a constant rate. Cash flow is usually erratic. As an example, examine total monthly cash receipts, total monthly cash payments, and monthly cash gain or loss in Figure 7-1. In the months of July, August, November, and December, Caremed Infusion Services estimates that it will have positive cash flow. More cash will come into the pharmacy than will be paid out. In September and October, it will have negative cash flow. Notice that there is no direct relation between sales and cash flow. Specifically:

- In July, sales are estimated at $137,800 and monthly cash gain at a $2,221.
- In August, sales are estimated to be lower—$91,000—but cash flow is estimated to be higher—$6,012.
- In October, estimated sales are much higher—$161,200—and cash flow is a negative $4,840.

| Sales Forecast | April | May | June | July | Aug. | Sept. | Oct. | Nov. | Dec. | Jan. |
|---|---|---|---|---|---|---|---|---|---|---|
| Cash sales (3%) | $2,730 | $3,198 | $3,432 | $4,134 | $2,730 | $3,432 | $4,836 | $3,588 | $3,510 | $2,925 |
| Credit sales (97%) | 88,270 | 103,402 | 110,968 | 133,666 | 88,270 | 110,968 | 156,364 | 116,012 | 113,490 | 94,575 |
| Total | 91,000 | 106,600 | 114,400 | 137,800 | 91,000 | 114,400 | 161,200 | 119,600 | 117,000 | 97,500 |
| Cash receipts | | | | | | | | | | |
| Cash sales (this month) | | | | 4,134 | 2,730 | 3,432 | 4,836 | 3,588 | 3,510 | |
| 25% of last month's credit sales | | | | 27,742 | 33,417 | 22,068 | 27,742 | 39,091 | 29,003 | |
| 35% of credit sales 2 months ago | | | | 36,191 | 38,839 | 46,783 | 30,895 | 38,839 | 54,727 | |
| 35% of credit sales 3 months ago | | | | 30,895 | 36,191 | 38,839 | 46,783 | 30,895 | 38,839 | |
| Total monthly cash receipts | | | | 98,961 | 111,176 | 111,121 | 110,256 | 112,412 | 126,079 | |
| Cash payments | | | | | | | | | | |
| Purchases (56% of next month's sales) | | | | 50,960 | 64,064 | 90,272 | 66,976 | 65,520 | 54,600 | |
| Salaries | | | | 32,000 | 32,000 | 32,000 | 32,000 | 32,000 | 32,000 | |
| Other expenses (10% of monthly sales) | | | | 13,780 | 9,100 | 11,440 | 16,120 | 11,960 | 11,700 | |
| Total monthly cash payments | | | | 96,740 | 105,164 | 133,712 | 115,096 | 109,480 | 98,300 | |
| Monthly cash gain (loss) | | | | 2,221 | 6,012 | (22,591) | (4,840) | 2,932 | 27,779 | |
| Financing | | | | | | | | | | |
| Cash balance: beginning of month | | | | 5,000 | 7,221 | 13,233 | 5,643 | 5,802 | 5,734 | |
| Monthly cash gain (loss) | | | | 2,221 | 6,012 | (22,591) | (4,840) | 2,932 | 27,779 | |
| Cash balance: end of month before financing | | | | 7,221 | 13,233 | (9,357) | 802 | 8,734 | 33,514 | |
| Borrowing | | | | 0 | 0 | 15,000 | 5,000 | 0 | 0 | |
| Repayment | | | | 0 | 0 | 0 | 0 | 3,000 | 17,000 | |
| Cash balance: end of month after financing | | | | 7,221 | 13,233 | 5,643 | 5,802 | 5,734 | 16,514 | |

**FIGURE 7-1** Cash budget for Caremed Infusion Services.

Cash flow varies from month to month for several reasons. First, many pharmacies' sales are not constant from month to month. Prescription sales in community pharmacies, for example, are higher during the winter and lower during the summer. Second, as a general rule, purchases must *precede* sales. Merchandise must be bought before it can be sold. Finally, when sales are made on credit, cash is not received until weeks or months after the merchandise is sold. Most pharmacies have high volumes of credit sales. Consequently, the lag between when a sale is made and when payment is received is a major cause of cash flow problems in pharmacies.

Because cash flow is erratic, there are months when the pharmacy needs additional cash to operate the business, and there are months when it will have excess cash. A cash budget allows the manager to anticipate when the pharmacy will need cash so he or she can arrange for financing before it is needed, and to anticipate when the pharmacy will be able to repay the loans or will have idle cash to invest. For example, the data in Figure 7-1 indicate that Caremed Infusion Services will need to borrow in September and October and can repay the loans in November and December.

## PREPARING THE CASH BUDGET

This section describes the process of preparing a cash budget. Information for Caremed Infusion Services, a home IV infusion pharmacy, will be used to illustrate the process. A home IV infusion pharmacy is one that prepares, delivers, and assists patients in receiving IV therapy in their homes. Examples of types of drug therapy commonly provided by home IV infusion pharmacies include IV chemotherapy for cancer patients, IV antibiotics for patients with serious infections, and IV analgesics for patients with severe pain. Cash budgeting is especially important to home IV infusion pharmacies because almost all of their sales are made on credit and because the time lag between provision of the service and payment may be several months.

## Budget Period

The first step in preparing a cash budget is selection of the *budget period*. This is the period of time that the budget will cover. A cash budget will normally cover a 6- to 12-month period. Shorter periods may not take into account seasonal shifts in cash flow. It is difficult to develop reliable estimates of sales for longer periods. The cash budget shown in Figure 7-1 covers the 6-month period from July to December.

## Monthly Sales Forecast

The next step is to forecast monthly sales for the budget period. This is the most important and difficult step in the process. *Monthly* sales are estimated in much the same manner as yearly sales. (Sales forecasting has been discussed previously in the chapter on budgeting.) If the pharmacy offers credit, the manager must also estimate the percent of monthly sales that will be made on credit and the percent that will be made for cash. The first section of Figure 7-1 shows the sales forecast for Caremed Infusion Services. The manager has estimated that 3% of the pharmacy's sales are cash and 97% are credit.

## Cash Receipts

Once the sales forecast is made, the manager can calculate monthly *cash receipts*. Cash receipts consist of cash sales for the month plus collections of accounts receivable from credit sales made in prior months. Any other income the pharmacy has, such as interest on savings accounts or other investments, should also be included.

To determine monthly credit collections, the manager must estimate the *lag time* between credit sales and payment. The manager of Caremed Infusion Services has estimated that the pharmacy will collect 25% of credit sales in the month following the sale, 35% 2 months after the sale, and an additional 35% 3 months after the sale. The manager has also estimated that 5% of credit sales will become bad debt.

For Caremed Infusion Services, July's cash receipts consist of:

- Cash sales for July—$4,134
- 25% of credit sales for June—$27,742
- 35% of credit sales for May—$36,191
- 35% of credit sales for April—$30,895

So, the manager estimates that Caremed's total cash receipts for July will be $98,961.

## Cash Payments

Next, monthly *cash payments* must be calculated. A major part of monthly payments consists of purchases of merchandise for resale. Purchase payments are estimated by multiplying sales by the pharmacy's cost of goods sold percent. The cost of goods sold percent is estimated from the pharmacy's historical gross margin adjusted for any anticipated changes in pricing or purchasing.

In calculating monthly purchase payments, the manager must determine the *timing* of purchase, payment, and sale of merchandise. Some pharmacies purchase merchandise in the same month that they sell it and pay for purchases the following month. For these pharmacies, merchandise sold in June is purchased in June and paid for in July. The situation will differ from pharmacy to pharmacy. Caremed Infusion Services estimates that purchases are made a month in advance of sales and are paid for in the month they are made. So, Caremed Infusion Services would make and pay for purchases in July to cover sales in August. To calculate Caremed Infusion Services' purchase payments for July, the manager would multiply estimated sales for August—$91,000—by the estimated cost of goods sold percent—56%. This yields the estimated purchase payments for July of $50,960.

Other normal monthly expenses must also be estimated. Fixed costs are estimated as a set dollar amount per month; variable costs are estimated as a percentage of sales. Caremed Infusion Services has estimated salaries at $32,000 per month and all other expenses at 10% of monthly sales. Finally, payments other than those made every month must be estimated. These would include payments for purchase of fixed assets, loan payoffs, or income taxes. Caremed Infusion Services expects to have no such payments for the budget period. Caremed's total monthly cash payments for July are estimated to be $96,740.

## Financing

Comparing monthly receipts and payments yields the monthly *cash gain or loss*. This is added to (if a gain) or subtracted from (if a loss) the beginning monthly cash balance to yield the *cash balance, end of month, before financing*. This amount is then compared with the pharmacy's *minimum cash balance*. The minimum cash balance is the minimum amount of cash that the pharmacy needs in its cash account. A pharmacy maintains a minimum cash balance as insurance against mistakes in cash budgeting and to cover unexpected emergencies. If the cash balance before financing is less than the minimum cash balance, the pharmacy will need to borrow enough cash to raise the balance to the minimum. If the cash balance before financing is greater than the minimum, the pharmacy may be able to repay past borrowing or to invest the excess cash.

For July, Caremed Infusion Services estimates cash receipts of $98,961 and cash payments of $96,740. Thus, the pharmacy expects a $2,221 cash gain in July. The cash balance at the beginning of July is $5,000. This amount plus the cash gain yields the cash balance before financing of $7,221. Caremed maintains a $5,000 minimum cash balance. Since the cash balance before financing is more than the minimum, borrowing is not necessary. Because no borrowing is necessary, the cash balance before financing is the same as the *cash balance, end of month, after financing*. This amount becomes the beginning balance for August.

For September, Caremed Infusion Services estimates cash receipts of $111,121 and cash payments of $133,712. Thus, the pharmacy expects a $22,591 cash loss in September. The cash balance at the beginning of September is $13,233. This amount less the cash loss yields the cash balance before financing of ($9,357). (Remember that accountants use parentheses to indicate negative numbers.) Caremed maintains a $5,000 minimum cash balance. Since the cash balance before financing is less than the minimum, borrowing is necessary. We will assume that the bank requires that Caremed borrow in $1,000 increments. Consequently, Caremed must borrow $15,000 in September to maintain its cash balance. Adding this sum to the cash balance before financing gives the *cash balance, end of month, after financing*. In this case, the amount is $5,643. This becomes the beginning balance for October.

A cash budget will also record the cumulative amount borrowed for each month. From this information, the manager can estimate, in advance, when, during the year, he or she will need to borrow and when he or she will be able to repay loans or invest excess cash.

## USING THE CASH BUDGET

Caremed Infusion Services will need to borrow in September and October. Repayments can be made in November and December. There will be an excess of cash (above the minimum cash balance) in December. The excess cash could be invested in an interest-bearing bank account. Knowing in advance when borrowing will be necessary and when repayment can be made is helpful. It allows the manager to arrange for financing well in advance of when it is actually needed. This improves peace of mind and allows the manager to negotiate lower finance charges and interest rates. It also helps the manager avoid the cost and embarrassment of losing discounts or being late with payments because he or she was unable to borrow on the spur of the moment.

## PROBLEMS

1. Prepare a cash budget for Urbana Pharmacy for the 6 months of August 20X1 through January 20X2. Make the following assumptions:
   a. Sales for 20X1 and 20X2 are as estimated in the example.
   b. The pharmacy has 70% credit sales and 30% cash sales.

    c. Assume that 75% of credit sales are collected the month following the sale and the remaining 25% is collected 2 months after the sale.

    d. Purchases are made and paid for 1 month in advance of sales (i.e., purchases to cover February sales are made and paid for in January.)

    e. Assume a 30% gross margin.

    f. Monthly salary expenses are as shown. Rent is a fixed $1,750 per month. Other monthly operating expenses are estimated to be equal to 5% of sales.

    g. Beginning cash balance is $10,000 and minimum cash balance is $5,000.

| Month | Estimated Sales | Estimated Salaries |
|---|---|---|
| June | $53,000 | NA |
| July | 48,000 | NA |
| Aug. | 59,000 | $11,000 |
| Sep. | 93,000 | 12,000 |
| Oct. | 81,000 | 12,000 |
| Nov. | 126,000 | 15,000 |
| Dec. | 155,000 | 15,000 |
| Jan. | 70,000 | 11,000 |
| Feb. | 65,000 | NA |

2. Williams Pharmacy is a community pharmacy. Prepare a cash budget for Williams Pharmacy for 20X2. Make the following assumptions:

    a. Sales for 20X2 are as shown.

    b. Credit sales are 15% of total sales.

    c. Assume bad debt is zero.

    d. Credit collections will be made:
        80% in the month after the sale.
        20% in the second month after the sale.

    e. Sales for the last 2 months of 20X1:
        November $36,000
        December $40,000

    f. Purchases are made the same month they are sold and are paid for the following month (i.e., purchases to cover January sales are made and received in January and paid in February).

    g. Assume a 36% gross margin.

    h. Total operating expenses = $13,150 per month.

    i. Beginning cash balance is $12,000, minimum cash balance is $10,000, and borrowing must be done in $1,000 increments.

| Month | Estimated Sales |
|---|---|
| Jan. | $ 50,000 |
| Feb. | 45,000 |
| March | 50,000 |
| April | 40,000 |
| May | 35,000 |

| | |
|---|---|
| June | 35,000 |
| July | 20,000 |
| Aug. | 20,000 |
| Sept. | 25,000 |
| Oct. | 40,000 |
| Nov. | 40,000 |
| Dec. | 50,000 |

3. Cooper-Con is a long-term care consulting pharmacy. The business provides no drug products to long-term care patients; rather it provides consulting services to assess and make recommendations about the adequacy and appropriateness of their drug therapy. Prepare a cash budget for Cooper-Con for the first 6 months of 20X9. Make the following assumptions:
   a. Sales for 20X9 are as shown.
   b. All sales are credit sales.
   c. Assume bad debt is zero.
   d. Credit collections will be made:
      60% in the month following the sale.
      40% in the second month after the sale.
   e. Salaries are $6,000 per month. Rent and utilities are $4,000 per month. Other operating expenses are estimated to be 14% of monthly sales.
   f. The beginning cash balance is $2,000, minimum cash balance is $2,000, and borrowing must be done in $1,000 increments.

| Month | Estimated Sales |
|---|---|
| Nov. | $15,000 |
| Dec. | 12,000 |
| Jan. | 15,000 |
| Feb. | 12,000 |
| March | 8,000 |
| April | 8,000 |
| May | 10,000 |
| June | 12,000 |

CHAPTER 8

# Break-even Analysis*

## OBJECTIVES

After reading this chapter, the student should be able to:

1. Define and identify fixed, variable, and semivariable costs,
2. Conduct and interpret the results of a break-even analysis using the contribution margin approach,
3. Conduct and interpret the results of a break-even analysis using the graphical approach,
4. Use break-even analysis to estimate the effects of changes in costs and prices on pharmacy profitability, and
5. Discuss the assumptions of break-even analysis.

P harmacy managers often are faced with decisions that involve predicting the effects of changes in costs, prices, or revenues on pharmacy profits. Examples of these situations include:

1. What volume of patient consultations is required to make a cholesterol counseling and monitoring service financially feasible?
2. Should advertising be increased to stimulate sales? If so, will the increase in sales volume be sufficient to cover the cost of the additional advertising?
3. Should prices be discounted to attract more business? If such a program is offered, will the additional sales resulting from the discount exceed the loss of revenue on individual sales?

---

*This chapter was based on the article "Break-even Analysis for Predicting Profit Margins," which appeared in *Current Concepts in Retail Pharmacy Management* 1984;2:3. The material is used with the permission of MacMillan Healthcare Information.

Break-even analysis (BEA) is a technique that can aid managers in making better decisions about these and similar problems. BEA is useful in these situations because it explicitly shows the relationship between costs and profits over a range of sales and for a variety of assumptions about costs, prices, and revenues. Before BEA can be used, it is first necessary to understand three types of costs.

## CLASSIFICATION OF COSTS

Pharmacy costs may be classified as fixed, variable, or semivariable over some relevant range of sales volume (relevant range will be defined later).

### Fixed Costs

Fixed costs remain the same regardless of volume. For example, depreciation is a fixed cost. No matter how high the pharmacy's sales go during a given year, the depreciation expense will not change. This is because depreciation is based on the value of fixed assets, which are not directly affected by changes in sales. Other examples of fixed costs include property taxes and business licenses. Fixed costs can be plotted as shown in Figure 8-1.

### Variable Costs

Variable costs increase in direct proportion to increases in volume. The largest variable cost for a pharmacy is the cost of goods sold. As sales increase, the cost of goods

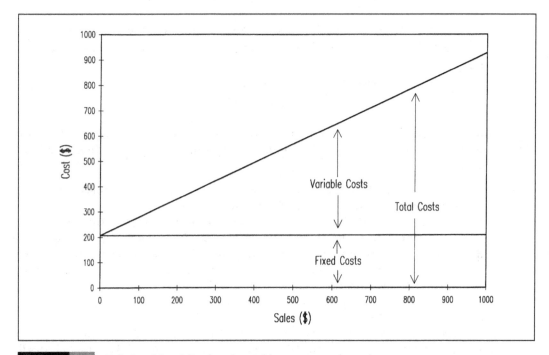

**FIGURE 8-1**    Relationship of fixed and variable costs to sales volume.

sold increases proportionately. Other examples of variable costs include cost of supplies (e.g., prescription bottles and labels) and any commissions or franchise fees based on sales volume. Variable costs can be plotted as shown in Figure 8-1.

## Semivariable Costs

Semivariable costs include both a fixed and a variable component. Examples include rent that is based on a fixed monthly fee plus some percentage of sales and utility rates that include a set fee for provision of the service plus an additional charge based on extent of usage.

## Relevant Range

Fixed costs may be classified as fixed only over some defined, relatively restricted range of sales volume. This is known as the relevant range of sales. Many fixed costs vary at levels of volume either above or below the relevant range. For example, consider a pharmacy that dispenses an average of 100 prescriptions per day. The relevant range of volume for this pharmacy might be 75 to 200 prescriptions per day. As long as the average prescription volume remained within this range, dispensing could be handled adequately by one pharmacist and one clerk. Consequently, salaries would be a fixed cost. But, if volume decreased to 50 prescriptions a day, the technician would no longer be needed. If volume were to exceed 200 prescriptions per day, another pharmacist or technician would be needed. Hence, at levels of volume outside the relevant range, the salaries expense would no longer be fixed.

## PURPOSE AND METHODS OF BREAK-EVEN ANALYSIS

The purpose of BEA is to find the pharmacy's break-even point (BEP). This is the volume at which total revenues, or sales, equal total costs. At the BEP, the pharmacy does not make a profit or suffer a loss.

The BEP for a pharmacy operation that produces only one product can be calculated in either dollars of sales or in units of the product produced. For example, the prescription department in a community pharmacy could be considered as a pharmacy operation that produced only one product. This product would be dispensed prescriptions. The BEP for the prescription department could be calculated as either the dollar sales volume at which total revenues (or sales) equaled total costs or the total number of prescriptions dispensed that would make total revenues equal to total costs. (To make either calculation, separate cost and revenue figures for the prescription department would be needed.) As another example, the IV room in a hospital pharmacy could be considered a pharmacy operation that produced only one product—IV solutions. The BEP for the IV room could be calculated as either the number of IV solutions dispensed or the sales volume at which total revenues equaled total costs.

Pharmacy operations that produce several products must calculate the BEP as the sales volume at which total revenues equal total costs. Because more than one type of product is produced, there is no way to calculate a BEP in number of units of product produced. A chain pharmacy is an example of a pharmacy operation that produces several products. A chain pharmacy sells not only prescriptions, but also over-the-counter (OTC) products, health and beauty aids, and cosmetics. Similarly, the pharmacy in a large hospital is a multiproduct operation. The hospital pharmacy produces

| Surrywood Pharmacy Income Statements Year Ended 12/31/X5 | | | | |
|---|---|---|---|---|
| | Pharmacy | | Prescription Department | |
| | $ | % | $ | % |
| *Sales:* | | | | |
| Prescription | 803,000 | | | |
| Other | 89,000 | | | |
| Total sales | 892,000 | 100.0 | 803,000 | 100.0 |
| Cost of goods sold | 628,500 | 70.5 | 602,300 | 75.0 |
| Gross margin | 263,500 | 29.5 | 200,700 | 25.0 |
| *Operating expenses:* | | | | |
| Manager's salary | 66,500 | 7.5 | 58,000 | 7.2 |
| Employee wages | 64,000 | 7.2 | 57,600 | 7.2 |
| Rent | 19,000 | 2.1 | 17,100 | 2.1 |
| Utilities | 7,500 | 0.8 | 6,800 | 0.8 |
| Prescription | | | | |
| Containers | 4,900 | 0.5 | 4,900 | 0.6 |
| Delivery costs | 3,500 | 0.4 | 3,500 | 0.4 |
| Computer | 4,100 | 0.5 | 4,100 | 0.5 |
| Advertising | 6,400 | 0.7 | 5,200 | 0.6 |
| Security | 1,100 | 0.1 | 1,000 | 0.1 |
| Other expenses | 45,100 | 5.1 | 40,500 | 5.0 |
| Total operating expenses | 222,100 | 24.9 | 198,700 | 24.7 |
| Net income | 41,400 | 4.6 | 2,000 | 0.2 |

**FIGURE 8-2**    Income statements for Surrywood Pharmacy: Pharmacy and Prescription Department.

medication orders for inpatients, IV solutions, prescriptions for outpatients, educational services for nurses and physicians, and clinical services for inpatients.

The BEP for either type of pharmacy operation can be calculated using either a graphic or a contribution margin approach. The data needed for a BEP are found in the pharmacy's income statement. Income statements for Surrywood Pharmacy, a small community pharmacy, and for Surrywood Pharmacy's prescription department are shown in Figure 8-2. These data will be used to calculate BEPs for the pharmacy and the prescription department using both graphic and contribution margin approaches.

## Graphic Approach to Break-even Analysis

The BEP may be found for either a multiproduct pharmacy or a single product pharmacy by plotting a break-even graph.

## Break-even Graph for a Multiproduct Pharmacy

A break-even graph for Surrywood Pharmacy is shown in Figure 8-3. The method of constructing the graph is explained below.

The first step in a break-even analysis is to classify all costs as either fixed or variable. Semivariable costs must be broken into their fixed and variable components. The manager of Surrywood Pharmacy estimates that only prescription containers, delivery costs, and advertising change in direct proportion to sales. These amounted to $14,800 for the year shown. The remainder of operating expenses are fixed with respect to sales volume. So, for Surrywood Pharmacy, fixed costs (FCs) are $207,300. Variable costs (VCs) consist of $14,800 in variable operating expenses and $628,500 in cost of goods sold. Total variable costs therefore amount to $643,300.

Once costs are classified, the break-even graph can be plotted. As shown in Figure 8-3, both X and Y axes are calibrated in dollars. The X axis represents sales. The Y axis represents either revenues or costs. The *total revenue line* is plotted as a line beginning at the origin ($0, $0) and having a slope of 1. The slope of the total revenue line will always be 1 because both axes are calibrated in dollars.

The *total cost line* is plotted by determining two of its points and joining them with a straight line. When the pharmacy has zero sales volume, its total costs are equal to its fixed costs. This determines the first point on the total cost line. For Surrywood Pharmacy, this point is ($0, $207,300). The other point that can be determined from the income statement is identified by the pharmacy's total costs and sales volume for the year. Surrywood Pharmacy's sales volume for the year was $892,000. Total costs amounted to $850,600. These consisted of $207,300 of fixed costs plus $643,300 in

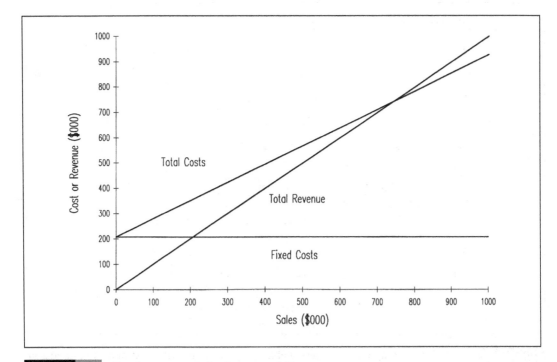

**FIGURE 8-3**    Break-even graph for Surrywood Pharmacy.

variable costs. Hence, the second point for the total cost line is ($892,000, $850,600). A straight line through these two points yields the total cost line.

The BEP is the point at which the total revenue line intersects the total cost line. The BEP for Surrywood Pharmacy occurs at a sales volume of about $744,000. At sales greater than $744,000, the pharmacy makes a profit. At sales less than $744,000, the pharmacy has a loss.

The amount of profit or loss can be estimated from the break-even graph as the vertical distance between the total revenue and total cost lines. The break-even graph shown in Figure 8-4 illustrates how this is done. The total cost line indicates that if Surrywood Pharmacy achieves a sales volume of $1,000,000, its total costs will be about $930,000. The total revenue line indicates that total revenues will be $1,000,000 at a sales volume of $1,000,000. The vertical difference between the two lines, $70,000, is profit. For sales less than $744,000, the amount of loss can be estimated in a similar manner. Figure 8.4 indicates that if Surrywood Pharmacy achieves only $600,000 in sales, it will have a loss of about $40,000. Thus, the break-even graph allows the manager to estimate pharmacy profits or losses over a range of sales volume.

## Break-even Graph for a Pharmacy Producing a Single Product

The graphic approach also can be used to find the BEP for a pharmacy operation producing a single type of product. For a prescription department, the BEP could be found in either sales volume or number of prescriptions dispensed. The method of calculating the prescription department's BEP in sales is identical to that used to find the pharmacy's BEP. A graph of the BEP for Surrywood Pharmacy's prescription

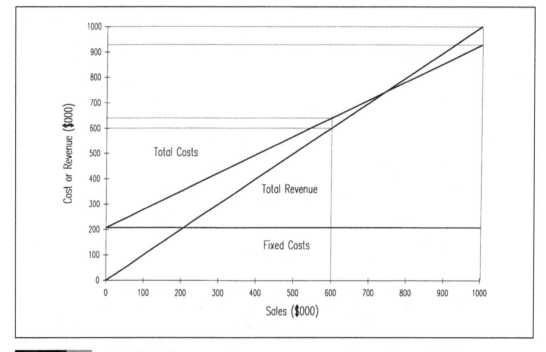

**FIGURE 8-4**  Break-even graph for Surrywood Pharmacy showing estimation of profit and loss at various sales volumes.

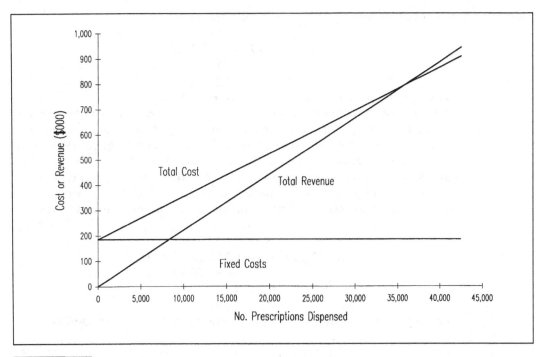

FIGURE 8-5 Break-even graph for Surrywood Pharmacy's Prescription Department.

department in numbers of prescriptions dispensed is shown in Figure 8-5. The BEP graph in prescriptions is constructed as follows:

1. The X axis is calibrated in number of prescriptions dispensed. As before, the Y axis is calibrated in dollars of revenue or cost.

2. Total revenue at several levels of prescription volume is calculated as the product of average prescription price and number of prescriptions dispensed. For the year, Surrywood Pharmacy's prescription department had sales of $803,000 and dispensed 36,100 prescriptions. Thus, the average prescription price (Ave. Rx price) is calculated as:

$$\text{Ave. Rx Price} = \text{Rx sales}/\# \text{ Rxs dispensed}$$
$$= \$803,000/36,100$$
$$= \$22.24$$

At each level of prescription volume, total revenue (TR) is calculated as:

$$\text{TR} = \text{Rx. Volume} \times \text{Ave. Rx Price}$$

So, when 5,000 prescriptions have been dispensed, total revenues are calculated as:

$$\text{TR} = \text{Rx. Volume} \times \text{Ave. Rx Price}$$
$$= 5,000 \times \$22.24$$
$$= \$111,200$$

When 10,000 prescriptions have been dispensed:

$$TR = 10,000 \times \$22.24$$
$$= \$222,400$$

Plotting these points defined the total revenue line.

3. The total cost line is defined by the sum of fixed costs and variable costs at several levels of prescription volume. Surrywood Pharmacy's prescription department had total variable costs of $615,900 and total fixed costs of $185,100. The variable costs consisted of cost of goods sold, prescription containers, delivery costs, and advertising. All other operating expenses were fixed costs. The prescription department dispensed 36,100 prescriptions for the year. The average variable cost per prescription (Ave. VC/RX) is calculated as:

$$Ave.\ VC/Rx = Total\ VC/Rxs\ dispensed$$
$$= \$615,900/36,100$$
$$= \$17.06$$

Total costs (TCs) at each level of prescription volume are calculated as:

$$TC = FC + VC$$
$$= FC + (Rx.\ Volume \times Ave.\ VC/Rx)$$

So, when no prescriptions have been dispensed:

$$TC = FC + (Rx.\ Volume \times Ave.\ VC/Rx)$$
$$TC = \$185,100 + (0 \times \$17.06)$$
$$TC = \$185,100$$

When 5,000 prescriptions have been dispensed:

$$TC = \$185,100 + (5,000 \times \$17.06)$$
$$= \$270,400$$

When 10,000 prescriptions have been dispensed:

$$TC = \$185,100 + (10,000 \times \$17.06)$$
$$= \$355,700$$

Plotting these points generated the total cost line.

As shown in Figure 8-5, the BEP for Surrywood Pharmacy's prescription department occurred at a volume of about 36,000 prescriptions. At lesser volume, there was loss; at greater volume, there was profit. The amount of profit or loss can be determined from the graph as explained earlier.

## Contribution Margin Approach to Break-even Analysis

A pharmacy's, or a prescription department's, BEP can also be calculated using the contribution margin approach.

## Break-even Point for a Multiproduct Pharmacy

A pharmacy's contribution margin (CM) is defined as revenue minus variable costs. Thus, the contribution margin is the amount of revenue available to cover fixed costs and net income. The relationship of the CM to fixed costs, variable costs, and net income is shown by the following equation:

$$
\begin{array}{l}
\text{Revenue} \\
\underline{- \text{ Variable Costs}} \\
\text{Contribution Margin} \\
\underline{- \text{ Fixed Costs}} \\
\text{Net Income}
\end{array}
$$

Using figures from Surrywood Pharmacy's income statement, the relationships would be:

$$
\begin{array}{r}
\$892{,}000 \\
\underline{- \ 643{,}300} \\
248{,}700 \\
\underline{- \ 207{,}300} \\
\$41{,}400
\end{array}
$$

The calculation indicates that Surrywood Pharmacy had a contribution margin of $248,700. This was the amount of total sales available to cover fixed costs and net income. The contribution margin was large enough to cover the fixed costs of $207,300 and leave a net income of $41,400.

The CM as a *percent of sales,* or CM%, is used to calculate the pharmacy's BEP. The CM% is calculated for Surrywood Pharmacy as follows:

$$
\begin{aligned}
\text{CM\%} &= \frac{\text{Sales}}{\text{Sales}} - \frac{\text{VC}}{\text{Sales}} \\
&= \frac{892{,}000}{892{,}000} - \frac{643{,}300}{892{,}000} \\
&= 100\% - 72.1\% \\
&= 27.9\% \text{ or } 0.279
\end{aligned}
$$

The calculation indicates that 27.9 cents of every dollar of Surrywood Pharmacy's sales were available to cover fixed costs and profit. The remaining 72.1 cents went to cover variable costs.

The BEP is calculated by dividing FC by the CM%. The logic underlying this calculation is straightforward. The CM% is the part of every dollar of sales available to cover FC. Dividing the CM% into FC yields the total dollars of sales—or the sales volume—necessary to cover FC. Because the CM% has already accounted for VC, this is the sales volume that just covers both FC and VC. This, of course, is the BEP.

The BEP for Surrywood Pharmacy is calculated as:

$$
\begin{aligned}
\text{BEP} &= \text{FC/CM\%} \\
&= \$207{,}300/0.279 \\
&= \$743{,}011
\end{aligned}
$$

Surrywood Pharmacy must generate $743,011 in sales to break even. Every dollar of sales over $743,011 will generate 27.9 cents of profit; the remaining 72.1 cents covers variable costs. Every dollar of sales less than $743,011 will represent 27.9 cents of loss.

The exact answer one calculates using the CM% method is sensitive to how the CM% is rounded off. For example, in the example just discussed, rounding the CM to three decimal places yields a BEP of $743,011. Rounding to two decimal places gives a BEP of $740,357 and rounding to four places gives $743,544. In actual managerial practice, each of these answers would be sufficiently precise for the use to which they would be put. For consistency, the text will use answers based on rounding the CM to three decimal places.

## Break-even Point for a Pharmacy Producing a Single Product

The CM approach can also be used to determine the BEP in units produced for an operation producing only one type of product. In this case a per unit CM is calculated. In the case of Surrywood Pharmacy's prescription department, this would be a per prescription CM. The per prescription CM (Per Rx CM) is calculated as the average prescription price minus the average variable cost per prescription. The Per Rx CM is calculated as follows:

$$\text{Per Rx CM} = \text{Ave. Rx price} - \text{Ave. VC/Rx}$$
$$= \$22.24 - 17.06$$
$$= \$5.18$$

The BEP is found by dividing fixed costs (FC) by the Per Rx CM:

$$\text{BEP} = \text{FC/CM} = \$185,100/5.18 = 35,733$$

So, the prescription department breaks even when it dispenses 35,733 prescriptions. For every prescription over 35,733 dispensed, profit (net income) will increase by $5.18, which is the amount of the Per Rx CM. For every prescription less than 35,733 dispensed, the pharmacy will suffer a loss of $5.18.

## ADDITIONAL MANAGERIAL USES OF BREAK-EVEN ANALYSIS

A manager can use the concepts of BEA to determine how changes in costs, revenues, or prices would affect the pharmacy's BEP and its profitability. To illustrate, BEA will be used to analyze some of the problems raised at the beginning of this chapter. Although the following analyses can be conducted with either the graphic or CM approach, the CM method will be used here. The data are from Figure 8-2. Before this is done, it will be useful to introduce the concept of the *stay-even point*.

## Stay-even Point

When managers consider making changes to their pharmacies, they are seldom interested in just breaking even. At minimum, they would like to maintain the pharmacy's current profitability. This can be easily incorporated into the standard BEA by treating net income as an additional fixed cost. When the net income included in this way is the pharmacy's current net income, the quantity that is calculated is called the *stay-even point*. The stay-even point (SEP) for Surrywood Pharmacy is calculated as follows:

$$SEP = (FC + NI)/CM\%$$
$$= (\$207,300 + \$41,400)/0.279$$
$$= \$891,398$$

The SEP can also be calculated in terms of units for a one-product firm. For example, Surrywood Pharmacy's prescription department made a net income of $2,000. To calculate the SEP in numbers of prescriptions, we add the net income to the FC and divide the sum by the Per Rx CM:

$$SEP = (FC + NI)/\text{Per Rx CM}$$
$$= (\$185,100 + 2,000)/\$5.18$$
$$= 36,120 \text{ Rxs}$$

In both of the SEP cases presented, calculating the SEP provides little useful information because the SEP is the pharmacy's current volume. However, the SEP calculation is useful when it is used to determine how changes in prices or costs will affect the pharmacy in the future. The following examples illustrate this point. In addition, the SEP concept can be used to determine the volume the pharmacy must achieve to generate any given level of net income. It could, for example, be used to determine how much sales would have to increase for Surrywood Pharmacy to reach a target net income of $75,000.

## What Effect Would an Increase in Advertising Have on Profits?

Assume that the manager of Surrywood Pharmacy is considering increasing advertising by $500 per month, or $6,000 per year. BEA can be used to determine the amount that the pharmacy's sales must increase to cover the additional advertising expense.

First, recall that the sales volume (before the additional advertising) was calculated to be $892,000; CM percentage, 0.279; FC, $207,300; and net income, $41,400. The increase in advertising will affect only FC, which will increase by $6,000. Calculation of the SEP will show the sales volume necessary to just cover the costs of the additional advertising. The additional advertising is added to fixed costs.

$$SEP = (FC + NI)/CM\%$$
$$= (207,300 + 6,000 + 41,400)/0.279$$
$$= \$912,903$$

The SEP would be $912,903 if advertising were increased. This represents a sales increase of $912,903 − $891,398 = $21,505. If sales increased by less than $21,505, the pharmacy's profits would decrease. Thus, the SEP indicates that the additional advertising should be purchased only if the manager expected that it would increase sales by more than this amount.

A similar procedure can be used to determine how much prescription volume would have to increase to cover the costs of increased advertising. In this case, assume the manager was considering increasing prescription department advertising by $250 per month, or $3,000 per year. As in the previous example, this would increase FC.

Recall that prescription volume before the additional advertising was 36,100; Per Rx CM, $5.18; FC for the prescription department, $185,100; and net income for the prescription department, $2,000. The SEP would be:

$$SEP = (FC + NI)/Per\ Rx\ CM$$
$$= (\$185,100 + \$3,000 + \$2,000)/\$5.18$$
$$= 36,698\ Rxs$$

So, a prescription volume of 36,698 per year is needed to cover the additional advertising costs and maintain current net income. This represents an increase of 36,698 − 36,100 = 598 prescriptions per year.

## What Effect Would a Discount Have on Profitability?

Assume that Surrywood Pharmacy is considering a 10% discount on selected OTC drugs. Also, assume that 25% of total sales are sales of the selected OTC drugs. Thus, a 10% discount on these products would have the same effect as a 2.5% discount on all sales (10% × 25% = 2.5%). Such an action would be the equivalent of decreasing dollar sales (on the same *unit* volume of sales) by 2.5%, or to $869,700. The dollar amount of fixed and variable costs would not change, but the CM *percentage* would change. The new CM% is calculated as follows:

$$CM\% = \frac{Sales}{Sales} - \frac{VC}{Sales}$$
$$= \frac{869,700}{869,700} - \frac{643,300}{869,700} \times 100\%$$
$$= 100\% - 74.0\%$$
$$= 26.0\%\ or\ 0.260$$

So the SEP would be:

$$SEP = (FC + NI)/CM\%$$
$$= (\$207,300 + \$41,400)/0.260$$
$$= \$956,538$$

So, sales of $956,538 are needed to cover the cost of the discount while maintaining current profit. How much would the pharmacy's sales have to increase to achieve this volume of sales? The pharmacy's current sales volume is $892,000. If the pharmacy sold the same *amount* of merchandise, but at the discounted prices, the sales volume would be only $869,700. So, if the pharmacy implemented the discounts, its sales would have to increase by $956,538 − $869,700 = $86,838 per year to maintain its current level of profitability. The discount program should be implemented if the manager expected that it would increase sales by more than this amount.

## Calculating the Break-even Point for a Lipid Management Service

Assume that Surrywood Pharmacy was considering starting a pharmacist-run lipid management service. The service would monitor patients' blood lipid levels and counsel them about proper diet and drug therapy to control lipid levels. The service will operate for 4 hours per day for 300 days per year. The manager estimates the costs of the service as follows:

| | |
|---|---|
| Supply costs | $2.35 per visit |
| Analyzer (to measure blood lipid levels) | $950 annual lease |
| Share of overhead costs (such as manager's salary, rent, utilities, and insurance) | $3,000 per year |
| Pharmacist salary (4 hours per day for 300 days per year) | $60,000 per year |

The manager believes that the pharmacy will be able to charge $30 per 20-minute patient visit. With these costs and prices, will the service be financially feasible? Calculation of the BEP will help the manager answer this question.

The service's variable cost per patient visit is $2.35, the cost of supplies. All other costs are fixed. Total fixed costs are $63,950. At a price per visit of $30, the CM per visit is $30 − $2.35 = $27.65. The BEP is calculated as:

$$BEP = FC/CM \text{ per visit}$$
$$= \$63,950/\$27.65$$
$$= 2,313 \text{ visits}$$

The service will operate 4 hours per day, and each visit will take 20 minutes, so the service can accommodate 12 patient visits a day. It is open 300 days per year. Thus, it can accommodate 3,600 visits per year. Because only 2,313 visits are required to break even, the service is financially feasible.

## Calculating the Break-even Price for a Lipid Management Service

Assume that the manager of Surrywood Pharmacy is not sure what price to charge for the service, but he or she is fairly confident that demand for the service would be about 1,500 patient visits per year. The manager could use BEA to calculate the price required for the service to break even.

As before, total fixed costs are $63,950, and the VC per visit is $2.35. The BEP is set equal to 1,500, the anticipated number of patient visits. The calculation of the break-even price is as follows:

$$BEP = FC/CM \text{ per visit}$$
$$BEP = FC/(\text{Price per visit} - VC \text{ per visit})$$
$$1500 = \$63,950/(\text{Price per visit} - \$2.35)$$
$$\text{Price per visit} = \$44.98$$

Thus, the service will break even at its anticipated volume of 1,500 visits if it charges $44.98 per visit.

## ASSUMPTIONS OF BREAK-EVEN ANALYSIS

A BEA must meet several assumptions if it is to yield valid results:

1. Valid and reliable data on costs and revenues are available to the pharmacy manager.
2. All costs are correctly classified as fixed or variable.

3. Costs and revenues act in a linear manner over the relevant range of sales volume. This assumption implies that the results of BEA may be invalid during periods of high inflation, when productivity changes drastically, or when prices are changed frequently.
4. The BEA is applied to a restricted, relevant range of sales volume. This assumption implies that BEA is useful only for short-range decisions and not for long-range planning. (As a rule of thumb, short range refers to periods of a year or less whereas long range refers to periods of longer than a year.)
5. The pharmacy's product mix must not change over the period covered by BEA. A pharmacy's product mix refers to the mix of products sold with different contribution margins. A change in the product mix will change the pharmacy's overall contribution margin. This, in turn, changes the BEP.

An example may clarify the effect of product mix. Assume that Surrywood Pharmacy conducted a BEA at a time when few of its prescriptions were reimbursed by third-party payers. Over the course of the year, the proportion of its prescription volume covered by third parties increased substantially. Third-party payers typically pay much less than cash-paying patients. Thus, an increase in the proportion of third-party payment would result in a substantial decrease in the pharmacy's contribution margin. This, in turn, would substantially increase the pharmacy's BEP.

### Suggested Reading

Anthony RN, Welsh GA. Fundamentals of Management Accounting. 3rd Ed. Homewood, IL: Richard D. Irwin, Inc., 1981.
Keown AJ, Petty JW, Martin JD, et al. Foundations of Finance: The Logic and Practice of Financial Management. 3rd Ed. Upper Saddle River, NJ: Prentice Hall, 2001.
Levin RI, Kirkpatrick CA. Quantitative Approaches to Management. 2nd Ed. New York: McGraw Hill, 1986.

## QUESTIONS

1. If a pharmacy decided to increase advertising expenses by $600 per month, which of the following would be affected?
   a. Fixed costs
   b. Variable costs
   c. Contribution margin percent
2. If a pharmacy increased its prices by 10%, which of the following would *always* occur?
   a. Fixed costs would increase.
   b. Variable costs would increase.
   c. The contribution margin percent would increase.
   d. Both a and c
   e. Both b and c
3. If a pharmacy decreased its *markup* by 10%, what would the effect on its break-even point be?
   a. It would decrease the break-even point about 10%.
   b. It would decrease the break-even point substantially more than 10%.
   c. It would have little or no effect on the break-even point.

   **d.** It would increase the break-even point about 10%.
   **e.** It would increase the break-even point substantially more than 10%.
4. Which of the following would cause the results of a break-even analysis to be incorrect?
   **a.** The pharmacy's contribution margin decreased over the period covered by the analysis.
   **b.** The pharmacy's sales increased by 5% over the period covered by the analysis.
   **c.** Depreciation was classified as a fixed expense.
   **d.** All of the above would cause the analysis to be incorrect.
   **e.** Only a and b would cause the analysis to be incorrect.
5. A pharmacy pays rent of $500 per month. Rent would be considered a:
   **a.** fixed cost
   **b.** variable cost
   **c.** semivariable cost
6. A pharmacy spends an amount equal to 1% of monthly sales on advertising. Advertising would be considered a:
   **a.** fixed cost
   **b.** variable cost
   **c.** semivariable cost

## PROBLEMS

1. In the Problems following Chapter 5, *Financial Statement Analysis*, financial statements for Apple Blossom Pharmacy are presented. Compute the contribution margin percent and the break-even point for Apple Blossom Pharmacy. Assume that rent and miscellaneous expenses are variable costs and all other operating expenses are fixed costs.
2. Assume that Apple Blossom Pharmacy increased its marketing costs by $6,000 per year. What would the pharmacy's stay-even point be? How much would sales have to increase to cover the increased marketing costs?
3. Assume that Apple Blossom Pharmacy instituted a discount program that resulted in an overall 5% discount on sales. Assuming no increase in unit sales, what would the pharmacy's new sales volume be? What would the new contribution margin percent be? What would the stay-even point be? What volume of sales would be needed to cover the cost of the discount program and maintain current profits?
4. In the Problems following Chapter 5, *Financial Statement Analysis*, financial statements for Rivbo Drugs are presented. Compute the contribution margin percent and the break-even point for Rivbo Drugs for 20X4. Assume that 75% of operating expenses are fixed costs and that 25% are variable costs.
5. Assume Rivbo implemented a new pricing program that resulted in an overall discount of 2% on all prices. What would the new contribution margin percent be? What would the stay-even point be? How much would sales have to increase to allow Rivbo to maintain its current profit?
6. A hospital pharmacy is determining whether it should start an IV service. The pharmacy would like to operate the service 365 days per year. It intends to charge $25 per IV solution. The average cost of goods sold is estimated to be $7 per IV, and the average variable cost (other than cost of goods sold) is estimated to be $2 per IV. The fixed costs associated with the service will amount to $150,000 per

year. How many IV solutions will the service have to dispense to break even? If the service can only dispense 20 IV solutions per day, will it be profitable to run the service?

7. Assume the hospital pharmacy charges $30 per IV. How many IV solutions will it have to dispense to break even? If it can only dispense 20 IV solutions per day, will it be profitable to run it at the higher charge?

## CHAPTER 9

# Pricing Pharmaceutical Products and Services

After reading this chapter, the student should be able to:

1. Explain why pricing is important,
2. List and discuss the effects of consumer-related factors, competition, pharmacy objectives, and costs on pricing decisions,
3. Calculate the cost of providing a pharmacist service and of dispensing a prescription,
4. Explain the relationships among price, cost, volume, and demand for a pharmacist service,
5. List and explain the steps involved in one strategy for pricing pharmacist services,
6. List and explain methods of presenting service prices to consumers,
7. Compare and contrast the methods for calculating prescription prices, and
8. Define AAC, AWP, EAC, WAC, and MAC.

Setting prices is critical to a pharmacy's success. Pricing is the mechanism by which the manager ensures that the pharmacy covers its costs and makes a satisfactory profit. If prices are set too high, consumers will take their business elsewhere. If they are set too low, the pharmacy will not be able to cover its cost of operation. Either way, the pharmacy will not be able to stay in business.

The price of a prescription consists of three components: the cost of the drug dispensed, the cost of dispensing the drug, and net income. The cost of the drug is usually referred to as the *ingredient cost* or *product cost*. The cost of dispensing the drug covers such expenses as salaries, rent and utilities, depreciation, and insurance. In general, we will refer to such costs as *service costs* because they relate to the service provided rather than to the product. The service cost of dispensing a prescription is called the *cost to dispense*. The net income is the amount of profit the pharmacy earns on the prescription.

The price of a pharmaceutical service, such as diabetic education and counseling, consists of the same components. While the service cost is likely to be the largest component, there may also be product costs related to supplies used to provide the service. For example, glucometer test strips and reagents may be used in providing services to diabetics.

If the pharmacy is to earn a satisfactory profit, its prices must cover its costs plus some surplus for net income. This suggests that pricing should be based primarily on cost factors. While costs are important, other factors play a major role in determining prices. The most important consideration in setting prices is the product or service's value *to the consumer*. The optimal price is the one that is less than the product or service's perceived value to consumers and greater than the pharmacy's cost of providing the product or service. The cost and noncost factors that affect pricing decisions are important because of their effect on the product or service's perceived value to consumers.

## SERVICE COSTS

To correctly set the price of a product or service, the pharmacy must have an accurate estimate of the average, or per unit, cost of providing it. As will be discussed later, calculating service costs is complicated because the service cost usually changes as the volume of service provided changes. Service costs include the expenses directly incurred in providing the product or service and a fair share of expenses incurred indirectly.

### Calculating Service Costs

To accurately calculate service costs, a manager must understand several different kinds of costs and how they are related.

### Types of Costs

All of a pharmacy's expenses can be classified as either direct or indirect costs. *Direct* costs are those that are directly caused by or result from providing the service. Direct costs of dispensing prescriptions include the costs of prescription labels and containers, patient education materials, pharmacy licenses, and continuing education costs for pharmacists. Direct costs of providing a diabetic education service include pharmacists' time spent counseling, educating, and monitoring patients; patient education materials; and equipment and supplies used to monitor patients' blood sugar levels. Direct costs may also be thought of as those costs that the pharmacy would *not* incur if it did not provide the service. For example, if the pharmacy did not dispense prescriptions, it would not incur the costs of prescription containers or pharmacy licenses.

*Indirect* costs are those that are not directly caused by or that do not directly result from providing the service. They are costs that the pharmacy would incur even if it did not provide the service in question. Examples include rent, utilities, and manager's salary. These costs are shared costs or joint costs. They are shared, or joint, in the sense that they are costs necessary to the sale of all the pharmacy's products and services.

If the pharmacy did not dispense, or if it did not provide diabetic education, it would continue to incur indirect costs.

The cost of providing a particular service includes all direct costs and a "fair share" of indirect costs. A basic problem of calculating a service cost is that of determining what is a "fair share." For example, how much of the rent should be recognized as part of the cost of dispensing and how much should be recognized as an expense of the rest of the pharmacy?

## Allocating Indirect Costs

Determining how much of an indirect cost should be recognized, or assigned to, a particular service is a problem of *allocating costs*. Cost allocation is a subjective procedure. There is no single, universally accepted method of allocating indirect costs. The general rules stipulate only that (a) the basis of allocation should be logical and rational and (b) the method of allocation should be based on a causal relationship.

For example, in deciding how much of the rent expense should be recognized as a cost of dispensing, several methods could be considered. Rent could be assigned based on the proportion of total floor space occupied by the prescription department, by the proportion of total sales accounted for by prescription sales, or by the proportion of total inventory accounted for by prescription inventory. All three methods might be considered rational and logical. However, assuming that rent is paid as a fixed, monthly amount, only the first reflects a causal relationship. Rent is usually based on the amount of space the pharmacy occupies. The larger a store is in a shopping center, for instance, the more rent it pays. Because of this, it is reasonable to conclude that the larger the prescription department is, the more of the rent expense should be allocated to it. Thus, allocating the rent expense based on a proportion of floor space is logical and rational and reflects the causal relationship between size and rental expense.

Some pharmacies' rent expense is not paid as a fixed monthly amount. It is instead based on a percentage of sales. For example, a pharmacy's rent may be charged as 2% of its monthly sales. In this case, allocating the amount of rent to be recognized as a cost of dispensing based on a proportion of floor space would not reflect a causal relationship. It would be more appropriate to allocate rent based on the ratio of prescription sales to total sales. This would recognize the causal relationship between sales and the amount of the rent expense.

## An Example of Estimating a Service Cost: The Cost to Dispense

During 2003, over 85% of all prescriptions dispensed in community pharmacies in the United States were paid for by third-party payers.[1] This figure is expected to increase when the Medicare prescription drug benefit is implemented. A third-party payer is an organization that pays the pharmacy for a patient's prescription. Insurance companies, large employers, health maintenance organizations (HMOs), and state Medicaid agencies are examples of third-party payers. The majority of third-party payers reimburse pharmacies on the basis of ingredient cost plus a fixed fee. For example, in 2003 the Virginia Medicaid program reimbursed pharmacies product cost plus a fixed $3.75 fee for each prescription dispensed.

In negotiating with third-party payers, managers need to know what it costs them to dispense a prescription. If they do not, they cannot make informed decisions about the adequacy of the fees offered by these payers.

The following is an example of how a pharmacy's cost of dispensing a prescription could be estimated. The method presented meets the criteria of being logical, being rational, and reflecting causal relationships. It should not, however, be regarded as the one correct method. Because of the subjective nature of cost allocations, other methods could be equally correct.

Much of the data for a cost-to-dispense calculation comes from the pharmacy's income statement. Income statement data reflect *past* costs. The cost to dispense is done to aid decision making for the *future*. Because of this, the manager should not use data from past years' income statements. Rather, the manager must estimate an income statement for the next year (this is called a *pro forma income statement*). Because of changes in the way the pharmacy may be operated and because of inflation, use of income statement data from past years may underestimate future costs. Consequently, use of past years' income statements for cost data could result in erroneous pricing decisions.

## Classification of Expenses

Each of the pharmacy's operating expenses, as shown on its pro forma income statement, must be classified into one of four categories: direct costs, salary expense, housing-related indirect costs, and other indirect costs.

Direct costs are those that result directly from dispensing prescriptions. These include labels and containers for prescriptions; dues and subscriptions; professional liability insurance; interest, depreciation, and maintenance fees on prescription department equipment (such as computers and software); and pharmacists' continuing education costs. The salary expense includes all salaries, fringe benefits (such as health and life insurance or pharmacists' liability insurance), and payroll taxes paid by the employer for each employee. Housing-related indirect costs include rent that is paid as a fixed dollar amount, repairs and maintenance on buildings and fixtures, and utilities. Other indirect costs include all other expenses incurred jointly by the prescription and nonprescription departments. They include such costs as advertising, bad debt, supplies, depreciation (on equipment and fixtures used in both dispensing and nondispensing functions), and rent that is paid as a percentage of sales.

## Allocating Costs to the Prescription Department

Direct costs are those that result directly from dispensing. As a result, *all* direct costs are charged to the prescription department.

Salary expenses are allocated based on time spent performing dispensing-related duties. The portion of each employee's salary expense that is allocated to the dispensing function is found by multiplying each employee's salary-including fringe benefits and payroll taxes-by the ratio of hours worked in dispensing-related functions to total hours worked. Dispensing-related functions include not only receiving and processing prescriptions, but also such tasks as ordering, stocking, and maintaining the inventory of prescriptions drugs; managing the prescription department; rectifying third-party prescription claims; and counseling patients about their prescriptions. A calculation is made separately for each employee. The amounts allocated to the dispensing function for each employee are then summed to find the total salary expense for dispensing.

Housing-related indirect costs are allocated according to a floor space ratio. This is done by multiplying total housing-related indirect costs by the ratio of prescription department size to total pharmacy selling space. Total pharmacy selling space includes only space used for selling and dispensing. Office space and storage areas are excluded.

Other indirect costs are allocated according to a sales ratio. The amount allocated to the prescription department is calculated by multiplying total other indirect costs by the ratio of prescription sales to total sales.

## Calculation of Cost to Dispense

Having classified all costs and allocated them to the prescription department, the cost to dispense can be calculated. The total cost of operating the prescription department is the sum of allocated costs in each of the four categories. The cost to dispense a prescription is found by dividing the total cost of operating the prescription department by the total number of prescriptions to be dispensed in the next year. The formula used to calculate the cost to dispense is shown in Figure 9-1.

## An Example Calculation

Green Cross Pharmacy is a unit of a major chain of pharmacies. Green Cross's pro forma income statement is shown in Figure 9-2. The income statement provides most of the data needed to calculate Green Cross's cost to dispense. Additional data needed are as follows:

1. The pharmacy employs two pharmacists who work, on average, a total of 90 hours per week. Both make the same salary. Of the 90 hours they work, 80

$$CTD = \frac{DC + \Sigma\,(RXS \times HW/TH) + HRC \times \dfrac{RXSF}{TSF} + IOC \times \dfrac{RXSA}{TSA}}{RXV}$$

CTD  = Cost to dispense a prescription
DC   = Direct costs
RXS  = Each employee's salary expense
HW   = Number of hours the employee works in prescription-related functions
TH   = Total hours the employee works in pharmacy
HRC  = Housing-related indirect costs
RXSF = Prescription department area, in square feet
TSF  = Pharmacy total area, in square feet
IOC  = Indirect other costs
RXSA = Prescription department sales
TSA  = Total sales of pharmacy
RXV  = Number of prescriptions dispensed

**FIGURE 9–1**  Recommended formula for calculating cost to dispense.

**Pro Forma Income Statement**
**Green Cross Pharmacy**
**Year Ending 12-31-0X**

| | | |
|---|---|---|
| Prescription sales | $3,285,000 | |
| Nonprescription sales | 3,000,000 | |
| Total sales | | $6,285,000 |
| Cost of goods sold | | 4,713,750 |
| | | 1,571,250 |
| Operating expenses | | |
| Pharmacists salaries and benefits | 304,200 | |
| Pharmacy technician salaries and benefits | 124,800 | |
| Store manager salary and benefits | 95,000 | |
| Other salaries and benefits | 312,000 | |
| Lease | 75,000 | |
| Repairs | 8,000 | |
| Housekeeping | 5,000 | |
| Utilities | 45,000 | |
| Pharmacy computer | 25,000 | |
| Prescription containers | 19,000 | |
| Supplies | 15,000 | |
| Advertising | 32,000 | |
| Depreciation | 30,000 | |
| Miscellaneous | 220,000 | |
| Total expenses | | 1,310,000 |
| Net profit | | $  261,250 |

**FIGURE 9-2**  Pro forma income statement for Green Cross Pharmacy.

    hours are devoted to dispensing-related duties and 10 are related to management and nonprescription merchandising and sales functions.

2. Pharmacy technicians work all of their time in the prescription department. The store manager works 60 hours per week. Of this, 6 hours are devoted to managing the prescription department. Other personnel work a total of 600 hours per week, of which 60 hours are worked in the prescription department.

3. The prescription department takes up 500 square feet of floor space. The entire pharmacy contains 10,000 square feet of selling space.

4. The manager estimates that the pharmacy will dispense 65,700 prescriptions in the coming year.

    Using these data, Green Cross's cost to dispense can be calculated using the method discussed earlier.

*Classification of Expenses*   The income statement shows two expenses that are direct costs of dispensing: prescription computer and prescription containers. Technicians' salaries are allocated completely to the prescription department. Pharmacists' salaries, store manager salary, and other salaries are joint salary expenses. Housing-related indirect costs include the lease, utilities, housekeeping, and repairs. Other indirect costs include supplies, advertising, depreciation, and miscellaneous.

*Allocation of Costs to the Prescription Department*   Direct costs include $25,000 for the prescription department computer and $19,000 for prescription containers. The sum, $44,000, is allocated to the prescription department.

Technicians' salaries of $124,800 are allocated completely to the prescription department. Joint salaries are allocated to the prescription department based on the percentage of time spent in dispensing-related functions. At Green Cross, pharmacists spend 80 of their 90 hours a week on these functions. Total pharmacist salaries are $304,200. The pharmacist salary expense allocated to the prescription department is calculated as:

$$304,200 \times 80/90 = \$270,400$$

The store manager earns $95,000 per year, works 60 hours per week, and works 6 of these in duties related to the dispensing function. So, store manager salary allocated to the prescription department is:

$$95,000 \times 6/60 = \$9,500$$

Sixty of the 600 other employees' hours per week are devoted to dispensing-related duties. Total other salaries are $312,000. The other salary expense of the prescription department is therefore:

$$\$312,000 \times 60/600 = \$31,200$$

Total salary expense allocated to the prescription department is the sum of these four, which amounts to $435,900.

Housing-related indirect costs are allocated using the ratio of prescription department size to total selling space. Green Cross has $133,000 in housing-related indirect costs, its prescription department takes up 500 square feet, and total pharmacy selling space amounts to 10,000 square feet. Indirect fixed costs allocated to the pharmacy are calculated as:

$$\$133,000 \times 500/10,000 = \$6,650$$

Other indirect costs are allocated using the ratio of prescription to total sales. Green Cross has $297,000 in other indirect costs, its estimated prescription sales are $3,285,000, and estimated total sales are $6,285,000. Other indirect costs allocated to the pharmacy are:

$$\$297,000 \times 3,285,000/6,285,000 = \$155,234$$

*Calculation of Cost to Dispense*   The cost to dispense is calculated as the sum of prescription department costs in each category—direct costs, salary expenses, housing-related indirect costs, and other indirect costs—divided by the number of prescriptions to be dispensed. Green Cross's cost to dispense is:

$$CTD = \frac{(44,000 + 435,900 + 6,650 + 155,234)}{65,700}$$

$$CTD = \$9.77$$

Thus, based on the estimates given, it should cost Green Cross Pharmacy an average of $9.77 to dispense a prescription during the coming year.

## Use and Interpretation of the Cost to Dispense

The cost to dispense is the *average* amount it costs the pharmacy to dispense a prescription. Consequently, it is the average amount that must be added to the ingredient cost to ensure that the prescription department breaks even. For example, if Green Cross Pharmacy's average ingredient cost was $50.00, its average prescription price would have to be at least $59.77 to ensure that the prescription department broke even. The price would have to be higher if the pharmacy wished to make a profit on prescription sales.

Because the cost to dispense is an average cost, and because many of a pharmacy's costs are fixed, the cost to dispense is sensitive to the *volume* of prescriptions dispensed. That is, within the relevant range, increases in volume will lead to a decrease in the cost to dispense, while decreases in volume will lead to increases. The greater the proportion of costs that are fixed costs, the more sensitive the cost to dispense will be to changes in volume. This leads to a circular relationship between demand, volume sold, cost to dispense, and price: price is frequently based on the cost to dispense, the cost to dispense is a function of the volume sold, which is a function of demand, and demand is a function of price.

## Another Example of Service Costs: Diabetic Care Center[2]

Pharmacist Jones wants to start a diabetic care center (DCC) in his retail pharmacy. The diabetic care center will provide counseling, educational, and monitoring services to diabetic patients. Pharmacist Jones plans for the basic unit of service in the DCC to be a 15-minute counseling/education/monitoring session. As a first step in setting a reasonable price, he needs to estimate the cost of a session.

Jones Pharmacy's pro forma income statement for the coming year is shown in Figure 9-3. This statement includes the estimated costs of operating the DCC. Additional information needed to estimate the cost of a session is given below:

1.  The DCC will be open for a total of 6 hours per week. Pharmacist Jones plans to hire a pharmacist to staff the DCC. The pharmacist's salary will be $45 per hour. Pharmacist Jones, the manager, figures he will spend about 3 hours a week managing the DCC. He typically works 60 hours per week.
2.  Two hours of technician time per week will be required by the DCC. The pharmacy's technician will cover this as part of the 40 hours per week she usually works.
3.  Opening the DCC will require renovation of the pharmacy and purchase of equipment. When renovation is completed, the DCC will occupy 150 square feet of floor space in the pharmacy. Total selling space occupied by

| Pro Forma Income Statement<br>Jones Pharmacy<br>Year Ending 12-31-0X | |
| --- | --- |
| Net sales | $ 2,000,000 |
| Cost of goods sold | 1,520,000 |
| Gross margin | 480,000 |
| Operating expenses | |
| Pharmacist manager's salary | 115,000 |
| Dispensing pharmacist's salary | 46,800 |
| Diabetic Care Center | |
|    Pharmacist's salary | 14,040 |
| Technician salary | 24,960 |
| Clerks' salaries | 80,000 |
| Rent and utilities | 34,000 |
| Promotion | 14,500 |
| Depreciation | 7,500 |
| Pharmacy computer | 9,000 |
| Miscellaneous | 53,000 |
| Total operating expenses | 398,800 |
| Net profit before taxes | $81,200 |

FIGURE 9-3   Pro forma income statement for Jones Pharmacy.

the pharmacy is 4,500 square feet. Renovation and equipment will cost $18,000 and will be depreciated over 6 years. This provides an annual depreciation of expense of $3,000.

4. Pharmacist Jones is budgeting $2,400 per year for promotion of the DCC to local physicians.

5. Pharmacist Jones estimates that the DCC will provide 1,000 sessions in the coming year.

## Classification of Expenses

Direct costs of operating the DCC include depreciation on the DCC and promotion of the DCC to physicians. Salary expenses are needed for the additional pharmacist and for the time the technician and manager spend on DCC work. Housing-related indirect costs include rent and utilities. Of the remaining expenses, depreciation, promotion, and clerks' salaries do not need to be considered. The part of depreciation and promotion attributable to the DCC have already been identified and allocated as direct costs. None of the clerks spend time working in the DCC.

## Allocation of Costs to the Diabetic Care Center

Direct costs of operating the DCC include $3,000 for depreciation on the DCC and $2,400 per year for promotion of the DCC to physicians. Thus, total direct costs amount to $5,400.

Salaries are allocated to the DCC according to the amount of time worked there. The pharmacist works there 6 hours a week and is paid $45 per hour. So, annual pharmacist expense for the DCC is:

$$6 \text{ hours per week} \times \$45 \text{ per hour} \times 52 \text{ weeks per year} = \$14,040$$

The technician works in the DCC 2 hours per week out of the total of 40 hours she works at the pharmacy. She is paid $24,960 per year. Annual technician expense for the DCC is:

$$\$24,960 \times 2/40 = \$1,248$$

Pharmacist Jones, the manager, spends about 3 hours per week managing the DCC. He works a total of 60 hours per week and draws a salary of $115,000 per year. Annual manager expense for the DCC is:

$$\$115,000 \times 3/60 = \$5,750$$

This gives a total salary expense for the DCC of $14,040 + $1,248 + $5,750 = $21,038.

Housing-related indirect costs include rent and utilities of $34,000. The DCC occupies 150 square feet of the 4,500-square-foot pharmacy. Housing-related expenses for the DCC are:

$$\$34,000 \times 150/4,500 = \$1,113$$

This leaves other indirect expenses of pharmacy computer and miscellaneous. These expenses total $62,000. Allocating these expenses, in this situation, is a problem. Normally, we would use the ratio of DCC sales to total pharmacy sales. However, we do not know what DCC sales will be because we have not yet decided what to charge for them. A reasonable approach in this situation would be to develop a rough estimate of DCC sales and then allocate other indirect expenses based on the sales ratio. If the estimate turns out to be substantially different than the estimate we get once the price is estimated, then we can repeat this step using a closer estimate. The manager has estimated that the pharmacy will provide about 1,000 counseling sessions in the next year. As a beginning estimate, we will assume the DCC will charge $30 per session. Therefore, estimated sales in the DCC will be $30,000. The portion of indirect other expenses allocated to the DCC is:

$$\$62,000 \times 30,000/2,000,000 = \$930$$

## Calculation of Service Cost of a Session in the Diabetic Care Center

The service cost for a session is calculated as the sum of costs in each category divided by the number of sessions to be provided. The service cost for a session is:

$$\text{Service Cost} = \frac{(\$5,400 + \$21,038 + \$1133 + \$930)}{1,000}$$
$$= \$28.50$$

The service cost is very close to our initial estimate of the price. Because of this, and because DCC sales are only a small percentage of total sales, it is not necessary to redo the estimate of DCC-related other indirect costs.

## Use and Interpretation of the Service Cost

At a volume of 1,000 sessions per year, the price of a session in the DCC must be at least $28.50 (plus the cost of any supplies used) for the service to break even. A higher price is needed to make a profit.

As with the cost to dispense, the average service cost of a session in the DCC is sensitive to the volume of sessions offered. The DCC's service cost is even more sensitive to volume because all costs of offering the service are fixed costs. This can be seen by examining the effects of changes in the volume of sessions provided on the service cost: if 500 sessions were provided, the service cost would rise to $57.00; if 1,500 sessions were provided, the service cost would be $19.00. Because of this, it is essential that the manager accurately forecast demand for the service.

## DEFINITIONS OF INGREDIENT COST

In regard to calculating prescription prices, the ingredient cost is the cost to the pharmacy of the drug product dispensed to the patient. In theory, this is a simple concept. In practice, actually defining and measuring a prescription's ingredient cost is not so simple. Several terms are used to define a prescription's ingredient cost. The price at which the pharmacy actually purchases the product is referred to as the *actual acquisition cost (AAC)*. This is the true ingredient cost of the product. It is very difficult to determine the AAC of a given product. The AAC of a given product is dependent upon several factors. One is the source from which the product was purchased. The product may have a lower AAC if purchased direct from the manufacturer than if purchased from a wholesaler. (The price at which a product may be purchased directly from the manufacturer is referred to as its *direct* price.) The product's price may depend on the total volume of purchases the pharmacy makes from the supplier. Pharmacies with larger volumes of purchases are typically given larger discounts. In addition, at certain times of the year the manufacturer may offer various incentives to encourage purchase of its products. The manufacturer may, for example, give one bottle of the product free with every 12 purchased. All of these factors make it difficult to reliably determine AAC.

The pharmacy receives an invoice that lists the actual amount it paid for the product. Because of this, it is possible for a pharmacy to determine its AAC on a given product at a given time. While this may change somewhat over the course of a year, for a given pharmacy it is unlikely to change dramatically. On the other hand, the AAC of a given product for different pharmacies is likely to be highly variable. Small-volume pharmacies are likely to pay more than large-volume pharmacies. Pharmacies that use a great deal of the product will pay less than those that use only a little. As a result, it is quite difficult for an outside party-such as a third-party payer-to determine an AAC for a given product that would accurately reflect the prices paid by all, or even most, pharmacies.

As a result of this, third-party payers have historically based their reimbursement for a prescription's ingredient cost on the *average wholesale price (AWP)* of the product dispensed. The AWP is *not* the average price at which the drug is sold by wholesalers.

The AWP is a cost assigned to the product by the manufacturer and listed as the AWP in a regularly published source such as *Drug Topic's Red Book*. While the AWP of a product will be the same for all pharmacies, it will not accurately measure the AAC. The Department of Health and Human Services has estimated that, for community pharmacies, the AWP is about 17% higher than AAC for brand-name drugs with no generic competition, 24% higher than AAC for multiple source brand-name drugs, and between 54% and 72% higher than AAC for generic drugs.[3] For a hospital, long-term care, or HMO pharmacy, the difference is typically much greater.

In an attempt to establish a standard cost figure that more accurately reflects the price pharmacies actually pay, third-party payers typically define a product's ingredient cost as its *estimated acquisition cost (EAC)*. The EAC is frequently defined as AWP less some percentage discount. The EAC may be defined, for example, as AWP less 10%.

Another measure of the cost of the drug product is *wholesale acquisition cost (WAC)*. This is defined as the "price paid by the wholesaler for drugs purchased from the wholesaler's suppliers (manufacturers)."[4] Like AWP, WAC prices are publicly available. However, like the AWP, the listed WAC does not reflect the wholesaler's true cost. As a rough estimate, AWP is equal to somewhere between WAC + 20% and WAC + 25%.

The *maximum allowable cost (MAC)* is a measure of the cost of multisource prescription products. Multisource products are those that are available from more than one manufacturer or distributor. This includes primarily generic drugs but also patented products that are sold by more than one company. Examples of the latter category include Ventolin and Proventil. The MAC is the maximum amount that the third-party payer will reimburse the pharmacy for the ingredient cost of a particular multisource product. For example, assume that generic diazepam is available for $10 per 100 tablets while the brand-name product, Valium, costs $30 per 100 tablets. A third-party payer would establish the MAC for diazepam at $10 per 100 tablets. Regardless of which product the pharmacist dispensed—either the generic diazepam or the brand-name Valium—the third party would only reimburse the pharmacy the MAC rate of $10 per 100 tablets for ingredient cost. Third parties use MAC pricing to give pharmacists a strong economic incentive to use lower-cost products. The MAC pricing system was developed by and is still used by the federal government for Medicaid. The MAC prices set by the federal government are referred to as federal upper limits (FULs).

## NONCOST FACTORS AFFECTING PRICES

While an understanding of costs is critical to rational pricing, several other factors must also be considered. The most important of these are discussed below.

### Demand

Demand refers to the quantity of a product or service consumers will buy at a given price. Demand is different from need. The need for pharmaceutical products and services can be objectively determined by medical experts based on the prevalence of disease in the population. Demand, on the other hand, is based on consumer perceptions. The need for diabetic counseling and education, for example, is based on the prevalence of diabetes. The demand is based on the value diabetics believe they will receive from counseling and educational services.

Because demand is based on consumer perceptions, it can be affected by marketing activities. Skillful advertising and promotion can increase the demand for a product or

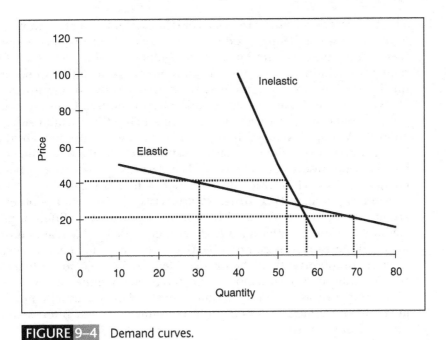

FIGURE 9–4 Demand curves.

service. As an example, skillful and heavy promotion has induced a substantial demand for cigarettes, even though there is no need for the product.

Demand is also affected by price. As the price of a product or service rises, the quantity demanded by consumers falls. The extent to which quantity demanded changes in response to price is known as the *price elasticity of demand*. It is a measure of how sensitive consumers are to different price levels. Different products and services will have different levels of elasticity or price sensitivity. Knowing how sensitive consumers are to prices for a service or product is critical to setting an appropriate price.

Figure 9-4 illustrates different price elasticities of demand. The flatter line illustrates the price elasticity of a product with *elastic demand*. Notice that a change in price—from $40 to $20—leads to a more than proportionate change in the quantity demanded—from 30 units to 69 units. Elastic demand means that consumers are very sensitive to price differences. The steeper line illustrates *inelastic demand*. Here, a change in price leads to a less than proportionate change in the quantity demanded. A change in price from $40 to $20 leads to an increase in quantity from 52 to 58 units. Inelastic demand means consumers are much less sensitive to price differences.

Dolan[5] and Nagel and Holden[6] suggest the following guidelines managers can use to estimate consumers' price sensitivity for a specific product or service:

1. The consumer's sensitivity to price rises as the price of the product or service becomes a greater part of the total cost of therapy. The total cost of treating coughs and colds is low. Thus, consumers are quite sensitive to the price of pharmacist counseling for cough and cold products. A high price for this service will likely result in little or no demand. The total treatment costs of asthma, on the other hand, are quite high. They include expensive drug therapy, frequent physician monitoring, trips to the emergency room, and hospitalizations. Compared with the total costs of treating asthma, the costs of asthma-related counseling provided by pharmacists are small. Therefore, consumers are likely to be much less sensitive to the price of asthma counseling services.

2.  The consumer's sensitivity to price is higher when there are minimal differences among competing products and services. Further, price sensitivity increases as consumers find it easier to compare products and services. This depends on both how competent consumers are to judge differences in quality and on how convenient it is for them to do so. Over-the-counter (OTC) drugs, for example, are standardized products. Consumers get the same product whether they buy it at a supermarket, a discount store, or an apothecary shop. Assuming there are no meaningful differences in the services that accompany the products, consumers can make their choice based on price. Because the products are standardized, it is easy to obtain and compare prices. Thus, price differences can have a major effect on where consumers purchase OTC drugs. Pharmacists' services, on the other hand, are not standardized. The quality of services provided in different pharmacies and by different pharmacists varies a great deal. This makes it difficult for consumers to easily compare services. They have to actually receive the services, or observe them being provided, to be able to evaluate them. Further, consumers have a more difficult time judging the quality of services. While they can assess interpersonal aspects, they are usually not able to judge technical merit. Consequently, consumers are much less sensitive to the price of services.

3.  The consumer's price sensitivity increases as switching costs increase. Switching costs refer to the costs—both monetary and nonmonetary—that consumers incur when they change their source of supply for a product or service. For example, if a particular pharmacy is much more convenient for consumers, then they will incur significant time costs in switching their purchases to another pharmacy. Because of the time and trouble they would experience in using another pharmacy, they will be much less likely to change pharmacies solely because of differences in prescription prices. Services that require a relationship to be built between the consumer and the provider have high switching costs. If, for example, a consumer switched lawyers in the middle of a complicated case, he or she would have to repeat with the new lawyer the process of providing all relevant information about the case, developing rapport, and developing a strategy for the case. Patients who build relationships with pharmacists through receipt of patient-oriented services over a long period of time face similar switching costs.

The manager must have a good estimate of demand for a service before it can be priced. Considering consumers' price sensitivity aids the manager in estimating demand. Chapter 6, *Budgeting*, provides more information on estimating demand. A more in-depth discussion of demand estimation is provided by Simon[7] and Nagle and Holden.[6]

## Competition

A pharmacy must consider the prices charged by the pharmacies and health care practitioners with which it competes when setting prices. Unless a pharmacy has some major advantage over its competitors—such as more convenient location, larger or more extensive selection of merchandise, or better services—it will not be able to charge substantially higher prices. A pharmacy that has a distinct advantage will be able to charge higher prices only if it can convince consumers of the value of the advantage.

## Pharmacy Image

When consumers choose a pharmacy, their choices are based on what they *perceive* the pharmacy's prices to be, not necessarily what the pharmacy's prices actually are. Consumer perceptions are based largely on the pharmacy's *image*. The pharmacy's image is determined to some extent by the prices it charges. However, it is unlikely that most consumers will be familiar with a pharmacy's prices, or even with how one pharmacy's prices compare with another's. At most, consumers on chronic medications will know how much a few pharmacies charge for the medications they buy regularly.

Because consumers are generally unfamiliar with prices, a number of other factors are as important, if not more important, in establishing a pharmacy's image. These include the size and location of the pharmacy, the quality and variety of nonprescription merchandise carried, the variety and quality of services offered, the appearance and actions of personnel, and the types of promotions used.

For example, a small, apothecary-type pharmacy located in a medical center would probably have a high-quality, high-price image. If the pharmacists there spent a great deal of time counseling patients and if the pharmacy carried only drugs and health care supplies, consumers would be even more likely to have this image. On the other hand, a pharmacy located in a mass merchandiser, such as K-Mart or Wal-Mart, would probably be perceived as a low-price, discount pharmacy. Pharmacists who avoided talking with patients and weekly advertisements for sale-priced nonprescription merchandise would strengthen the low-price image.

Because pharmacy image determines consumer perceptions of prescription prices, a manager is well advised to offer prices that are consistent with the pharmacy's image. The small, apothecary pharmacy mentioned above will be expected, because of its image, to have higher prices. Even if it actually offers discount prices, few consumers will be aware of the low prices, and most will continue to perceive it as a high-price pharmacy. Because of this, the manager will have little incentive to offer discount prices. On the other hand, a pharmacy that appears to be a discount pharmacy but charges high prices will have little to offer to consumers who discover, as they ultimately will, that it does not offer discount prices.

## Price as a Signal of Quality[8]

Consumers sometimes use price as an indicator of quality. This is especially likely to occur for services because consumers have much greater problems judging the quality of services than of products. Compared with products, services tend to be intangible and infrequently advertised or associated with brand names. (Consumers use both brand names and frequency of advertising as indicators of quality.) As a result, consumers may rely on price as an indicator of service quality; that is, they may assume that higher-priced services are of higher quality. This is more likely to occur when there is great variability in the quality of service provided or when the service is seen as involving high risk to the consumer—as in the case of surgery. Many pharmacists' services fall into this category. There is likely to be a large variability in the quality of service provided and many—such as counseling and monitoring asthma patients— may be seen as high-risk services. In these situations, low prices may actually decrease demand for the service by signaling low quality to consumers.

## Pharmacy Goals

The pharmacy's prices should be consistent with its goals. The goal of most pharmacies will be to maximize long-term profits. To do this, the manager must set prices low enough to attract and retain customers and high enough to yield a profit. This strategy allows the pharmacy to make a reasonable profit over a long life. While maximizing long-term profit is the most common goal, others may be important in particular situations.

A new pharmacy, or a pharmacy offering a new service, might have the goal of rapidly building sales volume. To do this, it might offer low prices to attract business. This is a strategy that sacrifices short-term profits in order to build sales quickly. This is called a *penetration pricing* strategy. A penetration strategy is preferred in situations where demand is highly elastic (i.e., consumers are price sensitive), where there is strong competition, and/or where increased volume leads to economies of scale.

Some stores, especially units of large chains or mass merchandisers, use their prescription departments as *loss leaders*. These stores offer extremely low prices on prescriptions. They frequently sell products at or below cost. Their objective is to use low prescription prices to attract consumers into the store to buy other merchandise. The stores intend to make their profits on the other merchandise. This strategy can only be used by stores that have sufficient nonprescription volume and profits to be able to operate the prescription department at a break-even or loss.

Some pharmacies have a goal of attracting only those consumers who are willing to pay higher prices for special or high levels of services. The pricing strategy by which this goal is pursued is known as *price skimming*. This strategy requires offering a service that is not widely available or offering a level of overall service that other pharmacies cannot, or choose not, to provide. Many specialist physicians and lawyers use a price skimming strategy; they serve only those consumers who are willing to pay for their higher levels of training and expertise.

Price skimming can also be used to price a new product or service. This is done when the business would like to maximize its profits on the service quickly. Price skimming is most appropriate for pricing new products and services when there is a substantial number of price inelastic consumers and when there are few substitutes for the service. Pharmaceutical companies that develop therapeutically unique products, especially those that are the first products in a new therapeutic class, use price skimming when the product is first introduced. Businesses that introduce products and services at a skimming price typically lower the price over time. They do this to attract additional business by serving more price-sensitive markets.

## Nonmonetary Costs[8]

Patients incur a number of costs in addition to the prices they pay for pharmaceutical products and services. They incur time costs in traveling to the pharmacy and in waiting for services to be delivered. They incur search costs in trying to find pharmacists who provide the products and services they need. They incur psychic costs in worrying about whether their medicines will help or harm them. Zeithaml and Bitner[8] point out that for some patients, these costs may outweigh monetary costs. Consequently, managers need to carefully consider how the products and services they offer affect nonmonetary costs.

Many pharmacy services strongly affect nonmonetary costs. Delivery services, for example, decrease consumers' time costs. Patient education and counseling initially increase time costs because consumers must spend time interacting with pharmacists. On the other hand, these services reduce psychic costs and may, in the long run, reduce time costs. A few minutes spent discussing medications with the pharmacist may be more than compensated for by the time saved as a result of preventing adverse reactions or treatment failures. Good patient counseling can also dramatically decrease psychic costs by making patients aware of possible side effects and informing patients of how to deal with them.

## Pricing When the Pharmacy Is Offered a Set Price

During 2003, over 85% of all prescriptions dispensed in community pharmacies (including chains, independents, supermarket and discount store pharmacies, and mail-order pharmacies) in the United States were paid for by third-party payers.[1] In almost all cases the third-party payer, not the pharmacy, sets the price. As third-party reimbursement for patient care services grows, pharmacies may find themselves in the same situation in regard to the pricing of services.

Marketers refer to this situation as *demand backward* pricing. The pharmacy's goal in demand backward pricing is not to determine an optimal price for its services, but to determine how it can profitably provide the service at the offered price. Much of the literature and training material on providing patient care services has assumed a demand backwards framework. For example, most programs to assist pharmacists in implementing patient care services in community pharmacies include a substantial discussion of changing the pharmacy's workflow so that pharmacists have more time to care for patients. Usually this involves turning more dispensing-related tasks over to technicians and increasing automation in the pharmacy. The goal is to allow pharmacies to be able to provide patient care services without increasing the pharmacy's costs. The implicit assumption behind this goal is that the reimbursement that pharmacies receive will be sufficiently low that they will have to change the way they operate in order to profitably provide the services.

## Interaction of Factors Affecting Pricing

The prices a pharmacy charges should be based on careful consideration of cost and noncost factors. The manager must consider not only the effects of these factors independently, but also the interactions among them.

This may be seen through consideration of a pharmacy that has the goal of quickly increasing sales. A pricing strategy consistent with this goal would have the pharmacy charge low prices. Assume that prices were set below cost. If the pharmacy's potential clientele were highly price sensitive, the low-price strategy would result in high demand—that is, the pharmacy would be successful in attracting new patients. Most pharmacies have substantial fixed costs (such as managers' salaries, rent and utilities, and depreciation). Fixed costs do not increase as volume increases. Because of this, increases in volume decrease *average* costs. If the pharmacy's clientele were sufficiently price sensitive, then volume could grow fast enough to force average costs below the pharmacy's prices. Thus, in time the pharmacy could make a profit at prices that were, originally, below its costs.

On the other hand, the pharmacy's clientele may not be particularly price sensitive. This might happen, for example, if competing pharmacies were much more convenient for consumers, if they provided markedly better service, or if most consumers had their prescriptions paid for by an insurance company or HMO. In this case, the pharmacy's lower prices would not lead to rapid increases in sales. Average costs would remain higher than prices and the pharmacy would suffer large financial losses.

Another example of the interaction of pricing factors is setting price based on cost. As we have seen, the demand for a product or service (the quantity demanded) has a major impact on the average cost of the product or service. Demand, in turn, is greatly affected by price. So, basing the price on the cost is difficult because of the interaction and circularity between price, cost, and demand. The various interactions between the factors that affect pricing suggest that setting proper prices requires a substantial amount of judgment in addition to technical skills.

## A RECOMMENDED STRATEGY FOR PRICING

A pharmacy needs an overall strategy for setting proper prices. The strategy should ensure that prices are high enough, in aggregate, to cover all costs and a reasonable profit. At the same time, the strategy must recognize that the prices the pharmacy can charge are constrained by demand, competition, pharmacy goals and image, and non-monetary costs. To illustrate the recommended strategy, we will continue the example of the Diabetic Counseling Center (DCC).

## Estimate Demand

The first step is to estimate demand for the service. For the DCC, the demand estimate is based on the number of diabetics the pharmacy serves, the number of diabetics who live in the area served by the pharmacy, the amount the pharmacy plans to spend to promote the DCC, and the prices of similar services charged by physicians in the area. The manager estimates that demand will be as shown below:

| Price | Quantity of Sessions Demanded Per Year |
|-------|----------------------------------------|
| $20 | 1,000 |
| $25 | 750 |
| $35 | 500 |
| $45 | 250 |

## Calculate the Pharmacy's Service Cost

The next step is to calculate the service cost. This will let the manager know how much, on average, the pharmacy must make on each unit of service to break even. Because of the dependency of costs on volume, the manager should calculate the cost of providing the service over a range of sales volume. The service cost for a session of diabetic counseling (as calculated earlier in the chapter) is as follows:

| Volume | Service Cost |
|--------|--------------|
| 500 | $57.00 |
| 1,000 | $28.50 |
| 1,500 | $19.10 |

## Determine the Net Income

Next, the manager must determine the average amount of net income the pharmacy must make on each unit of service to meet its overall profit objective. The profit objective is based on the pharmacy's desired return on assets, then adjusted for competition and the pharmacy's image.

The DCC has $18,000 in assets. A reasonable rate of return on assets is 12%. To attain this return, the DCC would need to earn a $18,000 × 0.12 = $2,160 profit. If the pharmacy expected to provide 1,000 sessions during the year, it would need an average net income of $2.16 per session to attain the $2,160. The amount of profit that is reasonable depends on the pharmacy's objectives and strategy. If it is following a penetration strategy, it may want to forgo all profits (initially) to increase sales more rapidly. If it has a skimming strategy, it will seek a higher profit.

## Set the Required Dollar Margin

The average dollar margin is the amount the pharmacy needs to cover its costs plus a reasonable profit. It is calculated as the sum of the service cost plus the average net income. (For the DCC the average dollar margin and the price are the same because there is no ingredient cost.) The DCC's service cost, net income per session, and average dollar margin at various levels of volume are:

| Volume | Service Cost | Average Net Income | Average Dollar Margin |
|--------|--------------|--------------------|-----------------------|
| 500 | $57.00 | $4.32 | $61.32 |
| 1,000 | $28.50 | $2.16 | $30.66 |
| 1,500 | $19.10 | $1.44 | $20.54 |

## Compare Demand and Price

At this point, the manager compares demand for the service with the price the pharmacy must charge to provide the service. The chart below shows the comparison for the DCC.

| Volume Assumed | Average Dollar Margin (Price) | Quantity Demanded at That Price |
|----------------|-------------------------------|----------------------------------|
| 500 | $61.32 | <250 |
| 1,000 | $30.66 | about 625 |
| 1,500 | $20.54 | about 1,000 |

The first column in the chart shows the volume that was assumed when calculating the service cost and net income. The second column shows the average dollar margin, which in this case is the price, and the final column shows the quantity of diabetic counseling sessions that would be demanded at that price.

The chart indicates that the DCC has a major problem—as currently planned, the pharmacy cannot provide the service for a price that a sufficient number of consumers would be willing to pay. For example, the pharmacy needs to provide 1,500 sessions to be able to provide the service for around $21. But at that price, only about 1,000 sessions will be demanded.

At this point the manager can either not provide the service or he can consider ways to increase demand or lower costs. It may be possible to increase demand for the service by increasing promotional expenditures. This could include advertising in local media and/or detailing local physicians about the service. Costs might be lowered by doing less extensive renovations or by decreasing the pharmacist expense. This might be accomplished by training staff pharmacists to provide the service in addition to their dispensing duties and by training technicians to assume more dispensing duties to free pharmacists' time for the DCC. Let us assume that the manager is able to cut costs to the point that the price required to earn the required profit is $18 per session at a volume of 1,000 sessions. Because estimated demand for the service is 1,000 sessions at $20, the pharmacy should be able to profitably provide the service.

## Monitor Patient and Competitor Reactions

Prices are initially based on *estimates* of demand, costs, and competitors' responses. After the price is implemented, the manager should carefully measure and document the actual response of patients and competitors to the service. Lower than anticipated demand may require lowering the price, increasing promotion, or re-evaluating the way the product or service is provided. Higher demand may allow raising the price to maximize profits or to limit demand to what the pharmacy can physically accommodate. The important point is that the manager needs to carefully monitor sales and competitors' responses to ensure that problems are quickly identified and addressed.

## Re-evaluate Periodically

The manager must periodically evaluate the system to ensure that the pharmacy is making its desired profit. The average dollar margin required should be recalculated at least every 6 months. Changes in competition may also require the manager to re-evaluate prices.

## ADDITIONAL CONSIDERATIONS FOR PRICING MULTIPLE PRODUCTS

The DCC pricing example is simplified in the sense that it deals with pricing only one service. The manager typically faces the task of pricing a group of products and services. This allows the manager to set different dollar margins for different types of products. The most common example is pricing prescriptions.

The example presented in this section describes how a manager can vary dollar margins across products to maintain a low-price image. As discussed earlier, the pharmacy's image is as critical to consumers as the pharmacy's actual prices. Consequently, the pharmacy should be as concerned with its price image as with its actual prices. It is difficult, if not impossible, to charge high prices and maintain a low-price image. However, it is possible to charge reasonable prices and maintain a low-price image. This is done by considering product-specific demand and competition. While the example uses prescription products, the principles apply to both products and services.

## Classifying Products

Consumers are unlikely to know the prices of many products. Many will, however, know the prices of a few high-demand prescription products such as insulin, oral antidiabetic agents, birth control pills, and many minor tranquilizers. A pharmacy must have low prices on these items if it is to maintain a low-price image. Frequently, it will be necessary to sell these products at or below their cost. Nelson refers to these high-demand, well-known products as *market priced* products, because the prices at which they can be sold are determined more by competition than by the pharmacy's cost of operation.[9] Zelnio and Nelson estimate that a pharmacy will have only 10 to 25 market-priced prescription products, but that they will account for roughly 30% of prescription sales.[10]

A second group of products are referred to as *staple* products. These products are used commonly, but not as frequently as the market-priced products. Consequently, the chances of consumers knowing the prices of staple products is much less than for market-priced drugs. Zelnio and Nelson estimate that the staple category for a typical pharmacy will contain up to 75 products and account for 25% of prescription sales.

The remaining products are known as *premium* products. These are drugs that are prescribed infrequently. Because of this, consumers are unlikely to know their prices. As a result, the pharmacy, rather than the competitive market, can set their prices. Premium products account for the vast majority of the pharmacy's products and for around 45% of its sales.

## Pricing by Product Category

The manager should charge a different dollar margin for each of these groups. The margin for market-priced products should be low because of consumer familiarity with the prices of these products. To maintain a reasonable price image, the pharmacy may have to sell these products at or only slightly above acquisition cost. Thus, the pharmacy will lose money on market-priced products. The pharmacy recovers the loss on market-priced products by charging a higher dollar margin on premium products. Prices of premium products are not well known, so the pharmacy can charge higher prices for them without damaging its price image. The pharmacy should charge the average dollar margin—that covers the cost to dispense plus a reasonable profit—for staple products.

This is consistent with a return on equity approach to pricing. The DuPont Model (Chapter 5) shows that return on equity is equal to net income multiplied by asset turnover. Fast-moving products have high turnover and can yield a given return on equity at lower levels of price and profit; slow-moving products have low turnover and require higher dollar margins to yield a target return on equity.

## Identifying Products in Each Category

The 10 to 25 products that account for 30% of the pharmacy's prescription sales comprise the market-priced category. To verify that these are the top-selling prescription products in the area in which the pharmacy competes, the manager should check the prices of these products at competing pharmacies. If the competition is selling them at or below cost, then the products should be included in the pharmacy's market-priced category. If not, they should be included in the staple category. The 75 or so products that account for the next 25% of sales volume are staples. The remaining products are the premiums.

Most pharmacy computer systems include report-writing features that allow the manager to identify the pharmacy's top-selling prescription products. Pharmacies that purchase all, or essentially all, prescription drugs from one wholesaler can get this information from wholesaler-generated product movement reports. Product movement reports tell how much of each prescription product the pharmacy has purchased from the wholesaler over some period of time.

## METHODS OF CALCULATING PRODUCT PRICES

The manager determines the pharmacy's pricing strategy based on the cost and non-cost considerations discussed above. Once the overall strategy has been selected, a method of calculating individual prices must be selected. Three methods are commonly used for pharmaceutical products: the markup method, the professional fee method, and the sliding scale.

### The Markup Method

The markup method bases price and dollar margin on the ingredient cost of the product dispensed. Consequently, as ingredient cost increases, both price and margin increase proportionately. The markup may be calculated as a percentage of either ingredient cost or price.

The following formula is used to calculate price using *markup on cost:*

$$Price = Ingredient\ cost + (Ingredient\ cost \times Markup\%)$$

If, for example, the cost of a drug were $20.00 and the markup were 50%, the price would be:

$$Price = \$20.00 + (\$20.00 \times .50) = \$30.00$$

Prices may also be calculated using a markup on the retail price, or *markup on retail,* as shown below:

$$Price = Ingredient\ cost + (Price \times Markup\%)$$

For actually calculating prices, the formula simplifies to:

$$Price = Ingredient\ cost/(1 - Markup\%/100)$$

For example, if the ingredient cost were $20.00 and the pharmacy used a markup on retail of 30%, the price would be calculated as:

$$
\begin{aligned}
Price &= Ingredient\ Cost/(1 - Markup\%/100) \\
&= \$20.00/\ (1 - 30/100) \\
&= \$20.00/.7 \\
&= \$28.57
\end{aligned}
$$

Most pharmacies use the markup on retail method because it is directly comparable to the gross margin percentage. That is, to get a 30% gross margin, a pharmacy would price products at a 30% markup on retail. (This assumes no discounts, bad debt, or shrinkage. These factors would lead to a gross margin lower than the markup on retail.)

A markup system automatically adjusts prices to accommodate changes in ingredient costs. If the cost of the product increases, the dollar margin increases proportionately. This protects the pharmacy from declining gross margin percentages in periods of inflation.

A disadvantage of the markup system is that it subsidizes low-cost products with high-cost ones. For example, if prescription prices are calculated using a markup, low-cost products have margins lower than the pharmacy's cost to dispense. Expensive drugs have high dollar margins. This may damage the pharmacy's price image because consumers are more likely to recognize and react to higher prices on expensive drugs than to lower prices on inexpensive ones.

An example may clarify this. Assume that Old-Tyme Pharmacy prices at a 33% markup on retail. A drug with a $5.00 ingredient cost would be sold for $7.46. The pharmacy would receive a dollar margin of $2.46 on the prescription. This is, in all likelihood, below the pharmacy's cost to dispense. As a result, the pharmacy loses money on this prescription. A drug with an $80.00 ingredient cost would be sold for $119.40. The pharmacy would receive a $39.40 margin, which is well above its cost to dispense plus a reasonable profit. Overall, the pharmacy's prescription profits are reasonable. But, the patient who must pay $39.40 over cost for the expensive prescription is probably going to be upset to the point that he or she may go elsewhere. The patient with the low price on the inexpensive drug, on the other hand, is unlikely to even notice that his prescription has been sold for an unusually low price. Thus, use of an unmodified markup system may result in a poor price image and loss of business.

## The Professional Fee Method

The professional fee method is frequently used to calculate prescription prices. Almost all third-party prescription programs use this method to reimburse pharmacies for prescriptions. The professional fee is a set dollar amount that is added to ingredient cost to determine the prescription price. It should be set at a level sufficient to cover the pharmacy's cost to dispense and net income. The fee is the same regardless of the cost of the drug dispensed. If, for example, the ingredient cost of a drug were $5.00 and the fee were $6.25, the prescription price would be $11.25. If the ingredient cost were $80.00, the price would be $86.25. Thus, the professional fee method avoids the markup system's disadvantage of subsidizing low-cost products with high-cost ones.

The professional fee system also calls attention to the service and professional aspects of pharmacy. The pharmacist performs the same professional functions on each prescription dispensed regardless of the cost of the drug. Whether it is an inexpensive or an expensive product, the pharmacist must go through the same process of selecting an appropriate product, packaging and labeling it correctly, counseling the patient, and checking for drug interactions. Because the amount of effort and expertise are the same for each prescription, the amount charged for effort and expertise should be the same. In the professional fee system, this is recognized by adding a set amount to the cost of each product. The markup system, on the other hand, emphasizes the importance of the product by basing the price and dollar margin on ingredient cost.

A disadvantage of the professional fee system is that it produces low gross margin percentages on expensive products. As the cost of prescription products rises, the pharmacy's gross margin percent declines. A related disadvantage is that the professional fee disregards the costs of carrying inventory. It costs the pharmacy more to invest in and carry expensive drugs. Consequently, the pharmacy requires a higher dollar margin on these items. The professional fee system—by adding the same dollar margin to all drugs—does not allow for this.

## The Sliding Scale Method

The markup method subsidizes low-cost drugs with expensive ones. The professional fee method disregards the higher inventory carrying costs associated with more expensive products. The sliding scale method overcomes both disadvantages by using *variable* markup percentages or professional fees to calculate prescription prices.

If a markup is used, the size of the percentage markup decreases as drug cost increases. A larger markup is added to the cost of cheaper drugs and a smaller markup is added to the cost of more expensive products. Thus, the amount by which expensive drugs subsidize cheaper ones is minimized and the effect of charging higher prices for expensive drugs is moderated.

If the professional fee method is used, a smaller fee is added to cheaper products and a larger fee to more expensive ones. This recognizes the higher inventory costs of carrying expensive drugs by providing the pharmacy with additional compensation for more expensive products.

A sliding scale system may also employ both a percentage markup and a professional fee. In such combination systems, either the fee or the markup or both may be varied. With any type of sliding scale the intent is the same—to trade off the conflicting demands of providing for inventory carrying costs with the necessity of offering reasonable prices on very expensive products. Because a sliding scale is the best method of optimizing pricing to meet these two demands, it is the system that most pharmacies use.

## SPECIAL CONSIDERATIONS IN PRICING SERVICES

In general, the manager considers the same factors in determining a price strategy for services as for products. However, once an overall pricing strategy has been selected, several different methods are available for presenting prices to buyers of pharmaceutical services.

Many pharmacists bill for their services based on *time and expenses*. The pharmacist's charge is based directly on the time it takes to provide the service plus the costs of any out-of-pocket expenses incurred. Typically, the number of hours required to provide the service is multiplied by some factor that is large enough to cover the pharmacy's salary costs and overhead and yield a reasonable profit. For example, a consultant pharmacist might charge a long-term care facility for doing drug regimen reviews for its patients on the basis of the number of hours he or she spent conducting the reviews plus the number of miles he or she had to drive to reach the facility. The charge might be presented, for example, as $100 per hour spent reviewing charts plus $0.40 per mile driven.

A special case of the time and expenses method is the *resource-based relative value scale (RBRVS)*. In general, the RBRVS method bases the charges for a service on both the time required to provide the service and the intensity of effort required. The Peters Institute of Pharmaceutical Care at the University of Minnesota has proposed a RBRVS for pharmaceutical care services.[11] The Peters Institute RBRVS allows the pharmacist to charge the patient or a purchaser of pharmaceutical care services based on the level of drug-related needs of the patient. The pharmacist is able to bill at five different levels. The level of payment is dependent upon seven different variables: the pharmacist's workup, the pharmacist's assessment, the level of care planning and eval-uation, the nature (risk) of the presenting drug therapy problems, counseling and coordination of care, and the face-to-face time involved in the encounter. These vari-ables reflect the level of the patient's drug-related needs and, consequently, the time and intensity of pharmaceutical services required by the patient.

Another method of presenting or billing for services is to charge a fixed fee. A con-sultant pharmacist using this method might charge the long-term care facility a set monthly fee, say $500, for conducting drug regimen reviews on all patients at the facility.

In some situations, pharmacists might bill for services on a *contingency* basis. Using this method, the pharmacist's fee is based on a percentage of the savings that the phar-macist generates for the payer. For example, some third-party payers reimburse phar-macies a percentage of the savings they generate through generic substitution. The savings are calculated as the difference in price between the brand-name product pre-scribed and the generic product dispensed. The contingency method has also been suggested as a way of charging third-party payers for pharmaceutical care services. Essentially, the pharmacist's fees would be based on how much he or she saved the third-party payer in total medical payments. This assumes that the provision of phar-maceutical care will contribute to better patient health and will, consequently, lead to lower costs for physicians and hospitalization.

## CAPITATION

Pharmacies have traditionally been paid on a *fee-for-service* basis. With fee-for-service reimbursement the pharmacy receives a separate payment for every unit of product or service provided. For example, the pharmacy is paid a fee for each prescription dis-pensed. The more prescriptions it dispenses, the more it is paid.

Some third-party payers have experimented with replacing fee-for-service reim-bursement with *capitation.* Under the capitation method, patients enroll with a specific pharmacy (or group of pharmacies) and agree to get all of their pharmaceutical serv-ices and products from that pharmacy (or group). The pharmacy is paid a set and pre-determined monthly fee for each patient enrolled. The fee is the same regardless of how many, or how few, prescriptions the patient gets during the month. As an exam-ple, an HMO might pay a pharmacy $50 a month for each enrolled patient. Whether the patient received no prescriptions during the month or whether he or she received 12 different prescriptions, the fee paid to the pharmacy would be $50.

Third-party payers have adopted capitated reimbursement to help control costs. Fee-for-service reimbursement gives pharmacies an incentive to provide more services. The more services they provide, the more revenue they receive. Thus, pharmacies have an economic incentive to dispense prescriptions and provide services that may be of little use to patients. Capitation, on the other hand, gives pharmacies an incentive *not* to supply unnecessary products and services. Providing more products and services in a capitated system simply raises the pharmacy's costs and lowers its profits. The incen-tive in a capitated system is to keep patients well. Healthy patients, in the long run, use fewer services and lead to higher profits. In addition, capitation provides pharmacies with an incentive to provide lower-cost products and services whenever possible. Thus, capitated pharmacies have a strong economic incentive to use generic drugs, to call physicians to persuade them to use lower-cost therapeutic alternates, and to suggest OTC products to patients who might otherwise use prescription products.

Capitation provides a number of other advantages for the payer. It is simpler to administer because there is no need to process a bill and generate a payment each time a service is provided. It allows for simpler and more accurate budgeting because payments to pharmacies are based on the number of patients enrolled and not the volume of products and services patients use. Most importantly (from the third-party payer's perspective), it shifts the risk of overutilization from the payer to the pharmacy. If patients get more prescriptions and use more services than anticipated, the payer is not responsible for additional payments. The pharmacy, rather than the payer, suffers financially when there is overutilization.

Individual pharmacies seldom take capitation contracts because of the risk of overutilization. An individual pharmacy is not likely to serve large numbers of patients from any one payer. Consequently, a single pharmacy is not able to spread the risk of overutilization over a large group of patients. Large chain pharmacies, such as Rite Aid or Walgreens, may accept capitated reimbursement. They can spread the risk of overutilization over the thousands of patients they serve. However, even large pharmacy organizations may not be willing to assume the total risk of a fully capitated contract. They are more likely to participate in *shared risk* arrangements. In shared risk contracts, as in capitation, the payer pays the provider a set fee per patient per month. However, in a shared risk contract, the payer and pharmacy agree to share the risk of overutilization and the rewards of controlling utilization. If the costs of caring for the patient exceed the fee, the pharmacy and payer each pay a part of the extra cost. If the patient's costs are less than the fee, the pharmacy and payer share the savings.

## SUMMARY

Pricing is an important managerial function. Proper pricing meets the dual objectives of providing prices that consumers will be willing to pay and profits the pharmacy needs to remain in business. The proper price for a pharmaceutical product or service is based on a number of cost and noncost considerations. However the major consideration in setting prices should be the perceived value of the product or service to the consumer.

### References

1. IMS Health Inc. DDD annual class-of-trade analysis 2003. Plymouth Meeting, PA: IMS Health Inc., 2004.
2. Zgarrick DP. Evaluation of cognitive services in a community pharmacy. AACP/Glaxo Management Resources Project, June 1, 1995.
3. Office of the Inspector General. Medicaid Pharmacy—Additional Analyses of the Actual Acquisition Cost of Prescription Drug Products (A-06-02-00041). Washington, DC: Department of Health and Human Services, 2002.
4. Kreling DH, Mott DA, Weiderholt JB. Prescription drug trends: a chartbook update. From Kaiser Family Foundation Website, http://www.kff.org/rxdrugs/upload/13796_1.pdf. Accessed December 23, 2004.
5. Dolan RJ. How do you know when the price is right? Harvard Bus Rev 1995;73: 174–183.
6. Nagle TT, Holden RK. The Strategy and Tactics of Pricing: A Guide to Profitable Decision Making. 3rd Ed. Upper Saddle River, NJ: Prentice Hall, 2002.
7. Simon H. Pricing opportunities—and how to exploit them. Sloan Manage Rev 1992;55-65.

8. Zeithaml VA, Bitner MJ. Pricing of services. In: Services Marketing. New York: McGraw-Hill, 1996:482–515.
9. Nelson AA Jr. Prescription pricing I: concepts and systems. Pharmacy Manage 1980;152:17
10. Zelnio RN, Nelson AA Jr. Prescription pricing II: computational methods. Pharmacy Manage 1980;152:57
11. Cipolle RJ, Strand LM, Morley PC. A reimbursement system for pharmaceutical care. In: Pharmaceutical Care Practice. New York: McGraw Hill, 1998:267–296.

### Suggested Readings

Carroll NV. Estimating a reasonable reimbursement rate for community pharmacies in third-party prescription programs. Managed Care Interface 1999;12(2):73–80.
Carroll NV. Pricing pharmacist services. In: Marketing for Pharmacists. Washington, DC: American Pharmaceutical Association, 2003.
Christensen DB, Fassett WE. Understanding capitation and pharmaceutical care. J Am Pharm Assoc 1996;NS36:374.
Gagnon JP, ed. Cost Accounting for Pharmaceutical Services, DHEW Publication No. (PHS) 80-3215. Hyattsville, MD: U.S. Department of Health, Education and Welfare, 1980.
Herman CH, Zabloski EJ. An assessment of prescription dispensing costs and related factors. Med Care Rev 1978;35:835.
Kotler P, Bloom PN. Setting fees. In: Marketing Professional Services. Englewood Cliffs, NJ: Prentice-Hall, 1984.
Tellis GJ. Beyond the many faces of price: an integration of pricing strategies. J Mktg 1986;50:146.
West DS, ed. 2004 NCPA-Pfizer Digest. Alexandria, VA: NCPA, 2004.

## QUESTIONS

1. The component of the prescription price that covers the cost of the drug to the pharmacy is called the:
   a. ingredient cost
   b. cost to dispense
   c. net cost
2. The component of the prescription price that covers the expense incurred in filling a prescription is called the:
   a. ingredient cost
   b. cost to dispense
   c. net cost
3. Costs that are shared by all departments in a pharmacy, such as rent and managers' wages, are known as:
   a. direct costs
   b. indirect costs
   c. fixed costs
   d. variable costs
4. Which of the following would be considered a direct cost to the prescription department?
   a. Housekeeping expense
   b. Prescription vials

    **c.** Manager's salary

    **d.** Depreciation

    **e.** All of the above

**5.** Wahoo Pharmacy's lease stipulates that the monthly rent expense is calculated as 1% of monthly sales. In calculating the pharmacy's cost to dispense, rent should be:

    **a.** charged as a direct cost to the prescription department

    **b.** allocated to the prescription department based on the space ratio

    **c.** allocated to the prescription department based on the sales ratio

**6.** The manager of Wahoo Pharmacy classifies the pharmacy's utility costs as a fixed expense. In calculating the pharmacy's cost to dispense, the utility expense should be:

    **a.** charged as a direct cost to the prescription department

    **b.** allocated to the prescription department based on the space ratio

    **c.** allocated to the prescription department based on the sales ratio

**7.** In calculating the cost of a session of asthma-related counseling and monitoring, the costs of prescription vials and containers:

    **a.** should be charged as a direct expense of the counseling and monitoring service

    **b.** should be allocated to the counseling and monitoring service based on the ratio of counseling and monitoring revenues to total sales

    **c.** should *not* be considered as a cost of the counseling and monitoring service

**8.** The data for calculation of service costs should come from:

    **a.** an income statement for the most recent year

    **b.** an income statement that averages the pharmacy's performance over the most recent 5-year period

    **c.** a pro forma income statement

**9.** A hospital pharmacist works 45 hours per week. Of this time, 15 hours are spent providing patient counseling, education, and monitoring in a hypertension clinic and 30 hours are spent in dispensing-related duties. How much of the pharmacist's salary should be allocated as a cost of the hypertension clinic?

    **a.** 15/45 of her salary

    **b.** 30/45 of her salary

    **c.** all of her salary

**10.** The manager of Wahoo Pharmacy calculates the pharmacy's cost of providing a session in the Diabetic Care Center to be $15.00. His calculation is based on an estimated volume of 2,000 sessions per year. If the Diabetic Care Center provides only 1,500 sessions and each is priced at $15.00, which of the following is true?

    **a.** The Diabetic Care Center will break even.

    **b.** The Diabetic Care Center will lose money.

**11.** When setting prescription prices, which of the following factors must a manager consider?

    **a.** Costs

    **b.** Competition

    **c.** The pharmacy's goals

    **d.** All of the above

    **e.** a and b only

**12.** Consumers are likely to know prescription prices for:

    **a.** most of the drugs dispensed by pharmacies

    **b.** many of the drugs dispensed by pharmacies

    **c.** a few of the drugs dispensed by pharmacies

13. To maintain a viable prescription business, pharmacies must maintain:
    a. low prescription prices on all items
    b. low prescription prices on most items
    c. low prescription prices on a select, few items
14. In setting a pricing strategy, managers should keep in mind that consumers' selection of pharmacies is based *primarily* upon:
    a. the pharmacy's actual prescription prices
    b. their perceptions of the pharmacy's prices
    c. the pharmacy's image
    d. a and c only
    e. b and c only
15. A lower price is most likely to result in lower demand for which of the following?
    a. A diabetic education and monitoring service
    b. An over-the-counter drug
    c. A market-priced prescription product
16. Stores that use the prescription department as a loss leader:
    a. make normal profits on prescription sales
    b. make high profits on prescription sales
    c. make little or no profit on prescription sales
17. Pharmacists can teach asthma sufferers to monitor their condition and modify their therapy using peak flow meters. Patients who learn these skills experience considerably less anxiety about their health. This is an example of decreasing patients':
    a. monetary costs
    b. search costs
    c. psychic costs
18. Large consultant pharmacy operations frequently offer long-term care facilities very low prices on patient drug regimen reviews in order to gain the facilities' drug distribution business. This is an example of:
    a. loss leader pricing
    b. penetration pricing
    c. price skimming
19. Pharmacies that use the pricing strategy outlined in the text will make the largest profits on:
    a. staple prescription items
    b. premium prescription items
    c. market-priced prescription items
20. An advantage of the markup method of pricing is that:
    a. it maintains the gross margin in times of inflation
    b. it calls attention to the professional aspects of pharmacy
    c. it simplifies third-party participation decisions
    d. all of the above
    e. b and c only
21. A disadvantage of the professional fee method of pricing is that it:
    a. yields higher than competitive prices on inexpensive drug products
    b. yields higher than competitive prices on expensive drug products
    c. may lead to lowered gross margins in times of inflation
    d. a and c only
    e. b and c only
22. The sliding scale method of prescription pricing:
    a. may be used as a variation of the markup method
    b. may be used as a variation of the professional fee method

    c. overcomes some of the disadvantages of the professional fee method

    d. all of the above

23. The average wholesale price is:

    a. also known as AWP

    b. a cost figure set by the manufacturer of the product

    c. the average price at which pharmacies can purchase the product from a wholesaler

    d. all of the above

    e. a and b only

24. The actual acquisition cost is:

    a. the amount the pharmacy actually paid for a product

    b. easily determined by pharmacies and third-party payers

    c. usually less than AWP

    d. all of the above

    e. a and c only

25. When a resource-based relative value scale is used, the price of a service is based on:

    a. the time spent in providing the service

    b. the intensity of physical and mental effort required

    c. the savings generated by the service

    d. all of the above

    e. a and b only

26. Allied Consultants charges long-term care facilities $30 per hour for conducting drug regimen reviews. This method of pricing is called:

    a. time and expenses

    b. fixed fee

    c. contingency based

27. In the capitation method of pricing, a pharmacy is reimbursed a fixed fee:

    a. for each patient enrolled with the pharmacy

    b. for each prescription dispensed

28. The capitation method of pricing shifts the risk of overutilization to the:

    a. patient

    b. pharmacy

    c. payer

29. Capitation reimbursement provides pharmacies with an economic incentive to:

    a. dispense more prescriptions

    b. use lower-priced generic products rather than their brand-name equivalents

    c. keep patients healthy

    d. all of the above

    e. a and b only

## PROBLEMS

1. A pro forma income statement for Winter's Pharmacy is shown. Using this statement and the following data, calculate Winter's Pharmacy's cost to dispense a prescription. The manager of the pharmacy works 60 hours per week; of this time, he works 50 hours in prescription-related duties. A relief pharmacist works 15 hours per week—all in prescription—related duties. Clerks work an average of 80 hours per week; half of this time is devoted to prescription-related duties. The

selling space in the pharmacy occupies 2,000 square feet; the prescription department occupies 500 of these. The manager anticipates that the pharmacy will dispense 22,500 prescriptions in the coming year. Only delivery and prescription supplies are direct costs. Other expenses are categorized as shown on the income statement.

2. The cost to dispense is sensitive to the volume of prescriptions that the pharmacy dispenses. What would Winter's Pharmacy's cost to dispense be if it only dispensed 18,000 prescriptions in the coming year? What if it dispensed 30,000? Assume that all operating expenses except prescription supplies, delivery, and other expenses are fixed. Assume for the three variable expenses that prescription supplies cost $0.16 per prescription, delivery costs $0.14 per prescription, and other expenses costs $0.20 per prescription.

3. Agee's Pharmacy offers a monitoring and counseling service for patients on drug therapy for high cholesterol. The pharmacist counsels patients about their disease, the consequences of not keeping it under control, and the importance of diet and compliance with drug therapy in controlling cholesterol. In addition, he measures, records, and monitors patients' blood cholesterol levels. The pharmacist currently counsels about five patients a day. Each session takes about 15 minutes. The cholesterol service is offered for 4 hours a day for 6 days a week. The pharmacy currently provides 1,500 counseling sessions per year. The annual budget for the service is shown below:

| | |
|---|---:|
| Supply costs: $2.35 per visit | $ 3,525 |
| Analyzer costs (annual lease) | 950 |
| Pharmacist salary | |
| ($20 per hour × 4 hours per day × 300 days) | 24,000 |
| Total annual budget | $28,475 |

    a. Given this information, what is the average cost of a counseling session?

    b. Assume that the pharmacist's salary and the analyzer lease are fixed costs and supplies are variable costs. What would it cost the pharmacy to provide one additional counseling session?

    c. What would the average cost of a session be if volume increased to 3,000 sessions a year?

    d. What would the average cost be if volume decreased to 500 sessions a year?

4. Ziglar Pharmacy has a calculated cost to dispense of $4.00, $250,000 in prescription department assets, and requires a 10% return on assets. The pharmacy is estimated to have an average ingredient cost of $10.00 and to dispense 25,000 prescriptions in the coming year. What should Ziglar's average prescription price be? What is the average percent markup on retail that this would yield? If the pharmacy required a 15% return on assets, what would its average prescription price and markup on retail be?

5. Given are five combinations of drug acquisition costs and markups. Calculate the prescription price that should be charged for each combination assuming, first, that the price is calculated as markup on retail price and, second, that price is calculated as markup on cost.

    a. $7.50 and 40%

    b. $2.00 and 45%

    c. $28.50 and 30%

    d. $69.00 and 35%

    e. $25.00 and 38%

**Pro Forma**
**Income Statement**
**Winter's Pharmacy**

| | |
|---|---:|
| Net sales | |
| Prescription | $ 562,500 |
| Nonprescription | 60,000 |
| Total sales | 622,500 |
| Cost of goods sold | 448,200 |
| Gross margin | 174,300 |
| Expenses | |
| Salary | |
| Manager's salary | 50,000 |
| Relief pharmacist salary | 23,400 |
| Clerks' salaries | 41,600 |
| Housing-related indirect | |
| Rent | 11,400 |
| Utilities | 3,900 |
| Repairs | 1,200 |
| Other indirect | |
| Accounting and legal | 1,200 |
| Taxes and licenses | 8,500 |
| Insurance | 4,200 |
| Interest | 2,000 |
| Depreciation | 6,200 |
| Telephone | 1,100 |
| Advertising | 2,500 |
| Other | 5,500 |
| Direct prescription | |
| Department expenses | |
| Delivery | 3,000 |
| Prescription supplies | 3,500 |
| Total expenses | 169,200 |
| Net income | $5,100 |

# Differential Analysis

After reading this chapter, the student should be able to:

1. Define and identify differential costs, sunk costs, and opportunity costs,
2. Conduct a differential analysis to assist in managerial decision making, and
3. Discuss the importance of and give examples of nonquantitative factors that should be considered in making decisions based on differential analysis.

In their capacity as managers, pharmacists must frequently make decisions that involve choices among several alternative courses of action. Community pharmacists face decisions about whether to dispense prescriptions to patients covered by insurance or Medicaid programs, which pay less than the pharmacy's normal prices. Hospital and health maintenance organization (HMO) pharmacists must decide about the advisability of expanding or eliminating services. All pharmacists face decisions about making the best use of existing resources. For example, should floor space be used to sell gift items or sick room supplies, or should it be used to house a patient counseling and education area? Or, should pharmacists' time be used to fill orders or to supervise technicians or to provide pharmaceutical care services? This chapter explains the use of *differential analysis* to evaluate the financial effects of alternatives. The focus of differential analysis is on those costs and revenues that *differ* among alternatives.

For example, Buckeye Pharmacy is considering whether to participate in a third-party prescription plan. The particular plan with which Buckeye Pharmacy is negotiating offers to reimburse the pharmacy the ingredient cost of the drug plus a $2.50 fee for each prescription dispensed. If Buckeye participates, it will gain new patients (who are covered by the plan) and additional prescription volume. The alternatives available to Buckeye's manager are (a) to participate in the plan and (b) to not participate.

One approach to the problem would be to consider the *full costs* of dispensing a prescription. The manager would calculate the pharmacy's cost to dispense a prescription. If this figure were less than $2.50, it would be profitable for the pharmacy to participate.

Full costs include *all* costs of dispensing a prescription. They include both the costs directly incurred in dispensing the prescription, such as pharmacists' salaries and prescription containers, and those costs incurred indirectly, such as rent, utilities, and manager's salary. If the amount that the plan will pay is greater than the pharmacy's full costs, it will be profitable to participate in the plan.

But what if the pharmacy's cost of dispensing was more than $2.50? Would this mean that it would be unprofitable for Buckeye Pharmacy to participate in the program? Not necessarily. Whether profits would increase would depend on the *differential costs* of dispensing prescriptions for the program and the *differential revenues* to be gained from the program. If differential costs were less than $2.50 per prescription and the pharmacy gained new patients and additional prescription volume as a result of participating, then Buckeye Pharmacy might find it profitable to participate.

## TYPES OF COSTS

In discussing differential analysis, several different types of costs need to be identified. These include differential costs, sunk costs, and opportunity costs.

### Differential Costs

Differential costs are those costs that differ among the alternative courses of action. Costs that are the same under either alternative are not differential. In Buckeye Pharmacy's case, the differential costs of participation would be the *additional* costs that the pharmacy incurred in dispensing prescriptions to patients covered by the third-party plan. Which costs are differential and which are not depends on the specific situation.

Some costs of dispensing prescriptions for the third-party program would be differential in any situation. The prescription department's variable costs, such as the costs of prescription containers and labels, would be differential costs. If the pharmacy dispensed additional prescriptions (which it would not otherwise have dispensed) as a result of participating in the third-party plan, variable costs would be higher than if it did not participate.

Variable costs are not always differential costs. If an alternative involves a change in sales, then variable costs will be differential costs. However, the alternatives associated with some decisions, such as whether to hire a clerk or to buy a computer program to process accounts receivable, do not involve increases in sales. For these, variable costs may not be differential costs.

In our example, Buckeye Pharmacy's fixed costs may not be differential. Whether they are depends on whether participation in the program would move the pharmacy above its relevant range of sales. As discussed in the chapter on break-even analysis, the relevant range of sales is that range of sales volume in which fixed costs remain fixed. If participation in a third-party prescription plan increased the pharmacy's prescription volume to such an extent that it moved the pharmacy above its relevant range, then certain of its fixed costs would increase. In this case, the increases in fixed costs would be differential costs.

For example, first assume that Buckeye Pharmacy had excess capacity. That is, it could handle the additional prescription volume from participating in the plan without adding additional staff and assets. In this case, fixed costs would not be differential costs because they would be the same whether the pharmacy participated in the plan or not.

But what if the increase in prescription volume were large enough to require the pharmacy to hire additional pharmacists or technicians? In this case, the pharmacy would have moved above its relevant range of sales and, consequently, some of its fixed costs—in this case, salary expenses—would have increased. In this situation, the costs of the additional staff would be differential costs. They would be differential because they would increase if the pharmacy participated in the plan.

In each case and for each situation, the manager must carefully consider which costs change and which do not. Only those that change for the alternative under consideration are differential costs.

## Sunk Costs

Sunk costs refer to costs that have already been incurred. Because they have already been incurred, sunk costs are not relevant to a differential analysis.

To illustrate, assume that the Bulldog Hospital Pharmacy has recently paid an annual fee of $1,000 to join a buying group. Membership in the buying group will allow Bulldog to purchase prescription drugs for about 10% less than it otherwise could. On annual purchases of $2,500,000, this will save Bulldog Pharmacy about $250,000 a year.

After joining the first group, Bulldog discovers another group that could save it 15% a year. It will cost $5,000 to join this group. In making the decision as to whether to join the second group, which costs are differential and which are not?

The $5,000 fee for joining the second buying group is a differential cost. If Bulldog joins the second group, it will incur this cost; if it does not join, it will not incur it. The $1,000 fee that Bulldog paid to join the original buying group is *not* a differential cost. The cost of the initial membership already has been incurred. It is a cost whether Bulldog joins the second group or whether it does not. Consequently, it is irrelevant to the analysis. The initial $1,000 fee is an example of a sunk cost.

## Opportunity Costs

Many decisions involve whether to put valuable resources such as capital, assets, or personnel to some particular use. Many times the resources could be put to other uses. The opportunity cost associated with a given use of a resource is the amount that could have been earned by putting the resource to the next best use.

For example, Gamecock Pharmacy uses a portion of its floor space for a patient education and counseling room. The gross profit it earns from patient education and counseling amounts to $5,000 per year. It could have used the space to display a line of gift items. If the gift items would yield a gross profit of $3,000 per year, then the opportunity cost associated with the patient education and counseling room is equal to $3,000 per year. This simply reflects that by choosing to use the space for patient counseling and education, the pharmacy gave up the opportunity to earn $3,000 on gift items.

## GENERAL FRAMEWORK FOR DIFFERENTIAL ANALYSIS

A differential analysis consists of four steps: identifying differential revenues, identifying differential costs, calculating the contribution margin, and considering nonquantitative factors.

First, the manager must identify the differential revenues associated with the alternative. The differential revenues are those that differ among the alternatives. For example, the differential revenues associated with Buckeye Pharmacy's participation in the third-party prescription plan would consist of the $2.50 per prescription fee multiplied by the number of prescriptions dispensed to patients covered by the plan. (This assumes that no patient who was covered by the plan would have a prescription dispensed at Buckeye unless Buckeye participated in the plan.)

Next, differential costs must be identified. These include only those costs that will change if the alternative is selected.

The contribution margin is the alternative's contribution to fixed costs and profits. It is calculated by subtracting the differential costs associated with the alternative from the differential revenues. If the contribution margin is positive—that is, if differential revenues exceed differential costs—then selection of the alternative will result in increased profit.

Finally, the manager must consider *nonquantitative factors* that may affect the decision. There are factors that are important to the decision, but that are not easily quantified. Although these cannot be included explicitly in the financial analysis, they should be considered in making the final decision.

For example, in deciding whether to participate in a third-party plan, the manager might consider the effect of participation on the level of service and counseling the pharmacy could provide. He or she might also want to consider whether the pharmacy wants to set a precedent of charging different prices to different groups of customers. Although such factors cannot be included in the calculations, they may be as important or more important than the quantitative factors.

## EXAMPLE OF DIFFERENTIAL ANALYSIS: PARTICIPATION IN A THIRD-PARTY PRESCRIPTION PROGRAM

Use of an example may clarify the procedure. As stated earlier, Buckeye Pharmacy must decide whether to participate in a third-party prescription program. The program will pay $2.50 plus ingredient cost for each prescription dispensed. Buckeye currently receives an average gross margin of $7.00 on private pay prescriptions.

### Situation #1—A Small Increase in Volume

The pharmacy could find itself in several different situations with regard to the participation decision. In the first situation we will analyze, assume that the manager anticipates that participation will increase prescription volume by about 600 prescriptions per year.

## Identification of Differential Revenues

The differential revenues (DRs) associated with participation are calculated as the number of prescriptions dispensed to plan members for the year multiplied by the $2.50 per prescription fee. Thus:

$$DR = 600 \text{ prescriptions per year} \times \$2.50 \text{ per prescription}$$
$$= \$1,500 \text{ per year}$$

(For simplicity, we will assume that the amount the plan pays for product cost is the same as the pharmacy's actual acquisition cost. This assumption allows us to ignore product cost for both differential revenues and differential costs.)

## Identification of Differential Costs

Participation in the plan will increase Buckeye Pharmacy's prescription volume by only 600 prescriptions per year. This is a small change. Consequently, it will not be necessary to hire additional pharmacists or technicians or to buy additional assets to handle the increased volume. The only costs that increase are the variable costs of dispensing a prescription. The manager estimates that these costs amount to about $0.50 per prescription. (The cost of the drugs dispensed is also a variable cost and would increase if the pharmacy participated in the plan. However, because we did not consider the cost of the product in calculating differential revenues, it is not necessary to include them as part of differential costs.) So, total differential costs (DCs) are calculated as:

$$DC = 600 \text{ prescriptions per year} \times \$0.50 \text{ per prescription}$$
$$= \$300 \text{ per year}$$

## Calculation of the Contribution Margin

The contribution margin (CM) for participation would be:

$$CM = DR - DC$$
$$= \$1,500 - \$300$$
$$= \$1,200$$

This indicates that Buckeye Pharmacy's profit would increase by $1,200 per year if it participated in the plan. This is true even though the full costs of dispensing a prescription may be more than $2.50. The reason for the discrepancy is that many of the costs included in the full cost—such as salary, rent, and utilities—would not increase if the pharmacy participated in the plan.

## Situation #2—A Large Increase in Volume

The differential costs of an alternative depend on the specific circumstances of the alternative. To demonstrate this, we will continue the Buckeye Pharmacy example using a different set of circumstances. As in the previous example, the third-party program will pay the pharmacy product cost plus $2.50 per prescription. But, now assume that participation will increase Buckeye's prescription volume by 600 prescriptions *per month* and that Buckeye Pharmacy is currently dispensing as many prescriptions as its staff can handle.

In this case, the differential revenue would be calculated as:

DR = 600 prescriptions per month $\times$ \$2.50 per prescription $\times$ 12 months per year
   = \$18,000

The differential costs in this situation, as in the previous one, include the increased variable costs of \$0.50 per prescription. In addition, the manager judges that the pharmacy cannot dispense the additional prescriptions generated by the plan unless another technician is hired. The technician will cost the pharmacy \$15,000 per year. So, the differential costs will be:

DC = \$15,000 + (600 prescriptions per month $\times$ \$0.50 per prescription)
   $\times$ 12 months per year
   = \$18,600

The contribution margin of participating in the plan will be \$18,000 minus \$18,600 or \$600. Thus, in this case, because fixed costs increased, Buckeye Pharmacy would decrease its profit if it participated in the plan.

## Situation #3—Converting Prescriptions

The preceding situations assumed that all of the prescriptions that Buckeye Pharmacy dispensed to patients covered by the plan would represent additional prescription volume. That is, Buckeye would dispense these prescriptions if it participated in the third-party plan, and it would not dispense them if it did not participate. This could happen if the insurance company had set up a restricted network of pharmacies and most of Buckeye's competitors were not part of the network. Volume would increase as patients switched their prescriptions from the other pharmacies (that did not accept these patients' insurance) to Buckeye.

Buckeye could find itself in a less happy situation. The new third-party plan may provide coverage for some of Buckeye's current private pay patients. This would happen if, for example, a large employer began offering insurance coverage for prescription drugs to its employees. Before the plan was implemented, prescriptions dispensed to these employees would have been paid for by the employees (private pay). After implementation, prescriptions dispensed to the employees would be paid for by a third party (the insurance company). In this situation, Buckeye Pharmacy will lose these patients if it does not participate in the new plan. The incentive of getting prescriptions at reduced cost will be sufficient to induce patients to take their prescriptions to a participating pharmacy. If Buckeye does participate, it will receive lower reimbursement on each prescription dispensed to current patients covered by the plan.

Assume that 500 prescriptions per year will be affected. That is, if Buckeye Pharmacy chooses not to participate, it will lose 500 prescriptions because patients will take them to a pharmacy that participates in the third-party plan. If Buckeye participates, it will keep these patients and their 500 prescriptions but will receive third-party, rather than private pay, reimbursement for them.

## Loss from Not Participating

If Buckeye Pharmacy does not participate, it will lose 500 prescriptions a year. The average gross margin received on each of these prescriptions is $7.00. So,

$$DR = 500 \text{ prescriptions lost} \times \$7.00 \text{ per prescription}$$
$$= (\$3,500)$$

Buckeye's costs will decrease as a result of dispensing fewer prescriptions. The differential costs of $0.50 per prescription will not be incurred for the prescriptions that are lost. Therefore,

$$DC = 500 \text{ prescriptions lost} \times \$0.50 \text{ per prescription}$$
$$= (\$250)$$

Buckeye's net income will decrease by the difference in differential revenues and costs—$3,250—if it does not participate in the plan.

## Loss from Participating

If Buckeye Pharmacy chooses to participate, its profit will also decline. It will do so because prescriptions dispensed to current patients covered by the program will be reimbursed at the lower third-party rate rather than at the higher private pay rate.

Buckeye Pharmacy receives a gross margin averaging $7.00 on each private pay prescription dispensed. The third-party program will pay a fee of $2.50 per prescription. Thus, Buckeye Pharmacy's revenue would decline by $7.00 − $2.50 = $4.50 for each prescription dispensed to a program member who was previously a private pay patient. So, the differential revenue associated with participating is:

$$DR = (\$4.50) \text{ per prescription} \times 500 \text{ prescriptions}$$
$$= (\$2,250)$$

Buckeye's costs would not change because it dispenses the same number of prescriptions. Consequently, Buckeye Pharmacy's net income would decrease by ($2,250) if it participated in the program. In this situation, Buckeye Pharmacy is financially better off—because it loses less money—if it participates.

## COMMON DIFFERENTIAL ANALYSIS SITUATIONS IN PHARMACY

Pharmacist managers commonly are faced with several situations that can be addressed with differential analysis. These include decisions as to whether to participate in third-party prescription programs, add a new service, or eliminate a product line or service. Each of these will be discussed and illustrated.

### Participation in a Third-Party Prescription Program

This situation has been illustrated with the Buckeye Pharmacy example. The general situation is one in which a third-party payer—such as an insurance company or state

Medicaid agency—offers the pharmacy the opportunity to dispense prescriptions to its members. The third party will reimburse the pharmacy less than it normally charges for prescriptions. The pharmacy's incentive to participate comes from the promise of increased prescription volume.

As demonstrated in the first example, participation in these programs can, in some situations, increase profit even though the amount paid by the third party is less than the pharmacy's full costs. Profit will increase as long as the differential revenues from the plan exceed the differential costs. This occurs because participation will make some contribution to covering the pharmacy's fixed costs and profit. However, pharmacists should not agree to participate solely on the basis of increased profits. Other factors must be considered.

First, the pharmacist must be sure that giving a lower price to one plan will not interfere with other plans or customers who pay higher prices. For example, the Gamecock Pharmacy currently participates in a plan sponsored by the Palmetto Insurance Company. This plan pays product cost plus a $4.00 fee. Gamecock is negotiating with a similar plan sponsored by Blue Cross of Carolina. This plan will pay only $2.50 plus product cost. If Gamecock Pharmacy agrees to participate in the Blue Cross plan, which pays a $2.50 fee, and the Palmetto Insurance Company becomes aware of it, then Palmetto may ask for a reduction in its fee. If it cannot get a reduction immediately, then it certainly will negotiate for the lower fee as soon as its current contract with the pharmacy expires.

In many states, the Medicaid contract stipulates that any pharmacy participating in the Medicaid program must charge Medicaid no more than its lowest price to any customer. So, if a pharmacy agrees to participate in a plan that provides a lower reimbursement than does Medicaid, the pharmacy is obligated to also lower its charges to Medicaid.

Second, the pharmacy manager must be sure that the total proportion of the pharmacy's prescription volume priced lower than full cost does not become too large. If it does, the pharmacy will not be able to cover its fixed costs or generate a profit.

For most pharmacies, the amount of prescriptions dispensed for any single third-party program will be small in relation to total prescription volume. Consequently, participation in any single plan is not likely to affect the pharmacy's fixed costs. And, as a result, the pharmacy is likely to find that its profit will increase if it participates in the plan. This will be true even if the reimbursement paid by the plan is lower than the pharmacy's full cost of dispensing a prescription. Again, this is because participation will result in some contribution to fixed costs and profits.

The problem arises when a pharmacy deals with dozens of different plans. Although no single plan accounts for a large proportion of the pharmacy's volume, cumulatively all programs together may represent the majority of its volume. Although each plan considered separately has no effect on fixed costs, all plans considered together have a dramatic effect. In this situation, the pharmacy must begin to recoup its full costs of dispensing from the majority of the plans, or it must drastically increase its prices to customers not covered by any plan, or it must lower its costs, or it will not make a profit.

This puts the pharmacy in a difficult situation. Participation in any one of the plans, even at lower reimbursement, results in increased profit. But participation in several plans, each of which individually looks profitable based on differential analysis, places the pharmacy in a losing situation. The only obvious safeguard is for the manager to carefully select the plans with which he or she deals. Participation in too many plans that pay less than full cost will lead to bankruptcy.

A related difficulty involves the time span of the decision. At a given point in time, the pharmacy may have excess capacity. Because of this, it will be able to increase its profit by participating in a third-party program that pays less than full cost. But, many pharmacies will have excess capacity only in the short run. Over longer periods, say 2 or 3 years, as the pharmacy's normal prescription volume increases, the excess capacity that once existed is used up. As this occurs, participation becomes less and less profitable. At some point, when there is no longer excess capacity, it will be profitable to participate only if the third-party program reimbursement covers full cost.

Third, participation in third-party prescription plans may affect the quality of service that the pharmacy offers its patients. When a pharmacy has a low to moderate prescription volume, there may be plenty of time for patient consultation and personalized service. Patients may become accustomed to such service. In fact, this may be a primary reason that they patronize the pharmacy. If participation in third-party plans increases the pharmacy's prescription volume, and if the pharmacy's staffing does not increase, pharmacists may no longer have time to counsel patients and provide the personalized service to which patients have become accustomed. This may result in a loss of more profitable, private pay prescriptions.

Finally, the manager must consider the opportunity costs of participating in the program. A pharmacy has a limited amount of time and resources available. By choosing to invest the pharmacy's time and resources in participation in a particular third-party plan, the pharmacy loses that amount of time and resources to other opportunities. A careful consideration of all opportunities available to the pharmacy may indicate that some of the alternatives, such as providing dispensing or consulting services to long-term care facilities, adding durable medical equipment, or increasing involvement in prescription compounding, are more profitable than participation in a given third-party prescription program. This becomes more likely as participation in third-party plans becomes less profitable.

Basing prices on differential costs is dangerous and should be done cautiously. Reimbursement in the community pharmacy market provides an example of the dangers of differential cost based pricing. In the 1970s, only about 25% of all prescriptions were reimbursed by third parties. The other 75% of prescriptions were paid for by the patients themselves or by their families. In this environment, most community pharmacies could increase their profits by participating in third-party programs that reimbursed them at less than their full costs. Over time, however, the situation has changed dramatically. In the current environment, upwards of 80% of prescriptions are paid for by third parties. And, reimbursement rates for prescriptions have actually decreased since the 1970s. This has dramatically decreased profits in community pharmacies and has resulted in thousands of pharmacies going out of business.

## Dropping an Unprofitable Product or Service

Many organizations produce or sell more than one type of product or service. A community pharmacy carries prescription drugs, over-the-counter drugs, and other health and beauty aids. A hospital pharmacy may provide medication orders, IV solutions, and clinical services to inpatients; home IV solutions to home health care patients; and prescriptions to walk-in outpatients. A nursing home pharmacist may provide both prescription drugs and consulting services to long-term care facilities.

| Income Statement Tar Heel Hospital Outpatient Pharmacy | |
| --- | --- |
| Revenues | $ 300,000 |
| Cost of goods sold | 200,000 |
| Gross margin | 100,000 |
| Salaries | 55,000 |
| Other direct costs | 25,000 |
| Indirect costs | 30,000 |
| Net income | $(10,000) |

**FIGURE 10–1**   Income statement for Tar Heel Hospital outpatient pharmacy.

In some cases, one type of service or line of products may be unprofitable. That is, the revenues earned from providing the product or service may be less than the full costs of providing it. An example of this situation is shown in Figure 10-1. The figure provides an income statement for Tar Heel Hospital's outpatient pharmacy. The income statement, which is based on full costs, indicates that the pharmacy operated at a loss of $10,000 for the year. The hospital as a whole, as shown in Figure 10-2, realized a profit of $500,000. At first glance, it would appear logical to close the outpatient pharmacy. Presumably, this would increase the hospital's net income by $10,000—the amount of the outpatient pharmacy's loss. But this is not necessarily so. As in all differential cost problems, it depends on the specific circumstances.

## No Alternative Use for the Resources Employed

To determine whether the hospital would increase its profit by closing the pharmacy, we must first examine the pharmacy's income statement more closely. The pharmacy generates $300,000 of revenues annually. The costs of generating the revenues include $200,000 for cost of goods sold, $55,000 for pharmacist and technician salaries, and $25,000 in other direct costs to the pharmacy. The direct costs refer to costs that the hospital would not incur if the pharmacy were not operating. These include, for example,

| Income Statement Tar Heel Hospital | |
| --- | --- |
| Revenues | $5,000,000 |
| Expenses | 4,500,000 |
| Net income | $ 500,000 |

**FIGURE 10–2**   Income statement for Tar Heel Hospital.

| | |
|---|---|
| Differential revenue | $300,000 |
| Differential costs | |
| Cost of goods sold | 200,000 |
| Salaries | 55,000 |
| Other direct costs | 25,000 |
| Contribution margin | $ 20,000 |

**FIGURE 10–3** Differential analysis for keeping outpatient pharmacy open assuming there is no alternative use of space.

the containers and labels used in dispensing prescriptions, depreciation expense on pharmacy equipment, and utilities expense incurred by the pharmacy. All of these costs—cost of goods sold, salaries, and other direct costs—would be eliminated if the pharmacy were closed.

The pharmacy also incurred $30,000 of indirect costs. This is the pharmacy's share of expenses that were incurred by the hospital as a unit rather than by any particular department. They include depreciation on the building, janitorial and laundry expense, maintenance, and general hospital administration. Payment of these expenses is shared by all departments that generate revenue. The $30,000 of indirect costs allocated to the pharmacy would *not* be eliminated if the pharmacy were closed. The hospital would have no decrease in, for example, depreciation on the building or administrators' salaries if the pharmacy were closed. Other revenue-generating departments would be allocated a larger share of indirect costs if the pharmacy were closed. As a result, closing the pharmacy would not necessarily result in increased profits for the hospital. Whether it would depends on whether and what types of alternative uses exist for the resources employed by the pharmacy.

Assume that the only resource in question is the space occupied by the pharmacy. If the hospital has no alternative use for the space, then it is better off leaving the pharmacy open. This is shown by the differential analysis in Figure 10-3. The analysis indicates that the pharmacy contributes $20,000 to the hospital's indirect costs. If the pharmacy were closed, the hospital's profits would not increase $10,000. Rather, because of the loss of the pharmacy's contribution, profit would decrease by $20,000. This is demonstrated by the data in Figure 10-4.

| Income Statement Tar Heel Hospital | |
|---|---|
| Revenues | $4,700,000 |
| Expenses | 4,220,000 |
| Net income | $ 480,000 |

**FIGURE 10–4** Income statement for Tar Heel Hospital if outpatient pharmacy is closed and assuming no alternative use for space.

| Differential revenue | $300,000 |
|---|---|
| Differential costs | |
|    Cost of goods sold | 200,000 |
|    Salaries | 55,000 |
|    Other direct costs | 25,000 |
|    Rent expense | 24,000 |
| Contribution margin | $ (4,000) |

**FIGURE 10-5**  Differential analysis for keeping outpatient pharmacy open assuming there is an alternative use of space.

## Alternative Use for Resources

The situation would be different if the hospital did have an alternative use for the space occupied by the hospital pharmacy. Assume that the hospital currently rents space in another building for its outpatient arthritis clinic. Rent for this space costs the hospital $24,000 per year. If the outpatient pharmacy were closed, the hospital could move the arthritis clinic into the vacated space. This would allow the hospital to avoid the $24,000 of rent in the other building.

In this situation, the $24,000 of rent payment is an *opportunity cost* for the outpatient pharmacy. It is the amount the hospital could make on its best alternative use of the space now occupied by the pharmacy. Consequently, the $24,000 of rent is a differential cost of keeping the pharmacy open. If the pharmacy remains open, the hospital must pay $24,000 in rent for space for the arthritis clinic. If the pharmacy is closed, the arthritis clinic can use its space and avoid the rent expense.

Figure 10-5 shows the differential analysis for this situation. Because of the additional $24,000 cost, the pharmacy has a negative contribution margin. That is, it does not contribute to covering indirect costs. Consequently, the hospital would find it more profitable to close the pharmacy and move the arthritis clinic. The effect of this move is shown by the hospital income statement in Figure 10-6. The statement indicates that the hospital's net income would increase by $4,000 if it closed the pharmacy.

| Income Statement<br>Tar Heel Hospital | |
|---|---|
| Revenues | $4,700,000 |
| Expenses | 4,196,000 |
| Net income | $ 504,000 |

**FIGURE 10-6**  Income statement for Tar Heel Hospital if pharmacy were closed and assuming there is an alternative use of space.

## Consideration of Nonquantitative Factors

In deciding whether to close the outpatient pharmacy—even if alternative uses for the space existed—the hospital administrator would not base his or her decision solely on the quantitative analysis. Other factors should and would be considered.

First, the outpatient pharmacy might provide a needed service to the community. If there were no community pharmacies in the hospital's neighborhood, or if they could not provide all the products and services the hospital pharmacy provided, then the administrator might decide that the advantages of providing a public service to the community outweighed the financial disadvantages. This would be an especially relevant consideration for a hospital owned by a municipal or religious organization.

Second, closing the outpatient pharmacy might have a deleterious effect on other services provided by the hospital. Some patients might use the hospital's medical outpatient clinics because of the convenience of seeing physicians and getting prescriptions at the same place. Closing the outpatient pharmacy could result in a loss of revenues from the clinics.

Finally, the administrator would have to consider the effects on employee morale of closing the hospital pharmacy. This action would involve firing pharmacists and technicians who were employed in the outpatient pharmacy. This would probably have a negative effect on the morale of other pharmacists and technicians employed in the hospital, as well as other hospital employees. The loss of morale, and the disruption associated with it, might outweigh profit considerations.

## Adding a New Service

Technology, consumer tastes and preferences, and the state of pharmacy practice are constantly changing. Because of this, pressure on pharmacy managers to add new products and provide new services is constant. Differential analysis is useful in estimating the financial impact of doing so.

In the last few years, hospitals have come under increasing financial pressures. Many have responded by attempting to increase revenues by adding new services. One of these services has been to add an outpatient pharmacy. The Tar Heel Hospital outpatient pharmacy, considered from a different perspective, provides an example of using differential analysis to assess the feasibility of adding a new service.

To reuse this example, assume that Tar Heel Hospital does not have an outpatient pharmacy and is considering opening one. Assuming the hospital has space that could be used for the pharmacy, and there is no alternative use for this space, the relevant analysis is shown in Figure 10-3. This indicates that the pharmacy would contribute $20,000 to the hospital's overhead. In this situation, the hospital would benefit from providing the new service.

If, on the other hand, the hospital would have to rent space for the pharmacy, and if the rent amounted to $24,000 a year, the relevant analysis is shown in Figure 10-5. This indicates that the hospital would lose money by adding an outpatient pharmacy.

### Suggested Reading

Carroll NV. Forecasting the impact of participation in third-party prescriptions on pharmacy profits. J Res Pharmaceut Econ 1991;3(3):3.

Larson LN. Selective contracting with third-party programs. Drug Topics 1986;130:35.

Warren CS, Reeve JM, Fess PE. Accounting. 21st Ed. Mason, OH: Thomson South-Western, 2005.

## QUESTIONS

1. Costs that are *not* the same for all of the alternatives under consideration are known as:
   a. opportunity costs
   b. sunk costs
   c. differential costs

2. Jones Hospital is considering whether to keep its current outpatient pharmacy or to use the space now occupied by the outpatient pharmacy for an outpatient physical therapy facility. In deciding what to do, the manager should consider the profit that the hospital could make on the physical therapy service as a(n) ———— of keeping the outpatient pharmacy.
   a. Opportunity cost
   b. Sunk cost
   c. Differential cost
   d. Both **a** and **c**

3. The contribution margin associated with a given alternative indicates how much that alternative would contribute to:
   a. covering the pharmacy's differential costs
   b. covering the pharmacy's nondifferential costs
   c. pharmacy's profits
   d. All of the above
   e. b and c only

4. An insurance program offers Gator Pharmacy a chance to participate in a third-party prescription program that reimburses pharmacies ingredient cost plus a $3.00 fee. The pharmacy's cost to dispense plus a reasonable profit is $5.50 and its variable costs of dispensing a prescription are $0.75. The manager estimates that the average ingredient cost for a prescription dispensed under the program would be $10.00. If the pharmacy had substantial excess capacity and participation would cause only a moderate increase in prescription volume, would the pharmacy increase its profits by participating in the plan?
   a. Yes
   b. No

5. Full costs are frequently greater than differential costs because differential costs do not include:
   a. direct costs
   b. indirect costs
   c. Both a and b

6. The Metro University Hospital Pharmacy provides a pharmacokinetics dosing service for the hospital. The service generates $200,000 a year in revenues. The costs of operating the service consist of $180,000 in direct costs and $35,000 in indirect costs. The indirect costs consist of the service's allocated share of the hospital's overhead costs. What effect would eliminating the pharmacokinetics service have on the hospital's profits?
   a. It would increase the hospital's profits.
   b. It would decrease the hospital's profits.
   c. It would have no effect on the hospital's profits.

7. The Metro University Hospital Pharmacy also provides a drug information service. It generates $50,000 a year in revenues. The costs of operating the service consist

of $55,000 in direct costs and $5,000 in indirect costs. What effect would eliminating the drug information service have on the hospital's profits?

**a.** It would increase the hospital's profits.

**b.** It would decrease the hospital's profits.

**c.** It would have no effect on the hospital's profits.

## PROBLEMS

1. Slow-go Drugstore has calculated that its full cost of dispensing a prescription is $4.00. (This does not include cost of goods sold.) A new factory has just opened in the town that Slow-go serves. The factory offers its employees insurance coverage for prescriptions. The factory benefits manager offers Slow-go Drugstore the following deal. The factory will pay Slow-go ingredient cost plus $3.00 for each prescription dispensed to factory employees. If Slow-go accepts the deal, it should dispense an additional 5,000 prescriptions each year. Slow-go's manager estimates that the additional variable costs of dispensing a prescription amount to $0.50 per prescription.

   **a.** If the pharmacy will have to hire a part-time technician at $5,000 per year to fill another 5,000 prescriptions a year, will it find it profitable to participate in the plan? Calculate the differential costs, differential revenues, and contribution margin of participating.

   **b.** If the pharmacy currently has enough staff and assets to handle an additional 5,000 prescriptions a year, will it find it profitable to participate in the plan? Calculate the differential costs, differential revenues, and contribution margin of participating.

   **c.** If the pharmacy will have to hire a full-time technician at $15,000 per year to fill another 5,000 prescriptions a year, will it find it profitable to participate in the plan? Calculate the differential costs, differential revenues, and contribution margin of participating.

2. The vice president of a small chain of pharmacies must decide whether to close one of the chain's stores. The store's income statement is shown:

| | |
|---|---:|
| Revenues | $750,000 |
| Cost of goods sold | 550,000 |
| Gross margin | 200,000 |
| Other direct costs | 175,000 |
| Indirect costs | 40,000 |
| Net income | $(15,000) |

   Would closing the store improve the chain's profits?

   Calculate the differential revenues, differential costs, and contribution margin associated with closing the store. How much would the chain's profits change as a result of closing the store?

3. Hazelton Pharmacy is offered the opportunity to participate in a third-party prescription program. The program will pay the pharmacy its actual product cost plus a $2.00 dispensing fee. The pharmacy's current cost to dispense is $4.50.

Variable dispensing costs amount to $0.25 per prescription. Its current gross margin on a private pay prescription is $6.00. Hazelton's pharmacists and clerks have a substantial amount of time when they are not dispensing prescriptions or dealing with patients.

a. If participation in the plan will increase Hazelton's prescription volume by 600 prescriptions a year, what will be the net effect of participation on Hazelton's annual net profit?

b. If the plan will cover 600 prescriptions a year, which Hazelton currently fills as private pay prescriptions, how will participation affect the pharmacy's net income?

c. If the plan will cover 600 prescriptions a year, which Hazelton currently fills as private pay prescriptions, how will *not* participating affect the pharmacy's net income?

CHAPTER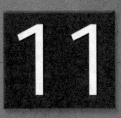

# Capital Investment Decisions

## OBJECTIVES

After completing the chapter, the student should be able to:

1. Define and give examples of capital budgeting decisions and explain how these decisions differ from operational decisions,
2. Explain why money has a time value,
3. Explain the concepts of present and future value, annuity, and compounding of interest,
4. Calculate the net present value of an investment,
5. Use the results of the net present value calculation to determine whether or not an investment should be made,
6. Explain the concept of required rate of return and discuss the factors that influence what the required rate of return of an investment should be, and
7. Explain why and how income taxes affect investment decisions and make net present value calculations which incorporate tax effects.

Sooner or later most pharmacies are faced with decisions that involve investments in noncurrent assets. Such decisions are known as *capital investment* or *capital budgeting* decisions. For a community pharmacy, examples include the purchase of a car or computer, or renovation of the building. A hospital or long-term care pharmacy may face decisions regarding whether to purchase an automated dispensing machine or establish an operating room pharmacy. Chain pharmacies must decide whether to open new units and whether to close or remodel existing units. As the capabilities and affordability of technology continue to improve, pharmacists are likely to be faced with capital budgeting decisions more frequently.

Capital budgeting decisions may also involve investments in human capital. From an economic point of view, the decision of whether to vaccinate children for polio is a capital investment decision. The decision involves whether substantial expenditures should be made to vaccinate children when they are young to prevent the occurrence and expense of treating polio in later years. Similarly, the decision of whether to treat patients for high cholesterol is a capital budgeting decision. The decision involves comparing the costs of treatment in the current time period with the costs (both monetary and humanistic) of strokes, myocardial infarctions, and other cardiovascular problems that untreated hypercholesterolemia may lead to in the future.

Capital investment decisions differ from more routine operating decisions in one important way. They involve cash inflows and outflows over a number of years. The decision to treat a patient for hypercholesterolemia involves the costs of treating the patient for many years as well as the savings that may occur as a result of preventing heart attacks and strokes. The decision to buy a dispensing robot involves initially paying out a great deal of money to purchase and install the robot, then realizing savings over several years as the robot replaces pharmacy technicians. Because capital budgeting decisions involve cash flows over several years, the *timing* of cash flows must be identified and considered when capital investment decisions are analyzed.

Consider the following example. The pharmacy director for the Tru-Care health maintenance organization (HMO) is considering whether to have the pharmacy become involved in disease management services. To make the change, the pharmacy will have to be remodeled to provide private consultation areas, new furniture and equipment will need to be purchased, and additional computer software will be required. A consultant has estimated that these costs will total $8,000. Provision of disease management services is expected to decrease total treatment costs for patients as a result of better management of drug therapy. The director has estimated that savings will average $2,000 per year for 5 years. In considering whether to make the investment, the manager makes the following analysis:

| | |
|---|---|
| Cost savings: | |
| $2,000 per year × 5 years | $10,000 |
| Cost of implementing services | 8,000 |
| Net savings | $ 2,000 |

Based on this analysis, the director might recommend that the HMO make the investment. But consider the assumption on which the analysis is based. The manager assumes that $10,000 to be saved over 5 years is worth as much as $10,000 received at the time the investment is made. The manager's assumption is not true. It ignores the *time value of money.*

The time value of money means that a dollar received today has more value than a dollar received sometime in the future. There are two reasons that money has a time value. First, there is *risk.* The further into the future that a given sum is to be received, the higher the risk is that it will not be received. Assume, for example, that a pharmacy dispenses a $75 prescription to one of its patients. If the patient pays for the prescription when he or she picks it up, then the pharmacy incurs no risk of the patient not paying. If the patient promises to pay by the end of the month, there is some risk that the patient will not pay. As the promised time of payment goes further into the future, the greater the risk is of nonpayment.

Money also has a time value because it can be *invested* to earn interest. A dollar received today is more valuable than one received a year from today because the dollar received today can be invested to earn interest. If it were invested in a passbook savings account paying 5% interest, it would be worth $1.05 in 1 year. To state it another way, the *future value* of $1.00 invested for a year at 5% interest is $1.05. Or, the *present value* of $1.05 to be received in 1 year at 5% interest is $1.00. Capital investment decisions—because they involve cash flows over several years—must consider the time value of money.

## CALCULATING TIME VALUE

Calculating the time value of an investment made for 1 year is straightforward. The future value—which is the amount to be received at the end of 1 year—is the amount invested multiplied by one plus the interest rate. For example, the future value of $1,000 invested for 1 year at 12% is:

$$\$1,000 \times (1 + 0.12) = \$1,120$$

Calculating the present value of a sum to be received in 1 year is equally simple. The present value is calculated by dividing the amount to be received by one plus the interest rate. The present value of $1,120 to be received in 1 year, assuming a 12% rate of interest, is:

$$\$1,120/1.12 = \$1,000$$

Calculating present and future values for periods greater than 1 year is more complicated. This is due to *compounding of interest*. Compounding of interest means that interest in later years is earned both on the original investment and on interest earned in earlier years. For example, $1,000 invested for 1 year at 12% earns $120 of interest per year. But, if it is invested for 3 years it earns *more* than $360 of interest. Why? Because the interest earned in year 1 draws interest in year 2, and the interest earned in years 1 and 2 draws interest in year 3. The following calculation shows how this occurs:

$$\text{Year 1: } \$1,000 \times 1.12 = \$1,120$$
$$\text{Year 2: } \$1,120 \times 1.12 = \$1,254$$
$$\text{Year 3: } \$1,254 \times 1.12 = \$1,405$$

The calculation indicates that $1,000 invested at 12% for 3 years will draw $405 of interest. The compounding of interest is responsible for the extra $45 of interest earned.

## Calculating Future and Present Values

The future value of an investment can be calculated as:

$FV = PV (1 + i)^n$, where
$FV$ = future value of the investment,
$PV$ = present value of the investment (the amount invested),
  $i$ = the interest rate, and
  $n$ = the number of years for which the investment is made.

Using the example of $1,000 invested for 3 years at 12%:

$$FV = PV \, (1 + i)^n$$
$$FV = 1,000 \, (1.12)^3$$
$$FV = \$1,405$$

Present value is calculated with a variation of the same formula:

$$PV = FV \, / \, (1 + i)^n$$

For example, what is the present value of $1,405 to be received in 3 years assuming an interest rate of 12%?

$$PV = FV \, / \, (1 + i)^n$$
$$PV = \$1,405 \, / \, (1.12)^3$$
$$PV = \$1,000$$

Present values can also be calculated from tables such as shown in Figure 11-1. The present value table shows the value of $1 to be received in a specified number of years in the future at a specified rate of interest. The tabled value for $1 to be received in 3 years at 12% is 0.712. This value is multiplied by the amount to be received to calculate the present value of the amount to be received. To find the present value of $1,405 to be received in 3 years at 12%, $1,405 is multiplied by 0.712. The result, $1,000, is the present value.

In the Tru-Care HMO example, the investment required to allow the pharmacy to provide disease management services would save the HMO $2,000 per year for 5 years.

| Years | 5% | 10% | 12% | 14% | 16% | 18% | 20% |
|-------|-------|-------|-------|-------|-------|-------|-------|
| 1 | 0.952 | 0.909 | 0.893 | 0.877 | 0.862 | 0.847 | 0.833 |
| 2 | 0.907 | 0.826 | 0.797 | 0.769 | 0.743 | 0.718 | 0.694 |
| 3 | 0.864 | 0.751 | 0.712 | 0.675 | 0.641 | 0.609 | 0.579 |
| 4 | 0.823 | 0.683 | 0.636 | 0.592 | 0.552 | 0.516 | 0.482 |
| 5 | 0.784 | 0.621 | 0.567 | 0.519 | 0.476 | 0.437 | 0.402 |
| 6 | 0.746 | 0.564 | 0.507 | 0.456 | 0.410 | 0.370 | 0.335 |
| 7 | 0.711 | 0.513 | 0.452 | 0.400 | 0.354 | 0.314 | 0.279 |
| 8 | 0.677 | 0.467 | 0.404 | 0.351 | 0.305 | 0.266 | 0.233 |
| 9 | 0.645 | 0.424 | 0.361 | 0.308 | 0.263 | 0.225 | 0.194 |
| 10 | 0.614 | 0.386 | 0.322 | 0.270 | 0.227 | 0.191 | 0.162 |
| 15 | 0.481 | 0.239 | 0.183 | 0.140 | 0.108 | 0.084 | 0.065 |
| 20 | 0.377 | 0.149 | 0.104 | 0.073 | 0.051 | 0.037 | 0.026 |
| 25 | 0.295 | 0.092 | 0.059 | 0.038 | 0.024 | 0.016 | 0.010 |
| 30 | 0.231 | 0.057 | 0.033 | 0.020 | 0.012 | 0.007 | 0.004 |

FIGURE 11-1    Present value of $1 received in N years.

The present value of the savings, assuming a 12% interest rate, can be calculated as follows:

PV of $2,000 to be received at end of:

| | |
|---|---|
| 1 year is 2,000 × 0.893 = | $1,786 |
| 2 years is 2,000 × 0.797 = | $1,594 |
| 3 years is 2,000 × 0.712 = | $1,424 |
| 4 years is 2,000 × 0.636 = | $1,272 |
| 5 years is 2,000 × 0.567 = | $1,134 |
| Total | $7,210 |

So, the PV of a savings of $2,000 per year for 5 years assuming a 12% interest rate is $7,210.

## Annuity Calculations

Capital investment decisions frequently involve payment or receipt of a fixed amount at the end of *every* year for some number of years. The director of Tru-Care HMO's pharmacy, for example, expects the investment in disease management to yield a savings of $2,000 per year for 5 years. (A savings of $2,000 per year has the same effect as receipt of $2,000 per year.) A series of payments of a fixed amount at the end of each year for a number of years is known as an *annuity*. The present value of an annuity can be calculated from the following formula:

$A_n = R \times [(1 - (1/(1 + i)^n))/i]$, where
$A_n$ = is the present value of the annuity,
$R$ = the amount to be paid (or received) at the end of each year,
$i$ = the interest rate, and
$n$ = the number of years the annuity will be received.

The present value of the savings Tru-Care HMO will realize, at a 12% rate of interest, may be calculated as follows:

$$A_n = R [(1 - (1/(1 + i)^n))/i]$$
$$A_4 = \$2,000 [(1 - (1/1.12^5))/.12]$$
$$A_4 = \$2,000 [(1 - (1/1.762))/.12]$$
$$A_4 = \$2,000 [(1 - 0.568)/.12]$$
$$A_4 = \$2,000 \times 3.600$$
$$A_4 = \$7,200$$

The calculation indicates that $2,000 to be received at the end of each year for 5 years at a 12% rate of interest is worth as much as $7,200 received immediately. (This is, within rounding error, the same answer as the one calculated with the year-by-year method.)

Tables may be used to calculate the present value of an annuity. Figure 11-2 shows an annuity table. The present value of Tru-Care's expected savings of $2,000 per year for 5 years at a 12% interest rate is calculated from Figure 11-2 using the following procedure. First, the table is consulted to find the present value of $1 to be received at the

| Years | 5% | 10% | 12% | 14% | 16% | 18% | 20% |
|---|---|---|---|---|---|---|---|
| 1 | 0.952 | 0.909 | 0.893 | 0.877 | 0.862 | 0.847 | 0.833 |
| 2 | 1.859 | 1.736 | 1.690 | 1.647 | 1.605 | 1.566 | 1.528 |
| 3 | 2.723 | 2.487 | 2.402 | 2.322 | 2.246 | 2.174 | 2.106 |
| 4 | 3.546 | 3.170 | 3.027 | 2.914 | 2.798 | 2.690 | 2.589 |
| 5 | 4.330 | 3.791 | 3.605 | 3.433 | 3.274 | 3.127 | 2.991 |
| 6 | 5.076 | 4.355 | 4.111 | 3.889 | 3.685 | 3.498 | 3.326 |
| 7 | 5.786 | 4.868 | 4.564 | 4.288 | 4.039 | 3.812 | 3.605 |
| 8 | 6.463 | 5.335 | 4.968 | 4.639 | 4.344 | 4.078 | 3.837 |
| 9 | 7.108 | 5.759 | 5.328 | 4.946 | 4.607 | 4.303 | 4.031 |
| 10 | 7.722 | 6.145 | 5.650 | 5.216 | 4.833 | 4.494 | 4.192 |
| 15 | 10.380 | 7.606 | 6.811 | 6.142 | 5.575 | 5.092 | 4.675 |
| 20 | 12.462 | 8.514 | 7.469 | 6.623 | 5.929 | 5.353 | 4.870 |
| 25 | 14.094 | 9.077 | 7.843 | 6.873 | 6.097 | 5.467 | 4.948 |
| 30 | 15.373 | 9.427 | 8.055 | 7.003 | 6.177 | 5.517 | 4.979 |

**FIGURE 11-2**  Present value of $1 received annually in N years.

end of *each year* for 5 years at a 12% rate of interest. This figure is 3.605. This is then multiplied by the amount to be received each year:

$$3.605 \times \$2,000 = \$7,210$$

## MAKING CAPITAL INVESTMENT DECISIONS—NET PRESENT VALUE

Capital investment decisions involve a large initial investment that yields cost savings or increased revenue in future years. Because of the time value of money, and because the cash inflows and outflows occur at different times, simply comparing the sum of inflows to the sum of outflows is not sufficient. A method is required that will adjust the cash flows for the time value of money so that they are comparable. The most common procedure is to calculate the present value of the inflows and outflows. The difference between the present value of the inflows and the present value of the outflows is known as the *net present value* (NPV) of the investment. If the NPV is greater than zero, the investment should be made. The larger the NPV, the more financially attractive is the project.

The NPV approach can be used to analyze Tru-Care's investment decision. Implementing disease management services will require an initial investment of $8,000. The period in which the investment is made is considered to be the present period. Thus, the present value of the initial investment is the amount of the initial investment—$8,000. The timing of subsequent cash flows is calculated with reference to this period. These consist of cash inflows of $2,000 per year for 5 years.

To calculate the present value of the inflows, an interest rate must be specified. In capital investment decisions, the interest rate is referred to as the *required rate of return* (RRR). It is the interest rate that the investment must earn to be financially attractive. For the Tru-Care HMO example, we assumed that the required rate of return was 12%. Earlier the present value of $2,000 annual savings for 5 years at a 12% RRR was calculated to be $7,210.

The net present value of the investment is:

| | |
|---|---|
| Cash inflows | $7,210 |
| Cash outflow | 8,000 |
| Net present value | (790) |

The NPV is negative and, therefore, the pharmacy should not invest. Why? Because the investment will not yield the 12% rate of return that the pharmacy requires. (To put it another way, the pharmacy would make more money by putting the $8,000 in an investment that yielded a 12% return on investment than by investing $8,000 in disease management services.)

But what if the pharmacy required a lower rate of return, say 5%? In this case, it should invest. The calculation is shown:

| | |
|---|---|
| PV of cash inflows = $2,000 × 4.33 = | $8,660 |
| PV of cash outflows = | 8,000 |
| NPV | $660 |

The positive NPV indicates that the investment would earn at least a 5% rate of return. If that is all the HMO requires, then it could earn it with this investment.

## Required Rate of Return

A business must estimate the RRR before making the NPV calculation. The RRR is the rate of return that an investment must earn to be financially attractive. As the Tru-Care HMO example demonstrates, the RRR selected has a dramatic effect on the calculated NPV of an investment. As the RRR increases, the present value of cash flows in future years decreases. Consequently, accurate estimation of the RRR is crucial to the accuracy of the NPV calculation.

## Estimating the RRR

The RRR for a *business* (that is, the average rate of return that it must earn when all of its individual investments are considered) should be set equal to its *cost of capital*. This is the cost of debt and equity to the business. Theoretically, the cost of capital is calculated as follows. First, the business's cost of debt, or the interest rate at which the business can borrow money, is determined. Then, the business's cost of equity, or the rate of interest that investors require to invest in the business, is determined. The business's cost of capital is then calculated as the *weighted* average of the cost of debt and equity. The average is weighted by the relative proportions of debt and equity on the business's balance sheet.

For example, Super-low Discount Drugs is financed with 40% equity and 60% debt. The firm's cost of debt (corrected for taxes) is 6%. Its cost of equity is 18%. The cost of capital for Super-low Discount Drugs is calculated as:

$$\text{Cost of capital} = (\text{Cost of debt} \times \text{Proportion of debt})$$
$$+ (\text{Cost of equity} \times \text{Proportion of equity})$$
$$\text{Cost of capital} = (6 \times .60) + (18 \times .4) = 10.8\%$$

So, on average, investments made by Super-low Discount Drugs should have a rate of return of 10.8%.

In practice, it is very difficult to actually determine a business's cost of capital.[1] The cost of debt can be reliably determined, but calculating the cost of equity is both complicated and unreliable.[1,2] Given the difficulty of estimating the cost of capital, Anthony and Welsch give two rules of thumb that can be used in estimating the RRR.[1] First, many organizations use a 10% RRR. Poterba and Summers found empirical evidence of this in a survey of 1,000 large businesses.[3] Twenty percent of the businesses used an RRR of 10%; 40% used an RRR between 10% and 15%. (These rates assume that NPV calculations will use cash flows for future years that have been corrected for the effects of inflation. Cash flows adjusted in this way are referred to as *constant-dollar* cash flows.)

Anthony and Welsch's second rule of thumb is that a business's RRR will always be higher than its cost of debt. Because of this, a pharmacy can estimate the lower limit of its RRR by calculating its cost of debt. The cost of debt will be the *tax-adjusted* interest rate at which the pharmacy can borrow money. The rate of borrowing must be tax adjusted because interest payments on loans are tax-deductible expenses. Thus, the interest payments lower the business's income taxes.

For example, assume Super-low Discount Drugs is in the 48% tax bracket and can borrow money from the bank at 12%. Super-low Discount Drugs must pay the bank 12% interest. But, the interest payments are tax deductible. Because of this (1-tax rate) or only 52% of the interest payments will represent additional cash payments for the pharmacy. The other 48% of interest payments would have been paid out in income taxes had the pharmacy not had the tax deduction for interest payments. Consequently, the business's net cost of borrowing is only 0.52 × 12% or 6.2%.

This calculation indicates that the RRR for Super-low Discount Drugs would be no less than 6.2%. It would have to be higher than 6.2% if any of the pharmacy's financing consisted of equity. The greater the percentage of equity financing, the higher the RRR would have to be.

Although it is difficult to calculate the RRR for the *business*, it is even more difficult to calculate the RRR for an individual *investment*. A major reason for this is that individual investments differ substantially in their riskiness. Some investments are safe; the pharmacy is sure of what the investment will cost and what return it will pay. Others are risky; that is, the pharmacy may be unsure of the final cost of the investment or of the return it will generate. Poterba and Summers found that the difference between the highest and lowest RRR used by a business averaged 11.2%.[3]

In estimating the RRR for an individual investment, the manager must consider the RRR for the business and the degree of risk for the individual investment. The business's RRR indicates the average return the business must make over all its investments. For risky investments, a higher rate must be earned. The higher the risk, the higher the RRR must be set.

Poterba and Summers also suggested that businesses use lower RRRs for projects that are critical to their strategy or mission.[3] For example, many managers believe that their pharmacies' future success depends on shifting from a dispensing-oriented to a pharmaceutical care–oriented style of practice. A manager who believes this should use a lower RRR for investments that facilitate moving the pharmacy to pharmaceutical care than for equally risky projects that are less critical to the pharmacy's mission.

## Sensitivity Analysis

Because of the difficulty of estimating the RRR, a manager usually will not have a great deal of confidence in the estimate. However, he or she might feel more confident about a range of estimates. For example, the manager might be unsure that the RRR was 12%; he or she might, however, feel confident that the RRR was between 10% and 14%. Because of this, the manager may be able to use sensitivity analysis to increase confidence in the results of an NPV calculation.

A sensitivity analysis consists of varying the estimates of an important, and uncertain, value to determine the effect on the final decision. For capital investment decisions, the manager can vary the estimate of the RRR to determine the effect on the NPV of the investment. If the manager is confident that the RRR is within some given range, he or she can use both ends of the range as estimates. If the NPV is positive (or negative) using either estimate, then the manager can have more confidence in his or her decision. If the NPV is positive with the lower RRR estimate and negative at the higher estimate, then the manager must devote more effort to more precisely estimating the RRR.

For example, assume that Triangle Hospital Pharmacy was considering the purchase of an automated dispensing system. The system would cost the pharmacy $100,000, would save $25,000 per year in personnel expense, and would last for 5 years. The director is not sure exactly what return the investment should yield, but feels confident it should be between 10% and 14%. The calculated NPVs are both negative: ($5,225) at 10% and ($14,175) at 14%. Consequently, the director can be confident that the investment should not be made, even though he or she is not exactly sure what the RRR should be.

## Tax Considerations in NPV Calculations

In determining the NPV of an investment, cash inflows and outflows must be adjusted for the effects of income taxes. The primary cash outflow—which is usually the purchase of a noncurrent asset—results in the business gaining a depreciable asset. In each year of the asset's useful life, it will be depreciated. The depreciation expense will result in lower income taxes. The additional cash inflows resulting from use of the asset are *pretax* inflows. They result in higher income tax payments. The inflows must be adjusted for the higher income taxes to calculate the *after-tax* inflows.

The following procedure can be used to adjust cash flows for taxes:

1.  Identify the pretax cash inflows.
2.  Calculate the annual depreciation expense.
3.  Calculate the additional tax payments. The calculation is made by subtracting the depreciation expense from the annual cash inflows, then multiplying the difference by the tax rate.
4.  Calculate after-tax cash inflows by subtracting the additional income tax payments from the pretax cash inflows.
5.  The NPV calculation is then made using the after-tax cash inflows.

In the Tru-Care HMO example presented earlier, the cash flows were not adjusted for taxes. In this example, the investments required to allow the pharmacy to provide disease management services totaled $8,000 and would generate $2,000 annually in savings for 5

years. Assume that Tru-Care was subject to a 30% tax rate and that straight-line depreciation was used. The tax adjustment is made by using the procedure outlined below:

1. Pretax cash inflows = $2,000 per year.
2. Calculate annual depreciation expense.

$$\text{Annual depreciation expense} = \text{Amount depreciated/years of life}$$
$$= \$8,000/5$$
$$= \$1,600$$

3. Additional income tax payments:

| | |
|---|---|
| Pretax cash inflows | $2,000 |
| Depreciation expense | 1,600 |
| Net income increase | $ 400 |
| Tax rate | × .30 |
| Additional tax payments | $ 120 |

4. After-tax cash inflows:

| | |
|---|---|
| Pretax cash inflows | $2,000 |
| Less additional taxes | 120 |
| After-tax cash inflow | $1,880 |

5. NPV calculation (tax adjusted)

| | |
|---|---|
| Cash inflows $1,880 per year for 5 years at 12% RRR | $6,777 |
| Cash outflow initial investment | 8,000 |
| Net present value | ($1,223) |

Consequently, consideration of taxes decreases the attractiveness of this investment.

## Another Example

Jeff Parker, a recent PharmD graduate, is interested in opening a home IV infusion
business in a rural part of the state in which he lives. After talking with several consultants and equipment vendors, he estimates that the capital investment required to
open the business will be $200,000. He also estimates that the business would earn an
annual, after-tax, net income of $45,000. Because this is a risky venture, Jeff estimates
that he must earn a 20% return on his investment. Assuming that Jeff has the $200,000
and that he believes he should be able to recover his investment in 5 years, should he
open the home IV infusion pharmacy?

The cash outflow for the investment is the initial $200,000 investment. The inflows
consist of $45,000 a year for 5 years. In this example, no additional consideration need
be given to tax effects because depreciation and taxes have already been taken into consideration in calculating the pharmacy's net income. The NPV calculation is as follows:

| | |
|---|---|
| Cash inflows = $45,000 × 2.991 = | $ 134,595 |
| Cash outflows = | 200,000 |
| NPV | $(65,405) |

The calculation indicates that opening the pharmacy, under these terms, will not generate the 20% return that Jeff requires. Consequently, he decides not to open the
pharmacy.

After additional thought, Jeff realizes that it might not be necessary to pay the entire $200,000 up front. He talks with the vendors of the inventory and equipment he will need to open the pharmacy and they agree to finance the investment over 4 years (with no interest charges). Under this agreement, Jeff must pay $50,000 per year for 4 years.

Jeff makes new calculations to see if this changes the expected return on the IV infusion business. The only change for the new offer is the calculation of cash outflows. The NPV is now calculated as:

$$
\begin{array}{llll}
\text{Cash inflows} & = \$45,000 \times 2.991 & = \$134,595 \\
\text{Cash outflows} & = \$50,000 \times 2.589 & = \underline{\phantom{0}129,450} \\
\text{NPV} & & \$ \quad 5,145
\end{array}
$$

The new NPV would be $5,145. Because of the change in the timing of cash outflows, the investment now returns better than 20%. Consequently, the new deal makes purchase of the pharmacy a more attractive investment. Jeff takes the offer.

## INTERNAL RATE OF RETURN

Another technique for analyzing capital investment decisions is based on the *internal rate of return* (IRR) of the investment. The IRR is defined as the interest rate at which the NPV of the investment is zero. If the IRR of an investment is greater than the RRR, the investment should be made. This is because the investment would yield a greater return than the firm requires.

As an example, assume that Chester's Pharmacy is considering purchase of a point-of-sale computer system. The IRR of investment in the system is calculated to be 15%. If Chester's Pharmacy's RRR is less than 15%, the computer system should be purchased. If its RRR is greater than 15%, the system should not be purchased.

The IRR is calculated by determining the interest rate that will set the PV of cash inflows from the investment equal to the PV of cash outflows of the investment. The calculation is usually made by trial and error; one tries different discount rates until he or she finds the one that makes outflows and inflows equal. In many cases, hand calculations of IRRs are tedious. Fortunately, financial calculators and computer spreadsheet packages usually include functions that automatically calculate IRRs for investments.

## References

1. Anthony RN, Welsch GA. Fundamentals of Management Accounting. 3rd Ed. Homewood, Illinois: Richard D. Irwin, 1981.
2. Maruca RF. The cost of capital—what's the best estimate? Harvard Bus Rev 1996;74:9.
3. Poterba JM, Summers LH. A CEO survey of US companies' time horizons and hurdle rates. Sloan Management Rev 1995;37:43.

## Suggested Readings

Besley S, Brigham EF. Essentials of Managerial Finance. 13th Ed. Mason, OH: Thomson South-Western, 2005.
Keown AJ, Petty JW, Martin JD, et al. Foundations of Finance: The Logic and Practice of Finance Management. 5th Ed. Upper Saddle River, NJ: Prentice Hall, 2006.

## QUESTIONS

1. Which of the following would be a capital investment decision?
   a. Renovation of the pharmacy
   b. Purchase of a computer
   c. Purchase of 1,000 bottles of Cefaclor
   d. Purchase of a line of generic drugs
   e. All of the above
   f. a and b only

2. A payment of $100 to be received in 5 years is worth _____ a payment of $100 to be received in 1 year.
   a. More than
   b. Less than
   c. The same as

3. The present value of $500 to be received in a year assuming a 10% interest rate RRR is _____ $500 to be received in a year at 15% interest rate.
   a. More than
   b. Less than
   c. The same as

4. Higher RRRs _____ the NPV of future cash flows.
   a. Increase
   b. Decrease
   c. Have no effect on

5. A capital investment should be made if its net present value is:
   a. positive
   b. negative

6. To estimate the pharmacy's RRR, the manager must consider:
   a. the interest rate at which the pharmacy can borrow money
   b. the rate of return required to attract investors
   c. the proportions of debt and equity on the pharmacy's balance sheet
   d. All of the above
   e. a and b only

7. The cost of equity for a pharmacy is:
   a. the interest rate at which the pharmacy can borrow money
   b. the rate of return required to attract investors
   c. the proportions of debt and equity on the pharmacy's balance sheet

8. Fidget Pharmacy uses an RRR of 15%. The internal rate of return of a project that would computerize inventory control for the pharmacy is 18%. Should the pharmacy make this investment?
   a. Yes—the IRR is greater than the RRR.
   b. No—the IRR is greater than the RRR.

9. The internal rate of return is defined as the interest rate at which the NPV of the investment is:
   a. greater than zero
   b. equal to zero
   c. less than zero

10. The most difficult step in estimating the NPV of an investment is:
    a. identifying the cash inflows and outflows
    b. estimating the RRR
    c. estimating the pharmacy's tax rate

## PROBLEMS

1. Calculate the present value of the following:
   a. $5,000 to be received in 4 years at an RRR of 12%
   b. $5,000 per year for 4 years at an RRR of 12%
   c. $5,000 to be received in 4 years at an RRR of 18%
   d. $5,000 per year for 4 years at an RRR of 18%
   e. $2,500 to be received in 10 years at an RRR of 10%
   f. $2,500 to be received in 5 years at an RRR of 10%
   g. $2,500 per year for 5 years at an RRR of 10%
   h. $2,500 per year for 10 years at an RRR of 10%
   i. $9,500 to be received in 10 years at an RRR of 10%
   j. $9,500 to be received in 10 years at an RRR of 18%
2. A hospital pharmacy is considering whether to establish an outpatient pharmacy. It will cost the hospital about $200,000 to set up and equip the outpatient facility. The hospital requires a minimum of 10% rate of return on all investment projects. The pharmacy director estimates the following cash inflows from the outpatient pharmacy:

| Year | Cash Inflow (per year) |
|------|------------------------|
| 1    | $5,000                 |
| 2    | 25,000                 |
| 3–10 | 50,000                 |

   Based on these assumptions, would the outpatient pharmacy be a profitable investment? (For this problem, ignore any income tax effects.)
3. A small chain of pharmacies is evaluating whether to invest $50,000 to computerize five of its busiest units (stores). The chain estimates that computerization will yield savings of $12,000 to $15,000 per year and the computer system will be used for 5 years. The chain's RRR is 10% and it is subject to a 40% income tax rate. Should the chain buy the computer system for its pharmacies? Use the straight-line method of depreciation and assume that the computer's residual value will be zero.
4. A chain pharmacy is planning to renovate one of its smaller units. The renovation will cost $80,000. The renovation is expected to increase the unit's net profit *before taxes* by $25,000 per year for 5 years. Assuming the chain's RRR is 12% and its tax rate is 30%, should it renovate the unit? Assume the renovation can be depreciated over 5 years and the residual value of the depreciation will be zero.

# 12

# Sources and Uses of Cash*

After reading this chapter, the student should be able to:

1. Explain the importance of cash to a pharmacy,
2. Explain why the income statement and balance sheet provide little cash-related information,
3. Construct a sources and uses statement from balance sheets and an income statement, and
4. Use a sources and uses statement to evaluate how well a pharmacy manages its cash and its ability to generate cash.

C ash is the lifeblood of a business. It is necessary for paying bills, making change, paying employees, and making any other financial transaction in which the pharmacy is involved. Consequently, proper management of cash is of vital importance to pharmacy managers. They must be aware of where the pharmacy gets its cash and how it uses it. Unfortunately, this information is not readily available to the managers of most pharmacies.

Most pharmacies receive annual income statements and balance sheets. Neither statement provides much information about the pharmacy's cash flow. This is apparent to the manager who wonders why the highly profitable pharmacy has no cash to pay this month's bills.

---

*Adapted from an article originally published in and copyrighted by CE PRN®, a publication of W-F Professional Associates, Inc., Deerfield, IL, 1986.

This chapter explains why the standard financial statements provide little information about cash, presents a simple method for developing statements that provide cash-related information, and shows how these statements are used.

## PROBLEMS WITH THE INCOME STATEMENT AND BALANCE SHEET

The standard financial statements—the income statement and balance sheet—are prepared using the accrual basis of accounting, not the cash basis. This means that revenues are recorded when sales are made, not when cash is received, and expenses are recorded when they are incurred, not when payment is made. Consequently, revenues and expenses for a given period are usually not the same as cash inflows and outflows for that same period.

A look at an income statement is helpful in understanding these concepts. The income statement shown in Figure 12-1 lists total sales of $37,250,000 for 20X6. This is the net amount of cash and credit sales the pharmacy made during the year. Because the pharmacy had accounts receivable, total sales would not be the same as the amount of cash taken in during the year. The income statement shows cost of goods sold of $26,800,000 for 20X6. This is the cost of merchandise sold during the year; it is not the amount of cash spent to purchase inventory during the year. The two amounts differ because of credit purchases and to the extent that the level of inventory increased or decreased over the year. Total operating expenses, including income tax, of $8,165,000 are shown. This is not the amount of cash paid out during the year. It is the amount of expenses incurred. These two amounts differ because of credit purchases and because some expenses are noncash expenses. For example, depreciation is listed as an $80,000 expense even though no cash was disbursed for payment of the depreciation expense. As a result of these differences, the income statement provides little information about the pharmacy's cash flow.

| | 20X5 | 20X6 |
|---|---|---|
| | $000 | $000 |
| Net sales | 36,600 | 37,250 |
| Cost of goods sold | 24,800 | 26,800 |
| Gross margin | 11,800 | 10,450 |
| Operating expenses | | |
| Rent | 625 | 640 |
| Utilities | 185 | 190 |
| Salaries and benefits | 4,200 | 4,300 |
| Depreciation | 80 | 80 |
| Delivery | 495 | 500 |
| Bad debt | 240 | 350 |
| Miscellaneous | 785 | 705 |
| Total | 6,610 | 6,765 |
| Net income before income taxes | 5,190 | 3,685 |
| Income tax | 1,972 | 1,400 |
| Net income after taxes | 3,218 | 2,285 |

**FIGURE 12-1**    Income statements for Goodcare Pharmacy, year ended 12/31.

## DEVELOPING SOURCES AND USES STATEMENTS

Although the standard, accrual-based financial statements provide little information about cash flows, they can be used to develop statements that do. To develop such statements, which are called *sources and uses statements*, for a given year, one must have balance sheets and income statements for both the current and previous years. Income statements and balance sheets for Goodcare Pharmacy, a long-term care pharmacy, are shown in Figures 12-1 and 12-2, respectively. These will be used to develop a sources and uses statement for Goodcare Pharmacy for 20X6.

### Statement of Balance Sheet Changes

The first step is to develop a *statement of balance sheet changes*. This is done by calculating the increase or decrease in each of the balance sheet accounts for the year (Fig. 12-2, column 4). Changes are calculated only for accounts, not for totals. The only change

|  | 20X5 $000 | 20X6 $000 | Change $000 |
|---|---|---|---|
| Assets |  |  |  |
| Cash | 35 | 25 | (10) |
| Accounts receivables | 4,950 | 5,800 | 850 |
| Inventory | 900 | 1,400 | 500 |
| Prepaid expenses | 75 | 50 | (25) |
| Total current assets | 5,960 | 7,275 |  |
| Property and equipment | 9,300 | 12,380 |  |
| Less accumulated depreciation | (1,300) | (1,380) |  |
| Net property and equipment | 8,000 | 11,000 | 3,000 |
| Total assets | 13,960 | 18,275 |  |
| Liabilities and equity |  |  |  |
| Accounts payable | 735 | 700 | (35) |
| Accrued expenses payable | 625 | 600 | (25) |
| Note payable (current) | 300 | 175 | (125) |
| Total current liabilities | 1,660 | 1,475 |  |
| Total long-term debt | 2,500 | 2,300 | (200) |
| Total liabilities | 4,160 | 3,775 |  |
| Owner equity | 9,800 | 14,500 | 4,700 |
| Total liabilities and owner equity | 13,960 | 18,275 |  |

**FIGURE 12–2**  Balance sheets for Goodcare Pharmacy, 12/31.

|  | ($000) |
|---|---:|
| Sources of cash |  |
| Decrease in cash account | 10 |
| Decrease in prepaid expenses | 25 |
| Increase in owner equity | 4,700 |
| Total sources | 4,735 |
| Uses of cash |  |
| Increase in accounts receivables | 850 |
| Increase in inventory | 500 |
| Increase in net property and equipment | 3,000 |
| Decrease in accounts payables | 35 |
| Decrease in accrued expenses payable | 25 |
| Decrease in note payable (current) | 125 |
| Decrease in long-term debt | 200 |
| Total uses | 4,735 |

**FIGURE 12-3**  Statement of balance sheet changes for Goodcare Pharmacy, year ended 12/31/20X6.

needed for fixed assets is the change in net fixed assets. Each change is classified as either a source or use of cash. Sources of cash include decreases in asset accounts and increases in liabilities or owners' equities. Uses of cash include increases in assets and decreases in liabilities and owners' equities. Total sources must always equal total uses. A statement of balance sheet changes for Goodcare Pharmacy is shown in Figure 12-3.

## A More Accurate Statement

The statement of balance sheet changes provides a rough estimate of the pharmacy's sources and uses of cash. To develop a more accurate statement, three changes must be made to the statement of balance sheet changes.

First, the change in the owner equity account is examined to determine how it occurred. Changes in owner equity come from net income or loss and from additional owner investment or withdrawal. Net income and owner investment increase owner equity and net losses, and owner withdrawals decrease it. The financial statements for Goodcare Pharmacy do not explicitly show the amount of owner withdrawals or investments. The amount can be estimated by comparing net income and the change in owner equity. For Goodcare Pharmacy, net income for 20X6 was $2,285,000. This is the amount by which owner equity would have increased if all profits had been left in the business and no owner investments or withdrawals had been made. However, owner equity increased by $4,700,000. Therefore, an owner investment of $4,700,000 − $2,285,000 = $2,415,000 must have been made during the year. To reflect these cash-related corrections, the change in retained earning is replaced by entries listing net income and owner investment as sources of cash.

The second adjustment converts accrual-based net income to cash generated from operation of the pharmacy. Net income is the starting point for estimating cash generated by operations. However, net income underestimates cash from operations. This occurs because noncash expenses—such as depreciation—are subtracted from revenues to calculate net income. As a result, all noncash expenses must be added back to net income to better estimate cash generated from operations.

For Goodcare Pharmacy, depreciation is the only noncash expense. Consequently, for Goodcare Pharmacy, the $80,000 depreciation expense must be added to the sources and uses statement as a source of cash. The sum of net income plus depreciation represents the amount of cash generated by operation of the pharmacy. This sum is frequently referred to as *cash from operations*.

The final adjustment estimates the amount of cash spent on fixed assets for the year. If the pharmacy had neither purchased nor sold fixed assets for the year, then the net value of fixed assets would have decreased by the amount of the annual depreciation expense. For Goodcare Pharmacy, this would be a decrease of $80,000. However, the statement of balance sheet changes shows that Goodcare Pharmacy's net fixed assets (which are listed here as property and equipment) actually increased by $3,000,000 over the year. Consequently, the pharmacy must have purchased fixed assets during the year. The amount the pharmacy spent to purchase fixed assets is estimated by adding the year's depreciation expense to the net change in fixed assets. For Goodcare Pharmacy, the sum of the $80,000 depreciation expense and the $3,000,000 increase in net fixed assets yields a $3,080,000 expenditure to purchase fixed assets. This amount replaces the net change in fixed assets as a use of cash. Figure 12-4 shows a completed sources and uses statement for Goodcare Pharmacy for 20X6.

| Sources and Uses Statement | |
|---|---|
| | ($000) |
| Sources of cash | |
| Decrease in cash account | 10 |
| Decrease in prepaid expenses | 25 |
| Net income | 2,285 |
| Plus depreciation | 80 |
| Increase in owner investment | 2,415 |
| Total sources | 4,815 |
| Uses of cash | |
| Increase in accounts receivables | 850 |
| Increase in inventory | 500 |
| Purchase of property and equipment | 3,080 |
| Decrease in accounts payables | 35 |
| Decrease in accrued expenses payable | 25 |
| Decrease in note payable (current) | 125 |
| Decrease in long-term debt | 200 |
| Total uses | 4,815 |

**FIGURE 12-4**    Sources and uses statement for Goodcare Pharmacy, year ended 12/31/20X6.

# USING THE SOURCES AND USES STATEMENT

The sources and uses statement can be used to evaluate how well the pharmacy's cash is managed and to evaluate the pharmacy's ability to generate sufficient cash to meet its needs. This can be done by using it to answer three questions of major importance to pharmacy managers:

1. What were the pharmacy's major sources and uses of cash for the year?
2. Were the major uses of cash financed by suitable and appropriate sources?
3. For the year, was the pharmacy a net user or provider of cash?

## Major Sources and Uses

The sources and uses statement shows where the pharmacy's cash came from and how it was used. The major sources of cash for Goodcare Pharmacy in 20X6 were net income plus depreciation (also called cash from operations) and owner investment. Major uses were purchase of property and equipment and increasing accounts receivables and inventory.

The major source of cash for a well-run pharmacy should be profitable operation of the pharmacy. We have referred to this as cash generated from operations and estimated it as net income plus depreciation. A pharmacy that generates its cash through profitable operations is more likely to have a constant and secure source of cash than one that must borrow, sell fixed assets, or depend on additional owner investment to meet its cash needs.

## Appropriateness of Sources and Uses

The question of appropriateness involves whether uses of cash were financed by appropriate sources. As a general rule, short-term uses should be financed by short-term sources and long-term uses by long-term sources. Net income plus depreciation, owner investment, increases in long-term debt, and net cash from sale of fixed assets are considered long-term sources. Net losses, owner withdrawals, decreases in long-term debt, and expenditures on fixed assets are long-term uses. Short-term sources of cash include increases in current liabilities or decreases in current assets. Short-term uses would be increases in current assets or decreases in current liabilities.

Using long-term sources to finance short-term uses, or vice versa, may cause cash flow problems. This is best seen through examples. The most straightforward is that of a short-term loan used to finance an owner withdrawal. The short-term loan is a temporary source. Owner withdrawal is a long-term use. At the end of the loan period, which is a year or less, cash must be found to repay the loan. But the cash from the loan is gone; it financed an owner withdrawal. Consequently, the pharmacy may have trouble repaying on time.

Other examples are less straightforward but, in practice, may be equally troublesome. Assume a long-term loan is taken to purchase inventory. The loan is a long-term source, but inventory is a temporary use. At the end of 30 or 60 days, the inventory will be sold. Most of the cash received from sales of the inventory will be used to purchase new inventory. When the loan comes due, after several cycles of buying and selling inventory, the pharmacy may not have the extra cash it needs to repay the loan. Finally, assume a 1-year loan is taken to purchase a truck that will be used for 5 years. At the end of 1 year, the loan is due and cash must be found to pay it off. The cash should come from the excess of cash over net income due to depreciation charges. (Depreciation decreases tax payments. This decreases cash outflow from the pharmacy.) But because only 1 year's depreciation has been charged, this excess would be inadequate.

Goodcare Pharmacy's long-term sources amount to $4,780,000 (from net income plus depreciation and owner investment). Long-term uses amount to $3,280,000 (from decrease in long-term debt and purchases of fixed assets). This indicates that long-term uses are financed by long-term sources. It also indicates that many short-term uses were financed by long-term sources.

The general rule is that long-term uses should be financed by long-term sources, and short-term uses should be financed by short-term uses. Some divergence from the rule is acceptable provided two conditions are met. First, all long-term uses must be financed with long-term sources. Second, long-term sources consist primarily of cash generated by operations. It is acceptable to finance short-term uses, or any type of uses, by means of cash from operations.

A closer look at the sources and uses statement reveals two additional problems. First, it shows a large increase in accounts receivables. The increase in accounts receivables is greater than the increase in sales in both dollar and percentage terms. This could indicate that a large percentage of sales shifted from cash to third-party payment in the past year, or it could indicate poor management of receivables. In any case, increases of this magnitude should be investigated. Second, the sources and uses statement shows that inventory increased substantially and that it increased proportionately much more than did sales. A large and disproportionate increase in inventory suggests a problem with inventory control. Again, increases of this magnitude should be further investigated. Ratio analysis can be used to better determine whether the pharmacy actually has problems with accounts receivables and inventory control.

## Net User or Provider

The sources and uses statement shows that Goodcare Pharmacy was a net user of cash for the year. During 20X6, the cash account decreased by $10,000. Thus, Goodcare Pharmacy used $10,000 more cash than it generated for the year. This cannot continue indefinitely. In a period of increasing sales the pharmacy needs more cash, not less.

### Suggested Readings

Coleman AR, Brownlee ER II, Smith CR. Financial Accounting and Statement Analysis: A Manager's Guide. Richmond, Virginia: Robert F. Dame, Inc., 1982.

Helfert EA. Financial Analysis Tools and Techniques: A Guide for Managers. 10th Ed. New York: McGraw-Hill, 2001.

Kreps CH Jr, Wacht RF. Analyzing Financial Statements. Washington, DC: American Bankers Association, 1978.

Viscione JA. Flow of Funds and Other Financial Concepts. New York: National Association of Credit Management, 1981.

# QUESTIONS

1.  The income statement shows:
    a.  the pharmacy's cash sales for the year
    b.  the pharmacy's cash and credit sales for the year
    c.  how much cash the pharmacy brought in for the year
    d.  All of the above
2.  Most pharmacies receive annual:
    a.  income statements
    b.  balance sheets
    c.  cash flow statements
    d.  All of the above
    e.  a and b only
3.  A pharmacy's major source of cash should be:
    a.  net income plus depreciation
    b.  sale of fixed assets
    c.  borrowing
    d.  All of the above
    e.  a and b only
4.  An increase in inventory should be financed through:
    a.  increased accounts payable
    b.  net income
    c.  a long-term loan
    d.  All of the above
    e.  a and b only
5.  A major renovation of the pharmacy should be financed by:
    a.  increased accounts payable
    b.  net income
    c.  a long-term loan
    d.  All of the above
    e.  b and c only
6.  Chester Pharmacy's cash account showed balances of $12,000 in 20X8 and $10,000 in 20X9. For 20X9, Chester Pharmacy was a:
    a.  net user of cash
    b.  net provider of cash
7.  The change in the owner equity account from one year to the next is directly affected by:
    a.  the pharmacy's net income for the year
    b.  owner withdrawals for the year
    c.  changes in the cash account for the year
    d.  All of the above
    e.  a and b only

# PROBLEMS

1.  Financial statements for Rose Pharmacy for 20X4 and 20X5 are shown. Using these data, construct a sources and uses statement for Rose Pharmacy for 20X5 and answer the following questions:

a. What were Rose Pharmacy's major sources and uses of cash during 20X5? What do the major sources of cash indicate about the pharmacy's ability to generate cash?

b. Were uses of cash financed by appropriate sources?

### Rose Pharmacy
### Balance Sheets for 12/31

|  | 20X5 | 20X4 |
|---|---|---|
| *Assets* | | |
| Cash | $17,500 | $15,100 |
| Accounts receivable | 17,650 | 16,650 |
| Inventory | 80,700 | 68,200 |
| Net property and equipment | 15,750 | 16,750 |
| Total assets | 131,600 | 116,700 |
| *Liabilities* | | |
| Accounts payable | 25,700 | 19,200 |
| Accrued expenses | 6,900 | 6,900 |
| Note payable (current) | 7,200 | 6,800 |
| Long-term debt | 16,800 | 19,800 |
| Total liabilities | 56,600 | 52,700 |
| *Owner equity* | | |
| Common stock | 32,000 | 32,000 |
| Retained earnings | 43,000 | 32,000 |
| Total owner equity | 75,000 | 64,000 |
| *Total liabilities and owner equity* | $131,600 | $116,700 |

### Rose Pharmacy
### Income Statements

|  | 20X5 | 20X4 |
|---|---|---|
| *Net sales* | | |
| Cash sales | $310,000 | $300,000 |
| Credit sales | 265,000 | 230,000 |
| Total sales | 575,000 | 530,000 |
| Cost of goods sold | 383,000 | 353,000 |
| *Gross margin* | *192,000* | *177,000* |
| *Expenses* | | |
| Depreciation expense | 1,000 | 1,000 |
| Other expenses | 173,625 | 161,000 |
| Total expenses | 174,625 | 162,000 |
| Net income | $17,375 | $15,000 |

2. Financial statements for King's Pharmacy for 20X0 and 20X1 are shown. Using these data, construct a sources and uses statement for King's Pharmacy for 20X1 and answer the following questions.
   a. What were King's Pharmacy's major sources and uses of cash during 20X1? What do the major sources indicate about the pharmacy's ability to generate cash?
   b. Were uses of cash financed by appropriate sources?

**King's Pharmacy**
**Balance Sheets for 12/31**

|  | 20X1 | 20X0 | Change |
|---|---|---|---|
| *Assets* |  |  |  |
| Cash | $ 30,414 | $ 11,075 | $19,339 |
| Accounts receivable | 8,810 | 4,979 | 3,831 |
| Inventory | 56,991 | 48,999 | 7,992 |
| Net property and equipment | 14,572 | 50,490 | −35,918 |
| Total assets | 110,787 | 115,543 |  |
| *Liabilities* |  |  |  |
| Accounts payable | 15,579 | 11,399 | 4,180 |
| Accrued expenses | 16 | 16 | 0 |
| Long-term debt | 14,613 | 30,476 | −15,863 |
| Total liabilities | 30,208 | 41,891 |  |
| *Owner equity* |  |  |  |
| Capital | 80,579 | 73,652 | 6,927 |
| *Total liabilities and owner equity* | $110,787 | $115,543 |  |

**King's Pharmacy**
**Income Statements**

|  | 20X1 | 20X0 | Change |
|---|---|---|---|
| *Net Sales* |  |  |  |
| Cash sales | $294,057 | $271,595 | $22,462 |
| Credit sales | 56,011 | 44,213 | 11,798 |
| Total sales | 350,068 | 315,808 | 34,260 |
| *Cost of goods sold* |  |  |  |
| Beginning inventory | 48,999 | 47,842 | 1,157 |
| Purchases | 223,472 | 196,856 | 26,616 |
| Cost of goods available for sale | 272,471 | 244,698 | 27,773 |
| Less ending inventory | 56,991 | 48,999 | 7,992 |
| Cost of goods sold | 215,480 | 195,699 | 19,781 |

| | | | |
|---|---|---|---|
| Gross margin | 134,588 | 120,109 | 14,479 |
| Depreciation | 1,825 | 2,500 | –675 |
| Other expenses | 84,512 | 82,243 | 2,269 |
| Total expenses | 86,337 | 84,743 | 1,594 |
| Net income | $48,251 | $35,366 | $12,885 |

3. Financial statements for Goodwill Pharmacy, a closed-shop, long-term care pharmacy, for 20X0 and 20X1 are shown. Using these data, construct a sources and uses statement for Goodwill Pharmacy for 20X1 and answer the following questions.
   a. What were Goodwill Pharmacy's major sources and uses of cash during 20X1? What do the major sources indicate about the pharmacy's ability to generate cash?
   b. Were uses of cash financed by appropriate sources?

**Goodwill Pharmacy**
**Balance Sheets for 12/31**

| | 20X0 | 20X1 | Change |
|---|---|---|---|
| Assets | | | |
| Cash | $178,943 | $ 153,380 | ($25,563) |
| Accounts receivable | 409,013 | 525,468 | 116,455 |
| Inventory | 284,985 | 286,525 | 1,540 |
| Prepaid expenses | 76,690 | 56,807 | (19,983) |
| Net property and equipment | 38,345 | 26,855 | (11,490) |
| Total assets | 987,976 | 1,049,035 | |
| Liabilities | | | |
| Accounts payable | 127,817 | 146,018 | 18,201 |
| Note payable (current) | 51,127 | 41,567 | (9,560) |
| Accrued expenses | 102,253 | 110,615 | 8,362 |
| Long-term debt | 148,267 | 135,485 | (12,782) |
| Total liabilities | 429,464 | 433,685 | |
| Owner equity | | | |
| Capital | 558,512 | 615,350 | 56,838 |
| Total liabilities and owner equity | $987,976 | $1,049,035 | |

**Goodwill Pharmacy**
**Income Statements**

| | 20X0 | 20X1 |
|---|---|---|
| Total sales | $2,556,332 | $2,840,368 |
| Cost of goods sold | 1,458,552 | 1,605,692 |
| Gross margin | 1,097,779 | 1,234,676 |
| Depreciation | 22,505 | 18,479 |
| Other expenses | 851,165 | 986,566 |
| Total expenses | 873,670 | 1,005,045 |
| Net income | $ 224,110 | $ 229,631 |

# Improving Cash Flow

After reading this chapter, the student should be able to:

1. Explain the cash flow cycle,
2. Explain how the following practices can improve cash flow:
   —proper control of inventory,
   —maintaining gross margin,
   —investing idle cash,
   —proper control of accounts receivable,
   —timing of purchases and payments, and
   —minimizing operating expenses, and
3. Monitor each of these practices to determine their effects on cash flow.

As emphasized in the last chapter, proper cash management is of vital importance to the operation of a pharmacy. The last chapter discussed means by which a manager could assess the pharmacy's cash flow. This chapter provides a framework that managers can use to improve cash flow.

Most authorities recommend thinking of cash flow as a cycle. A simplified cash flow cycle is shown in Figure 13-1. Cash flows out of the business to buy inventories. Inventories are then sold. This brings cash into the business. This simple scheme is complicated by several factors. First, the pharmacy usually buys inventory on credit. This creates a time lag between receipt of inventory and payment for it. Second, pharmacies frequently sell on credit. This creates a time lag between sale of merchandise and receipt of payment. Finally, cash flows out of the pharmacy to cover expenses such as salaries and utilities. Cash to cover these expenses must be generated from gross

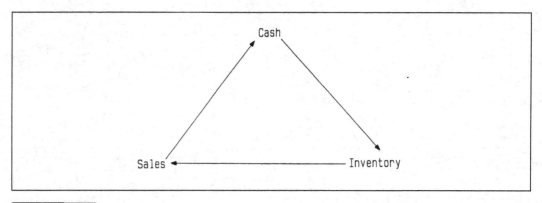

**FIGURE 13-1**    Simplified cash flow cycle.

margin. This more complex cash flow cycle is illustrated in Figure 13-2. (Much of what is referred to in this book as the cash flow cycle is referred to in institutional settings as the *revenue cycle*.)

The basic means of improving cash flow consist of decreasing the amount of cash invested in the pharmacy, slowing the amount and rate of cash flowing out of the pharmacy, and increasing the amount and rate of cash flowing in. Examining the cash flow cycle reveals six means by which this can be accomplished:

1. Properly controlling inventory
2. Maintaining gross margin
3. Investing idle cash
4. Properly controlling accounts receivable
5. Timing of purchases and payments
6. Minimizing operating expenses

## INVENTORY CONTROL

Proper inventory control consists of having only as much inventory as is needed, having the proper inventory, and minimizing shrinkage.

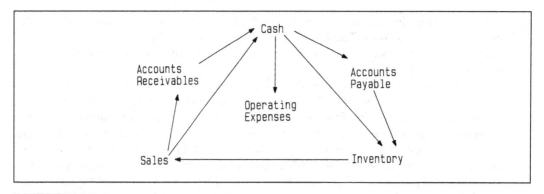

**FIGURE 13-2**    Realistic cash flow cycle.

## Inventory Size

A pharmacy that carries more inventory than it needs will have a larger amount of cash invested in inventory than is necessary to support sales. For example, a pharmacy that maintains a $100,000 inventory has $100,000 of cash invested in inventory. If the pharmacy could cut its inventory level to $75,000, it would free up $25,000 of cash and could decrease owner equity by $25,000. Although the total amount paid out for inventory purchases over the year would not change, the amount of cash that the pharmacy has invested would decrease substantially.

## Inventory Quality

Carrying the proper inventory has a similar effect. A large amount of unsalable inventory represents an unused source of cash. Unsalable inventory requires the same cash investment as salable merchandise. However, it decreases turnover and, therefore, increases total inventory investment. If possible, pharmacies should return unsalable merchandise for credit or for more salable merchandise. A credit would decrease cash outflow, whereas more salable merchandise would increase or speed up cash inflows.

## Shrinkage

Finally, shrinkage can hinder cash flow. *Shrinkage* refers to merchandise lost through breakage or theft. A high shrinkage rate indicates much lost merchandise. Because this merchandise must be paid for but generates no cash income, shrinkage has a direct and dramatic effect on cash flow.

## Monitoring Inventory

The inventory turnover ratio, which was discussed in Chapter 5, is a useful measure for monitoring inventory. A low inventory turnover may indicate either that the pharmacy has more inventory than it needs for its sales volume, that it has unsalable merchandise inventory, or both. The manager should monitor the inventory turnover ratio on a regular basis—monthly or weekly—to ensure that the pharmacy has an appropriate level and quality of inventory. The ratio needs to be monitored frequently, as do all ratios dealing with cash flow, because seasonal variations in sales can lead to seasonal variations in the amount of inventory (or accounts receivables or payables) needed. A decrease in the inventory turnover ratio indicates that the pharmacy may need to check the quality or decrease the size of inventory.

## MAINTAINING ADEQUATE GROSS MARGINS

The gross margin is the difference between the price at which pharmacies buy merchandise and the price at which they sell it. Consequently, the gross margin is the portion of sales that pharmacies have available to cover operating expenses and profits. Pharmacies must maintain adequate gross margins to ensure adequate cash flow.

Over the past several years, pharmacies have seen their gross margins decrease as competition has increased and as the proportion of reimbursement from third-party payers has grown. Consequently, pharmacies should pay close attention to their gross margins. Pharmacies can maintain, or improve, gross margins by emphasizing higher-margin products, carefully selecting the third-party contracts that they accept, reconciling third-party claims and payment, responding to suppliers' price increases in a timely manner, ensuring that payers are billed promptly, and decreasing product costs.

## Emphasize High-Margin Products

Pharmacies provide a range of products and services that differ in profit margins. Many community pharmacies sell house brands of popular over-the-counter (OTC) products. House brands contain the same active ingredients in the same dosages and dosage forms as name-brand products but are made or distributed by different companies and sold at much lower prices. For example, a local pharmacy sells "Top Care Nonaspirin Pain Reliever." This product contains the same active ingredients and is sold in the same dosage forms as Tylenol. The pharmacy makes a much higher gross margin on Top Care Nonaspirin Pain Reliever. Some pharmacies have found that certain lines of business—such as providing nursing home consulting services or durable medical equipment—are more profitable than other lines—such as dispensing. Long-term care pharmacies may find that patients with special needs—such as those requiring IV infusion services—are more profitable than their typical nursing home patients. In all of these cases, the pharmacy will increase its gross margin to the extent that it emphasizes the more profitable products and services.

## Selection of Third-Party Contracts

One of the major causes of decreasing gross margins in pharmacies is the growth of third-party reimbursement for pharmacy products and services. Third-party payers, such as insurance companies and managed-care organizations, almost always pay the pharmacy less than cash-paying patients. In addition, reimbursement rates vary substantially among third-party payers. Third-party dispensing fees, for example, can vary from zero (that is, no fee) to $4 or $5 per prescription. A pharmacy must carefully select among these programs if it is to maintain an adequate gross margin.

## Reconciling Third-Party Claims and Payments

The vast majority of pharmacies' prescription sales are reimbursed by third-party payers. It is not unusual for third-party payers to pay pharmacies less than the pharmacies have billed. This occurs when third party payers deny third-party claims or pay less than the pharmacy has billed them. Sometimes these denials or underpayments are made as a result of a mistake made by the third-party. Sometimes they are made because the pharmacy has submitted incomplete or erroneous patient or prescription information. In either case, pharmacies need to carefully compare and reconcile third-party claims and payments to determine why they were not reimbursed the full amount billed. In many cases, pharmacies can resubmit corrected or incorrectly denied claims and receive full reimbursement.

## Price Increases

A practice that causes cash flow problems for many pharmacies is that of not immediately passing on manufacturers' price increases to consumers. When merchandise costs the pharmacy more—due to manufacturers' price increases—and the pharmacy does not increase its prices to the consumer or third-party payer, its gross margin decreases. The decrease in gross margin reduces the amount of cash flowing into the pharmacy. This can be prevented by simply increasing prices to patients and payers as soon as suppliers initiate price increases. Because most pharmacy pricing and billing is now done by computer, this becomes a matter of updating drug costs in the pharmacy computer as quickly as possible.

## Billing

In most community pharmacies, making sure that payers are billed for all medications dispensed is not a major problem. This is because most pharmacies and payers are electronically linked so that third-party prescription claims can be adjudicated before the prescription is dispensed. *Claims adjudication* is the process by which each prescription is electronically checked by the third-party payer to ensure that both patient and prescription product are covered by the third-party, that the appropriate quantity is dispensed, that the pharmacy knows the appropriate copay to collect from the patient, and that the third-party agrees to pay the claim. In the vast majority of cases, this is done electronically as part of the normal dispensing process and before the prescription is dispensed to the patient.

Pharmacies may also subscribe to online services that perform additional edits to ensure that the pharmacy has not charged less than the amount to which it is entitled. This is useful because of the complexities of prescription pricing and the large number of third-party plans with which a typical pharmacy deals.

In institutional settings, dispensing and payment may not be as closely linked. In these situations, it is important that pharmacists document all prescriptions dispensed in such a way that the business office can send bills for the proper amount to the appropriate payer. In many institutional settings, this is referred to as *charge capture*.

## Product Costs

Decreasing the cost of products will, all other things equal, result in increased gross margins. Pharmacies can decrease product costs by taking cash discounts, searching out and utilizing the lowest-cost sources, and participating in buying groups. Pharmacies that have strong formularies, such as those in certain hospitals, long-term care facilities, health maintenance organization (HMOs), and mail-order facilities, can lower costs by negotiating larger discounts and rebates from manufacturers in return for including their products on formularies.

## Monitoring Gross Margin

Pharmacy managers can monitor gross margin through use of the gross margin percent ratio. In some pharmacies, the gross margin percent can be calculated for different lines of products. For example, pharmacies may calculate the gross margin percent for prescription products, for third-party prescriptions, for cash prescriptions, for home health care products, and for front merchandise. This allows the pharmacy manager to better monitor and control the gross margin of each line of products.

## INVESTING IDLE CASH

The typical pharmacy will have periods during the year when it needs more cash than it has and periods when it has more cash than it needs. The pharmacy can improve both profitability and cash flow by investing excess cash in interest-bearing accounts.

## Effects of Investing

The effects of investing idle cash can best be illustrated through use of an example. Assume that Cashmo Pharmacy has a balance of $25,000 in its cash account. Further, assume that Cashmo requires a cash balance of only $5,000 to operate. Thus, it has $20,000 of excess cash. This will not add to cash flow or profit if it is simply left in a checking account that pays no interest. However, it would contribute to both if invested in an interest-bearing account. Assume, for example, that the excess $20,000 is invested in a money market account paying 6% annual interest. That is about $\frac{1}{2}$% interest a month (it would be different depending on the compounding of interest, but $\frac{1}{2}$% a month is close enough for an example). Investment of the $20,000 of excess cash would earn $100 of interest each month. This would improve both cash flow and net profit.

## Selecting an Investment

The manager must consider risk, return, and liquidity when deciding where to invest excess cash.

The manager will want an investment with low risk if the excess cash will be needed to operate the pharmacy later in the year. Or, to put it another way, the manager will want to be sure that the investment will not be lost. As a general rule, common stocks are very risky.

Government-backed bonds and money market accounts are less risky. Bank savings accounts are virtually risk free.

The manager will also want a liquid investment. A liquid investment is one that can be rapidly, readily, and cheaply converted to cash. Savings accounts and many money market accounts are very liquid. They can be converted to cash on demand. Certificates of deposit are less liquid. They require that the cash remain in the account for some specified, minimum amount of time (e.g., a quarter or year) before interest will be paid. If the manager can accurately predict when the pharmacy will need the excess cash, then the lower liquidity of certificates of deposit is not a problem. Common stocks can be easily and rapidly converted to cash, but the conversion must be handled by a stock broker who will normally charge a fee for selling the stock.

A manager must also consider the potential return on the investment. As a general rule, the higher the *potential* return, the higher the risk associated with an investment. Common stocks offer the potential for a very high return. However, they are frequently risky; although there is the opportunity for a very high return, there is also opportunity to lose one's entire investment. Savings accounts offer lower, but surer, returns. When a manager is investing idle cash that will be needed later in the year, achieving a high return is less important than low risk and high liquidity.

A variety of investments offer acceptable risk and liquidity with a reasonable return. Examples include money market accounts, Treasury bills, bonds, and bank commercial paper. Accountants and bankers can aid in determining which is best for a particular pharmacy.

## ACCOUNTS RECEIVABLE MANAGEMENT

Operating a credit program hinders a pharmacy's cash flow in a number of ways. First, the pharmacy must invest a substantial amount of cash in the program. This is a long-term investment. As long as the pharmacy continues to offer credit, the initial investment will remain tied up in accounts receivable. If, for example, the pharmacy's average accounts receivable balance is $50,000, at some point, the pharmacy has invested $50,000 to finance its credit program. The pharmacy will continue to have $50,000 tied up in the credit program for as long as the accounts receivable balance stays at or above $50,000.

A basic cost of any investment is an *opportunity cost*. The opportunity cost of an investment is the amount that could be made on the next best investment. The opportunity cost of a credit program is at least as great as the interest that the pharmacy could earn by investing the cash tied up in the program in some interest-bearing account of comparable risk. For example, if the pharmacy has $50,000 in accounts receivable and long-term bonds pay 12% annually, the pharmacy has an opportunity cost for accounts receivable of at least $500 per month ($50,000 × 1% monthly interest = $500 monthly interest). This is the amount the pharmacy *could have made* if it had invested the $50,000 in a long-term bond rather than in a credit program.

Second, a credit program slows the rate of cash flowing into the pharmacy. Rather than receiving cash at the time of the sale, as it does with cash sales, the pharmacy must wait several weeks or months before receiving payment for credit sales.

Third, the pharmacy incurs a number of costs in operating a credit program. These include the costs of mailing bills, keeping records of charges and payments, and paying someone to do these tasks. Finally, most credit programs experience some bad debt.

## Minimizing Investment in Accounts Receivable

A pharmacy can minimize its opportunity costs, as well as the amount of bad debt it incurs, by minimizing the amount of cash it has invested in accounts receivable. This can be done by speeding up the collection of accounts receivable and by taking steps to minimize bad debt.

Application of the following procedures will minimize cash invested in accounts receivable.

1. Carefully screen credit applicants. Require customers to complete a credit application and have the applications checked by the local credit bureau before granting credit. This will decrease the number of nonpayers and late payers to whom credit is granted. To the extent possible, pharmacies should also screen third-party payers before they sign contracts with them. It is not unknown for third-party payers to go bankrupt and leave pharmacies with substantial amounts of unpaid prescription claims. Similarly, pharmacies should verify patients' eligibility for third-party payment before providing products or services to them. Patients frequently lose eligibility in third-party programs in which they have been enrolled as a result of changing insurers, changing jobs (most private health insurance is provided through one's employer), or, in the case of Medicaid, experiencing changes in financial status.

2. Send out bills promptly and regularly. Customers, both individual patients and third-party payers, will not pay until they get a bill.

3. Add a finance charge to overdue accounts. A finance charge is some extra amount that customers must pay if they do not pay their bills on time. Typically, the finance charge is some set percentage of the outstanding balance. Visa and Mastercard, for example, usually charge between 1% and 2% per month on unpaid balances. Use of a finance charge gives customers an incentive to pay on time.

4.  Follow up overdue accounts. The manager should increase the severity of his or her actions as the amount of time the account is past due increases. Actions could escalate from simply contacting accounts overdue for short periods, to revoking credit to accounts overdue for longer periods, to turning chronically overdue accounts over to a collection agency or taking them to court.

## Monitoring Accounts Receivable

The accounts receivables collection period is a ratio that indicates the average length of time it takes the pharmacy to collect for purchases made on credit by its customers. The manager should monitor this ratio weekly or monthly to assess how well accounts receivables are managed.

## TIMING OF PURCHASES AND PAYMENTS

A pharmacy can also improve cash flow by slowing payments to suppliers. Bills should be paid soon enough to receive cash discounts but no sooner. Paying early has the same effect as lending money to suppliers at no interest.

Cash flow may be improved by careful timing of purchases. For example, assume that a supplier closes his or her books and sends bills on the 25th of each month and that payment is due within 30 days of billing (or by the 25th of the following month). If the pharmacy orders on the 24th of June, the bill will be sent the next day and the pharmacy will have 30 days to pay. If the pharmacy orders on the 26th, the bill will not be sent until the 25th of July. This will give the pharmacy 59 days to pay. So, by ordering 2 days later, the pharmacy has use of its cash for an additional 29 days.

The accounts payable period ratio measures how quickly the pharmacy pays its suppliers for purchases made on credit. The pharmacy manager can use this ratio to monitor the pharmacy's performance at properly timing purchases and payments.

## DECREASING EXPENSES

Most expenses represent cash that must be paid out. If the pharmacy can decrease these expenses, it will pay out less cash. This, obviously, will improve cash flow. The income statement shows the dollar level of expenses and also expenses as a percent of sales. The manager should make sure that this measure is available not only for total expenses, but also for each of the pharmacy's major expenses. These might include, for example, rent, pharmacist salaries, technician salaries, computer expenses, and delivery expenses.

## AN EXAMPLE

Caremed Infusion Services has an impending cash flow problem. A large local health maintenance organization (HMO) has renegotiated its contract with Caremed. To keep the HMO's business, Caremed had to discount its fees. Caremed's manager estimates that this will reduce the pharmacy's gross margin from 64% to 62%. The reduced gross margin will have a major, negative effect on Caremed's cash flow.

Figure 13-3 shows Caremed's cash budget after taking account of the lower gross margin. As is obvious from this information, Caremed's manager must improve the

| Sales Forecast | Apr | May | June | July | Aug | Sep | Oct | Nov | Dec | Jan |
|---|---|---|---|---|---|---|---|---|---|---|
| Cash sales (3%) | 2,100 | 2,460 | 2,640 | 3,180 | 2,100 | 2,640 | 3,720 | 2,760 | 2,700 | 2,250 |
| Credit sales (97%) | 67,900 | 79,540 | 85,360 | 102,820 | 67,900 | 85,360 | 120,280 | 89,240 | 87,300 | 72,750 |
| Total sales | 70,000 | 82,000 | 88,000 | 106,000 | 70,000 | 88,000 | 124,000 | 92,000 | 90,000 | 75,000 |
| Cash receipts | | | | | | | | | | |
| Cash sales (this month) | | | | 3,180 | 2,100 | 2,640 | 3,720 | 2,760 | 2,700 | |
| 25% of last month's credit sales | | | | 21,340 | 25,705 | 16,975 | 21,340 | 30,070 | 22,310 | |
| 35% of credit sales 2 months ago | | | | 27,839 | 29,876 | 35,987 | 23,765 | 29,876 | 42,098 | |
| 35% of credit sales 3 months ago | | | | 23,765 | 27,839 | 29,876 | 35,987 | 23,765 | 29,876 | |
| Total monthly cash receipts | | | | 76,124 | 85,520 | 85,478 | 84,812 | 86,471 | 96,984 | |
| Cash payments | | | | | | | | | | |
| Purchases (38% of next month's sales) | | | | 26,600 | 33,440 | 47,120 | 34,960 | 34,200 | 28,500 | |
| Salaries | | | | 37,000 | 37,000 | 37,000 | 37,000 | 37,000 | 37,000 | |
| Other expenses (17% of monthly sales) | | | | 18,020 | 11,900 | 14,960 | 21,080 | 15,640 | 15,300 | |
| Total monthly cash payments | | | | 81,620 | 82,340 | 99,080 | 93,040 | 86,840 | 80,800 | |
| Monthly cash gain (loss) | | | | (5,496) | 3,180 | (13,602) | (8,228) | (369) | 16,184 | |
| Financing | | | | | | | | | | |
| Cash balance: beginning of month | | | | 5,000 | 5,504 | 5,684 | 5,082 | 5,854 | 5,485 | |
| Monthly cash gain (loss) | | | | (5,496) | 3,180 | (13,602) | (8,228) | (369) | 16,184 | |
| Cash balance: end of month before financing | | | | (496) | 8,684 | (7,918) | (3,146) | 5,485 | 21,669 | |
| Borrowing | | | | 6,000 | 0 | 13,000 | 9,000 | 0 | 0 | |
| Repayment | | | | 0 | 3,000 | 0 | 0 | 0 | 16,000 | |
| Cash balance: end of month after financing | | | | 5,504 | 5,684 | 5,082 | 5,854 | 5,485 | 5,669 | |
| Cumulative borrowing | | | | 6,000 | 3,000 | 16,000 | 25,000 | 25,000 | 9,000 | |

FIGURE 13-3 Cash budget for Caremed Infusion Services (reflects decrease in gross margin).

| | Jul | Aug | Sept | Oct | Nov | Dec |
|---|---|---|---|---|---|---|
| No changes | 6,000 | 3,000 | 16,000 | 25,000 | 25,000 | 9,000 |
| Decreased expenses[a] | 4,000 | 0 | 12,000 | 19,000 | 18,000 | 0 |
| Decreased inventory[b] | 1,000 | 0 | 11,000 | 20,000 | 20,000 | 4,000 |
| Improved accounts receivables management[c] | 4,000 | 0 | 11,000 | 18,000 | 14,000 | 0 |
| Improved accounts payables management[d] | 0 | 0 | 0 | 0 | 0 | 0 |

[a]Expenses are decreased from 17% to 15.5% of sales.
[b]Inventory is decreased by $5,000. The $5,000 freed up is then added to the pharmacy's cash balance.
[c]Bad debt is reduced from 5% to 2% of credit sales. Collections of accounts receivables are made sooner. The original budget assumed 25% of credit sales collected the month following the sale, 35% collected 2 months after the sale, and 35% collected 3 months after the sale. The revised budget assumes 30% collected the month after the sale, 35% collected 2 months after the sale, and 32% collected 3 months after the sale.
[d]Assumes that payment for merchandise purchases can be made the same month the merchandise is sold rather than the month before it is sold.

**FIGURE 13-4** Cumulative borrowing for Caremed Infusion Services following improvements in cash flow.

business's cash flow. To do so, she examines each of the areas we have discussed, considers how Caremed could make improvements in that area, and then uses the cash budget to estimate the effect of the improvements. The improvements and their estimated effects on cash flow are discussed below. Figure 13-4 summarizes the effects on cash flow by showing the cumulative borrowing for each improvement.

## Pricing and Maintaining Gross Margin

Almost all of Caremed's reimbursement comes from third-party payers. Caremed is not able to negotiate reimbursement rates with third-party payers. (In fact, Caremed's cash flow problem is a result of its inability to negotiate rates.) Caremed also believes that it is buying products at the lowest possible cost. Consequently, improving cash flow by increasing gross margin is not possible.

## Investing Idle Cash

The cash budget indicates that Caremed will have no idle cash during the coming 6 months. Therefore, investment of idle cash is not a reasonable means of improving Caremed's cash flow.

## Decreasing Expenses

The manager could decrease expenses by eliminating proposed salary increases for the budget period. This would decrease expenses from 17% to 15.5% of sales. As shown in Figure 13-4, this would resolve much of the pharmacy's cash flow problem. It would also be extremely detrimental to employee morale.

## Inventory Control

The pharmacy currently maintains a $50,000 inventory of pharmaceuticals. The manager thinks she may be able to cut the inventory by $5,000 by ordering more frequently and by eliminating some slower-moving products. If she is able to do so, the $5,000 of decreased investment in inventory can be added to the pharmacy's cash account. If this is done during June, the pharmacy's cash balance at the beginning of July (the first month of the budget period) will increase from $5,000 to $10,000. The increased cash balance decreases the amount that has to be borrowed each month (Fig. 13-4). However, the pharmacy will still need to borrow heavily.

## Accounts Receivables

The manager next considers tighter management of accounts receivables. More attention to billing on time, verifying patients' insurance status before providing services, and following up overdue accounts and denied claims should increase the rate of payment and decrease bad debt. She estimates that improvements in these areas would result in 30% of accounts receivables being collected the month after the sale, 35% being collected 2 months after the sale, and 32% being collected 3 months after the sale. As shown in Figure 13-4, these changes would have a dramatic effect on Caremed's cash flow. If the changes can be made, Caremed can pay off all borrowing by the end of the budget period.

## Timing of Purchases and Payments

Currently, Caremed purchases and pays for merchandise 1 month in advance of using it. The manager believes that tighter inventory control and paying more attention to when orders are placed would allow Caremed to pay for merchandise in the same month it is sold.

This would have two effects on cash flow. First, it would improve cash flow by decreasing the time between when the pharmacy paid for merchandise and when it sold and received payment for it. Second, it would result in the pharmacy having no purchase payments for 1 month. If the pharmacy successfully implemented the changes during June, for example, it would have no purchase payments in July. Why? Because merchandise for July's sales (under the current system of payment) is purchased and paid for in June. So, when July comes, the pharmacy will already have on hand and have paid for the merchandise needed in July. Under the new system of payment, merchandise for August's sales will not be paid for until August. Thus, no payment is required in July. The change in time of payment will have a major effect on cash flow; it will eliminate the need to borrow during the budget period (Fig. 13-4).

## Decision

After considering the effects of various improvements on the pharmacy's cash flow, the manager decides to concentrate on changing the timing of purchases and payments. This would eliminate much of the pharmacy's cash flow problems, eliminate the need for borrowing for the budget period, and cause the fewest disruptions to the pharmacy's workflow and workforce.

### Suggested Readings

Gagnon JP. Management of the community pharmacy: cash flow. In: Management Handbook for Pharmacy Practitioners. Chapel Hill, NC: Health Sciences Consortium, 1982.

Helfert EA. Managing operating funds. In: Financial Analysis Tools and Techniques: A Guide for Managers. New York: McGraw-Hill, 2001.

Henningsen J. Many happy returns: reverse distributors ease the pain associated with the reclamation and destruction of expired products. Drug Topics 2003;148(1):70.

Hunter RH. Accounts receivable management in the community pharmacy. In: Management Handbook for Pharmacy Practitioners. Chapel Hill, NC. Health Sciences Consortium, 1982.

Reeder CE, Dickson WM, Nelson AA Jr. Improve profitability with efficient cash management. Apothecary 1982;Sept/Oct:34.

Slezak M. Kmart exec outlines reconciliation system. Am Druggist 1997;214(4):24.

Vecchione A. Why managers should monitor revenue cycles. Drug Topics 2005;150(19)

## QUESTIONS

1. Which of the following types of investments would be most appropriate for a pharmacy to invest idle cash in?
   a. A common stock that, for the last 6 months, has yielded a return of 18% and on which the return has varied from 35% to a negative 10%.
   b. A certificate of deposit with a 1-year maturity (i.e., the cash must be left in for a minimum of 1 year to draw interest) and an interest rate of 12%.
   c. A savings account paying 6% interest and having no set maturity (i.e., cash can be deposited and withdrawn with no loss of interest).
2. Pharmacies offer credit to their customers with the expectation that the offer of credit will improve which of the following?
   a. Cash flow
   b. Sales
   c. Both a and b

For questions 3–5 please indicate the effect that each action will have on the pharmacy's cash flow:

3. The pharmacy institutes a 10% senior citizen discount program.
4. The pharmacy decides to participate in the state Medicaid prescription program.
5. The pharmacy closes the accounts of several customers who habitually pay their accounts late.

## CHAPTER 14

# Inventory

After reading this chapter, the student should be able to:

1. Define and give examples of the four types of inventory costs,
2. Define and give examples of opportunity costs,
3. Calculate the quantity of an item that should be ordered to minimize the total costs of inventory and determine the point at which an order should be placed,
4. Define and give the formula for the economic order quantity,
5. Calculate the total costs of carrying an item in inventory,
6. Define safety stock and discuss the factors that determine how large safety stock should be,
7. Explain the concept of ABC inventory analysis and discuss its use in inventory control,
8. Use gross margin return on investment to determine which items and lines to add to inventory, and
9. Explain how generic and therapeutic interchange, bid purchasing, and prime vendors are used to control inventory.

nventory control is of vital importance to pharmacies of all types. As indicated earlier in the book, inventory is typically a pharmacy's largest asset. Because so much is invested in inventory, proper inventory control has a strong and direct effect on a pharmacy's return on investment. Effective control results in smaller investment. For a given profit, this leads to a greater return on investment.

Inventory control is also important because a pharmacy must have the proper inventory to serve its patients. It must have those products that patients need in the quantities in which they need them. This aspect of inventory control is much harder to quantify and control, but equally important. If a community pharmacy does not have the products that its patients need at the time they need them, it will lose sales. If this happens frequently, the pharmacy will lose patients. If a hospital pharmacy does not have a needed item, the consequence can range from inconvenience—for items not needed immediately—to physical harm to patients in need of life-saving emergency drugs.

Thus, effective inventory control consists of optimizing two goals: minimizing total inventory investment and carrying the right mix of products to satisfy patient demand. This chapter will emphasize minimizing investment. This is not to imply that minimizing investment is the more important goal. Carrying the right mix of merchandise is equally important. The chapter will emphasize minimizing investment because that is the goal to which financial analysis can be applied. The task of selecting the appropriate products to carry is based on marketing considerations and is, consequently, less amenable to financial analysis.

As a result of computerization, inventory control systems in many pharmacies have become highly sophisticated. Computerized systems can maintain perpetual control of inventory. That is, inventory, cost of goods sold, and sales figures for individual products are updated constantly as purchases and sales are made. The result is that the computer keeps a continual count of the number of units of each product that the pharmacy has on hand. Many computerized systems calculate the quantities of products that need to be reordered based on past product usage. Some are sufficiently sophisticated to make seasonal adjustments to the quantities that need to be ordered. Most can generate and submit orders and provide detailed reports indicating the fastest- and slowest-selling products.[1-3] While a discussion of these systems is beyond the scope of this book, the principles on which they are based are the same ones discussed in this chapter.

## INVENTORY COSTS

There are four types of inventory costs: acquisition costs, carrying costs, procurement costs, and stockout costs.

A product's *acquisition cost* is the amount the pharmacy pays for the product. For example, if the pharmacy buys a bottle of cimetidine for $50 with no discount, then the acquisition cost is $50.

*Carrying costs* include all costs associated with carrying and maintaining inventories. They include such costs as obsolescence, deterioration, storage, inventory taxes, and insurance. The major component of carrying costs is the *opportunity cost* of the capital invested in inventory.

The opportunity cost of any investment is equal to the amount that could have been made by investing in the next best alternative of comparable risk. For a pharmacy, the opportunity cost of investing in inventory is the amount the pharmacy could have made by investing in some other asset instead. For example, if a pharmacy had $80,000 invested in inventory, and if it could have realized an annual return of 15% in some other investment of comparable risk (such as common stock), then the opportunity cost of carrying inventory would be equal to $80,000 × .15 = $12,000 per year. Carrying costs are usually expressed as a percentage of average inventory value. Most sources estimate annual carrying costs to be between 20% and 30%. So, for a pharmacy with an inventory valued at $75,000, inventory carrying costs would amount to $15,000 to $22,500 per year.

For a given annual usage of a product, carrying costs increase as the size of the average order increases and as the number of orders per year decreases. Making fewer, larger orders results in higher average inventory. Carrying costs (in dollar terms) are greater for larger inventories.

*Procurement costs* are costs of ordering and receiving goods. Procurement costs are also called ordering costs. They include the costs of placing the order; receiving, pricing, and placing goods in stock; and processing payment. Procurement costs are usually expressed as a dollar amount per order.

For a given annual usage of a product, procurement costs decrease as average order size increases and as the number of orders decreases. Hence, procurement costs would be minimized if only one order per year was placed and the size of that order was equal to the pharmacy's annual usage.

*Stockout costs* are the costs associated with being out of an item a patient needs or wants. The size of stockout costs is difficult to estimate. At minimum, it is the embarrassment and frustration of explaining to a patient or prescriber that the pharmacy is out of the item needed. At maximum, it is the cost of losing all a patient's future purchases or, in the case of life-saving emergency drugs, of causing physical harm to the patient.

## BASIC INVENTORY CONTROL QUESTIONS

Effective inventory control consists of finding correct answers to three questions:

1.  How much of an item should be ordered at one time?
2.  When should the item be reordered?
3.  How much attention should each item receive?

### How Much to Order?

The first problem in effective inventory control is determining how much of an item to order at one time. The quantity ordered should be the quantity that will minimize total inventory costs. The total cost of inventory is defined as:

$$TC = AC + CC + PC$$

where TC = total inventory costs,
     AC = acquisition costs,
     CC = carrying costs, and
     PC = procurement costs.

Stockout costs are not included. This is because the formula assumes a known and constant demand for the product and a known and constant lead time. *Demand* refers to the amount of the item the pharmacy's patients will purchase during some period of time. *Lead time* is the period of time required to place and receive an order. Lead time includes the time it takes the pharmacy to recognize that an order is needed, to process and place the order, to receive the order from the supplier, and to place it in inventory. There should never be a stockout if both demand and lead time are known and constant. The assumption of known and constant demand and lead time is unrealistic and will be dealt with later in the chapter.

The components of the total cost formula are calculated as follows:

$$AC = D \times C$$

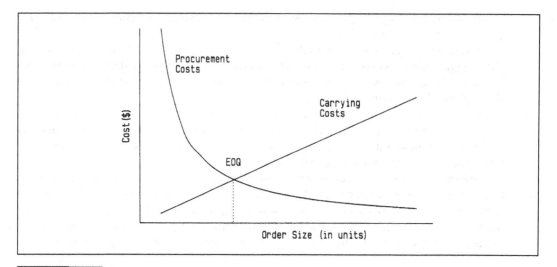

**FIGURE 14-1**    Inventory costs as a function of order size.

where D = annual demand for the item in units, and
      C = acquisition cost per unit.

$$PC = (D/Q) \times S$$

where Q = order size in units, and
      S = procurement cost per order.

$$CC = (Q/2) \times C \times I$$

where I = the carrying cost expressed as a percentage rate of interest.

As these formulas point out, procurement costs decrease and carrying costs increase as order size increases. A graph of this relationship is shown in Figure 14-1.

In deciding how much of an item to order at one time, the goal is to minimize total inventory costs. Total costs are minimized at the order size at which carrying costs are equal to procurement costs (Fig. 14-1). This order size can be calculated using the economic order quantity (EOQ) formula. The EOQ, which is the order size that minimizes total inventory costs, is calculated as:

$$EOQ = Q' = SQRT\ (2DS/CI)$$

where SQRT = square root,
          D = annual demand in units,
          S = procurement cost per order,
          I = the carrying cost interest rate, and
          C = acquisition cost per unit.

## An EOQ Example

St. Mary's Hospital Pharmacy uses 10,000 vials of Ceflyn per year. Ceflyn costs $50 per vial. St. Mary's estimates its carrying cost interest rate at 20% and its procurement cost to be $25 per order. The pharmacy director needs to know the order size (that is, how much she should order at one time) to minimize total inventory costs. The EOQ formula can be used to calculate this quantity:

$$EOQ = Q' = SQRT\ (2DS/CI)$$
$$= SQRT\ [(2 \times 10,000 \times \$25)/(\$50 \times .20)]$$
$$= 224\ vials$$

So, to minimize total inventory costs, St. Mary's should order 224 vials per order and place $10,000 / 224 = 45$ orders per year. We can use the total inventory cost formula to see that this really is the quantity that minimizes costs.

First, we compute the total costs of carrying Ceflyn at the EOQ. This is calculated as:

$$TC = AC + CC + PC$$
$$= (DC) + (Q/2) \times CI + (D/Q)S$$
$$= (10,000 \times 50) + (224/2) \times 50 \times .20 + (10,000/224) \times 25$$
$$= 500,000 + 1120 + 1116$$
$$= \$502,236$$

Next, we can check to see if the EOQ actually does minimize total inventory costs by calculating total costs at order sizes above and below the EOQ. First, we calculate total inventory costs for an order size of 500 vials:

$$TC = AC + CC + PC$$
$$TC = 10,000 \times \$50 + (500/2) \times \$50 + 0.2 + (10,000/500) \times \$25$$
$$TC = \$500,000 + \$2,500 + \$500$$
$$TC = \$503,000$$

Then we calculate total costs for an order size of 100 vials:

$$TC = AC + CC + PC$$
$$TC = 10,000 \times \$50 + (100/2) \times \$50 \times 0.2 + (10,000/100) + \$25$$
$$TC = \$500,000 + \$500 + \$2,500$$
$$TC = \$503,000$$

So, we see that ordering the EOQ does minimize total inventory costs.

## EOQ with Quantity Discounts

The situation is more complicated when quantity discounts are offered. In the normal case considered, the acquisition cost stays the same regardless of the quantity ordered. When quantity discounts are offered, the acquisition cost decreases when greater quantities are ordered. This, obviously, will affect total inventory costs.

There is a simple way to determine the quantity to order when quantity discounts are offered. First, calculate the EOQ using the nondiscounted price. If the EOQ is larger than the quantity needed to obtain the discount, then the EOQ is the order size that will minimize total costs. In this case, no further calculations are necessary. If, as frequently happens, the EOQ is smaller than the quantity required to get the discount, the following procedure must be used.

First, calculate the total costs of inventory using the EOQ at the nondiscounted price. Next, calculate total costs using the discounted price and the minimum order size required to obtain the discount. The quantity that minimizes total costs is the one that should be ordered.

## An Example of EOQ When Quantity Discounts Are Offered

In the example given earlier, St. Mary's Pharmacy's director found that the EOQ for Ceflyn was 224 vials and that using this order quantity resulted in total inventory costs of $502,236. Now, suppose the manufacturer of Ceflyn offered a 5% discount on orders of 1,000 vials or greater. Should St. Mary's take the discount?

The director knows that the EOQ at the nondiscounted price is 224 vials. This is less than the quantity required to obtain the discount. Consequently, she must compute the total costs using 1,000 as the order size and $47.50 as the discounted price ($50 less 5% yields the discounted price of $47.50).

$$
\begin{aligned}
TC &= AC + CC + PC \\
&= (DC) + (Q/2) \times CI + (D/Q) \times S \\
&= 10,000 \times \$47.50 + (1,000/2) \times \$47.50 \times 0.2 + 10,000/1,000 \times \$25 \\
&= \$475,000 + \$4,750 + \$250 \\
&= \$480,000
\end{aligned}
$$

The total costs are less using the larger order size and the discounted price. Consequently, the director should order 1,000 vials per order to obtain the discount and minimize total costs of Ceflyn.

## When to Reorder?

If demand and lead time were both known and constant, the question of when to reorder would be simple. The reorder point could be calculated as:

$$ROP = LD \times DD$$

where ROP = reorder point,
LD = lead time in days, and
DD = demand in units per day.

For example, continuing the St. Mary's example, assume that demand is 28 vials per day. That is, St. Mary's uses 28 vials per day every day. It never uses more or less; the demand is a constant 28 vials per day. Also assume that lead time is always 5 days. That is, it always takes 5 days to place and receive an order. In this situation, the order point would be:

$$
\begin{aligned}
ROP &= LD \times DD \\
&= 28 \text{ vials per day} \times 5 \text{ days} \\
&= 140 \text{ vials}
\end{aligned}
$$

In other words, when St. Mary's inventory of Ceflyn decreases to 140 vials, an order should be placed. Five days later, the order would be delivered just as the inventory decreased to zero. This situation is shown graphically in Figure 14-2.

Unfortunately, neither lead time nor demand is likely to be constant. Some days St. Mary's may use considerably more than 28 vials of Ceflyn. Other days, it may use none. Sometimes the order may come in 4 days; other times it may take 6 or 7 days. Because of the normal variability in both demand and lead time, the pharmacy must

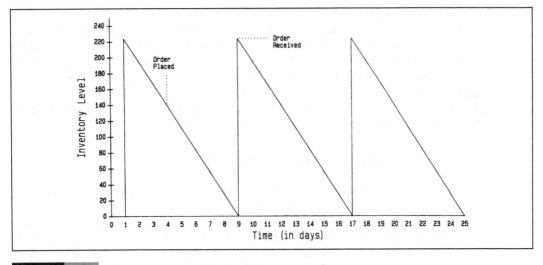

**FIGURE 14-2** Changes in inventory levels between orders.

maintain a *buffer* or *safety stock*. The safety stock is additional inventory, above the reorder point, that is maintained to cover the pharmacy in case demand is greater than expected or lead time is longer than expected.

The reorder point formula when either demand or lead time is not constant is calculated as:

$$ROP = (LD \times DD) + SS$$

where ROP = reorder point,
    LD = lead time in days,
    DD = demand in units per day, and
    SS = safety stock in units.

The situation of a reorder point with safety stock is shown in Figure 14-3. The reorder point for St. Mary's Hospital Pharmacy for Ceflyn would then be greater than

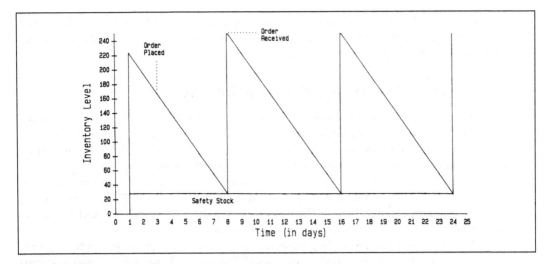

**FIGURE 14-3** Changes in inventory levels between orders when a safety stock is kept.

140 vials because of the need for a safety stock. The amount of safety stock needed depends on the variability in lead time and demand and the stockout costs associated with the product. Products with more erratic demand or lead time require greater safety stocks. Products with high stockout costs—such as drugs needed for emergency treatment of serious conditions—also require greater safety stocks. Safety stocks can be smaller when lead time and demand are less variable or when stockout costs are smaller. Levin et al. present a procedure for calculating the required level of safety stock based on historical variations in lead time and demand.[4]

## An Alternative Method—Fixed Review Periods

The methods of calculating reorder points just presented assume that inventory is constantly reviewed and that, consequently, orders can be placed whenever needed. Some pharmacies, such as chain pharmacies that order from chain warehouses, use *fixed review periods* for inventory. This means that inventory is reviewed and ordered at fixed time intervals. For example, a pharmacy may only check (or review) inventory and place orders once per week. If the quantity on hand is greater than the reorder point, no order is placed. If the quantity on hand is less than the reorder point, a sufficient quantity is ordered to bring the quantity on hand up to the reorder point.

The reorder point in a fixed review period system must be sufficient to cover not only product usage during the lead time, but also the amount of product that will be used between review periods. The reorder point must include this quantity because orders are placed only at the set review times. Thus, the reorder point for a fixed review period is higher than it would be in a system in which inventory were constantly reviewed.

For example, assume that Eckro Pharmacy places an order once weekly and that orders are usually received 3 days after they are placed. Further assume that Eckro uses, on average, two bottles of cimetidine per day and keeps a safety stock of six bottles. The reorder point for cimetidine is calculated as:

$$ROP = (LD \times DD) + SS + (RP \times DD), \text{ where RP is the review period in days}$$
$$= (3 \times 2) + 6 + (7 \times 2)$$
$$= 26 \text{ bottles}$$

If the quantity of cimetidine on hand were greater than 26 bottles, no order would be placed. If the quantity on hand were, say, 12 bottles then the greater of the EOQ – 12 or 26 – 12 bottles would be ordered.

## How Much Attention Should an Item Receive?

A typical pharmacy carries thousands of items. However, the great majority of a pharmacy's sales come from a much smaller number of items. These items need to be identified and carefully monitored. ABC inventory analysis is a way of determining which products merit frequent monitoring and which require monitoring less frequently.

According to the ABC system, all items in inventory are classified into one of three categories: "A" items represent 20% of items in inventory and 70% of total sales, "B" items represent 30% of items in inventory and 20% of total sales, and "C" items represent 50% of items but only about 10% of total sales.

"A" items consist of fast-selling products and, in some cases, very expensive products. There are few "A" items in a pharmacy's inventory. However, because they are high-demand, fast-moving products (or because they are very expensive), "A" items account for the majority of the pharmacy's sales. "A" items should be carefully monitored; reorder points and EOQs should be recalculated at least quarterly and inventory should be checked at least weekly. Certain other items—such as life-saving emergency drugs carried by hospital pharmacies—also demand close control even though they are not "A" items.

"B" and "C" items are slower-selling products. "B" items have average sales and inventory turnover. "C" items are the slowest-selling, least demanded products. Because "B" and "C" products constitute a much larger number of items and a smaller proportion of sales, it is not necessary, nor would it be efficient, to monitor them as closely as "A" items. For example, if the inventory of "A" items is monitored weekly, then "B" items should be checked every 2 weeks and "C" items every month.

Managers should periodically monitor "C" items to determine whether they should be dropped from stock. Dropping the slower-selling "C" items is a practical method of decreasing the number of items and dollar investment in inventory while having a minimal effect on sales and stockout costs. Typically, chain pharmacies carry few "C" items. As a result, they are able to attain higher inventory turnover and return on inventory investment.

Products can be classified as "A," "B," and "C" items through analysis of product movement reports (PMRs). PMRs indicate which items, and how much of each of these items, a pharmacy has purchased or used over some period of time. Most wholesalers will provide pharmacies with PMRs showing all products purchased from the wholesaler. Many pharmacy computer systems produce PMRs indicating the pharmacy's use of prescription items.

A basic type of PMR is an item analysis report. It lists all products purchased by the pharmacy for each class of products. An excerpt of the item analysis report for prescription items for Owens Pharmacy is shown in Figure 14-4. For each product, the report lists the purchase cost, retail price, gross profit, gross profit percentage, and rank by gross profit dollars for the year to date. The report indicates, for example, that Owens Pharmacy purchased $21,651 worth of Dyazide for the year to date. The Dyazide was sold for $40,330, yielding a gross profit of $18,679 or 46.3%. In terms of dollars of gross profit generated, Dyazide was the pharmacy's second most profitable product.

The manager can use PMRs to identify the fastest- and slowest-selling products and the most and least profitable products, in each class. This allows him or her to identify "A," "B," and "C" items. The PMR shown in Figure 14-4 indicates that the most profitable prescription items are Dyazide and E-Mycin 333-mg tablets in bottles of 500. These are the second and 66th most profitable prescription items sold by Owens Pharmacy for the year to date. The least profitable items are Eldercap 100, with a rank of 1,651 of the 1,776 items sold, and Elavil 10-mg tablets, with a rank of 1,429 of 1,776 products sold.

Some PMRs provide more sophisticated analyses. For example, two analyses from PMRs from a Walgreens pharmacy are shown in Figures 14-5a and 14-5b. The first is a drug location recommendation report. This report is used to increase the efficiency of dispensing in the pharmacy by placing faster-moving items in more convenient locations and slower-moving items in less convenient locations. The report recommends where an item should be placed in the pharmacy based on the number of prescriptions dispensed for that item in the past 120 days. The fastest movers—the "A" items—should be located in automated dispensing cells. A cell is an automated dispensing container electronically connected to the pharmacy computer. The cell automatically

**Owens Pharmacy**
**Item Analysis Report**
**Class 851 Pharmacy, Rx**

| Item Description | Rank | Year to Date | | | |
| --- | --- | --- | --- | --- | --- |
| | | Cost | Retail | Profit | % |
| Duricef 250 mg 100 mL | 298 | 523.14 | 969.05 | 445.91 | 46.0 |
| Dyazide CP 1 m | 2 | 21,651.45 | 40,330.77 | 18,679.32 | 46.3 |
| Dymelor TB 250 mg 200 | 938 | 91.28 | 174.61 | 83.33 | 47.7 |
| Dyrenium CP 100 mg 100 | 471 | 317.33 | 575.38 | 258.05 | 44.8 |
| E Mycin TB 250 mg 100 UP | 672 | 32.17 | 188.05 | 155.88 | 82.9 |
| E Mycin TB 333 mg 100 UP | 367 | 183.91 | 525.48 | 341.57 | 65.0 |
| E Mycin TB 333 mg 500 UP | 66 | 593.23 | 2,117.22 | 1,523.99 | 72.0 |
| E Pilo 2 pct 10 cc SMP | 1,366 | 33.05 | 61.36 | 28.31 | 46.1 |
| E Pilo 6 pct 10 cc SMP | 1,238 | 49.73 | 91.95 | 42.22 | 45.9 |
| EES CH TB 200 mg 50 ABB | 1,345 | 28.98 | 59.66 | 30.68 | 51.4 |
| EES TB 400 mg 100 ABB | 1,089 | 47.97 | 108.09 | 60.12 | 55.6 |
| EES 200 liq pt ABB | 751 | 91.55 | 221.33 | 129.78 | 58.6 |
| EES 400 liq pt ABB | 550 | 145.50 | 353.30 | 207.80 | 58.8 |
| Elase Chloromycet oint 10 g PD | 1,270 | 45.05 | 83.22 | 38.17 | 45.9 |
| Elase oint 30 g PD | 1,234 | 50.40 | 93.06 | 42.66 | 45.8 |
| Elavil TB 10 mg 100 | 1,429 | 24.30 | 46.92 | 22.62 | 48.2 |
| Elavil TB 25 mg 100 | 834 | 118.08 | 227.65 | 109.57 | 48.1 |
| Elavil TB 50 mg 100 | 679 | 163.36 | 316.74 | 153.38 | 48.4 |
| Elavil TB 75 mg 100 | 1,185 | 52.62 | 101.25 | 48.63 | 48.0 |
| Eldercap 100 | 1,651 | 11.75 | 21.79 | 10.04 | 46.1 |
| Eldoquin Forte CR 4% | 1,367 | 30.96 | 59.16 | 28.20 | 47.7 |
| Zyloprim TB 100 mg 100 | 984 | 62.84 | 136.41 | 73.57 | 53.9 |
| Zyloprim TB 300 mg 100 | 1,207 | 54.87 | 101.24 | 46.37 | 45.8 |

| | |
| --- | --- |
| Total items | 1,776 |
| Total retail | 1,153,649.45 |
| Total cost | 579,701.43 |
| Total profit | 573,948.02 |
| Total percent of profit | 49.8% |

**FIGURE 14–4**   Product movement report—item analysis report.

**Walgreens—Drug Location Recommendation Report**
**Store #: XXXX**
**Report Date: 02/28/20X6**

**Recommended Location: Cell**

| Drug Name | Manufacturer | NDC Number | # Rx | Current Location |
|---|---|---|---|---|
| Acetaminophen w/codeine #3 tablets | Teva | 00093-0150-10 | 105 | Cell |
| Amox-Clav 875-mg tablets | Geneva | 00781-1852-20 | 37 | Fast Rack |
| Azithromycin 250-mg tablets | Teva | 00093-7146-56 | 25 | Quick |
| Ciprofloxacin 500-mg tablets | Teva | 00093-0864-01 | 84 | Cell |
| Diovan 160-mg tablets | Novartis | 00078-0359-34 | 28 | Cell |
| Diovan 80-mg tablets | Novartis | 00078-0358-34 | 26 | Fast Rack |
| Hydrochlorothiazide 25-mg tablets | Purepac | 00228-2221-96 | 311 | Cell |
| Lorazepan 0.5-mg tablets | Panbaxy | 63304-0772-05 | 30 | Fast Rack |
| Naproxen 500-mg tablets | Mylan | 00378-0451-05 | 78 | Cell |
| Propoxyphene-N 100 w/APAP 650 tabs | Mallinckrodt | 00406-1721-05 | 37 | Alpha |
| Zyrtec 10-mg tablets | Pfizer | 00069-5510-66 | 25 | Cell |

**Recommended Location: Fast Rack**

| Drug Name | Manufacturer | NDC Number | # Rx | Current Location |
|---|---|---|---|---|
| Actos 30-mg tablets | Takeda | 64764-0301-14 | 21 | Fast Rack |
| Acyclovir 400-mg tablets | Zenith | 00172-4267-60 | 13 | Alpha |
| Albuterol inhaler (complete) 17 g | Warrick-Schering | 59930-1560-01 | 233 | Fast Rack |
| Alprazolam 0.25-mg tablets | Purepac | 00228-2027-96 | 21 | Cell |
| Amitriptyline 25-mg tablets | Mylan | 00378-2625-10 | 20 | Cell |
| Azithromycin 500-mg tablets 3-pak | Teva | 00093-7169-33 | 12 | Alpha |
| Benicar 40-mg tablets | Sankyo | 65597-0104-30 | 12 | Fast Rack |
| Bumetanide 1-mg tabs | Bon Labs | 00185-0129-01 | 13 | Fast Rack |
| Clonazepam 0.5-mg tablets | Purepac | 00228-3003-50 | 21 | Cell |
| Digoxin 0.125-mg tablets (yellow) | Bertek | 62794-0145-30 | 18 | Cell |
| Enalapril 10-mg tablets | Mylan | 00378-1053-01 | 17 | Fast Rack |
| Folic acid 1-mg tablets | Qualitest-Westward | 00603-3714-32 | 14 | Alpha |
| Fosinopril 10-mg tablets | Teva | 00093-7222-98 | 14 | Fast Rack |

**FIGURE 14–5a**  Product Movement Report—Drug Location Recommendation Report.

counts the number of units specified when the prescription is entered into the computer. The correct quantity is delivered into a prescription vial via a nozzle on the front of each cell. The pharmacy will have a cell for each of its 50 (or 100 or 200 depending on the pharmacy) fastest-moving prescription tablets or capsules. Because the automatic counting feature improves the speed of dispensing, the most frequently dispensed prescription products are kept in cells. The next fastest-moving products—the top "B" items—should be placed in the fast rack. This is a set of shelves (or wire racks) located over the dispensing counter. The pharmacist can easily reach up and access products in the fast rack without having to move away from the counter.

Walgreens—Rx Overstocked Report
Time: 10:09:49
Date: 02/28/X6

| WIC | Item Description | Drug Location | Excess Inventory (Packages) | On Hand (Units) | 120 Days Forecast Qty (Units) | NDC |
|-----|------------------|---------------|------------------------------|-----------------|-------------------------------|-----|
| 673359 | Accolate 10-mg tab (Zen) + 60 | Alpha | 1 | 60 | No Sales | 00310040160 |
| 673260 | Accuretic 20-mg/25-mg tab + 90 | Alpha | 2 | 261 | 23 | 00071022323 |
| 672956 | Albuterol INH AR REF (WR) 17 g | Alpha | 3 | 51 | No Sales | 59930156002 |
| 608848 | Amox-Clav 400-57 chew (Tev) + 20 | Alpha | 1 | 40 | 20 | 00093227234 |
| 599039 | Ampicillin 250-mg cap (Tev) + 100 | Alpha | 1 | 187 | 16 | 00093514501 |
| 673254 | Avandamet 1-mg/500-mg tab (SKB) + 60 | Alpha | 1 | 60 | No Sales | 00007316618 |
| 672452 | Buproban 150-mg ER tab (Tev) 100 | Alpha | 1 | 260 | 111 | 00093570301 |
| 674148 | But-Apap-Caf 50-500-40 tab (Q) + 100 | Alpha | 1 | 100 | No Sales | 00603254521 |
| 673822 | But-Apap-Caf-Cod 30-mg cap (Q) + 100 | Alpha | 2 | 316 | 71 | 00603255321 |
| 594246 | Carbinox 2-mg IR/8mg ER cap (B) + 60 | Alpha | 1 | 60 | 0 | 10914092006 |

**FIGURE 14 –5b** Product Movement Report—Prescription Overstocked Report

The slowest-moving products—slower "B" items and "C" items—should be located in the alpha section. These are the shelves behind the dispensing counter where the bulk of products are kept in alphabetical order. This is the least convenient area for the pharmacist to access, so the slower-moving products are kept here. (Drugs recommended to be placed in the alpha section are not shown on the report; if a drug is not recommended for cell or fast rack, then it is an alpha item.)

Figure 14-5B shows an overstock report. This report compares the amount of an item on hand with projected sales of the item for the next 120 days. Based on the comparison, the report indicates the number of excess, or overstocked, packages that the pharmacy has on hand. This allows the manager to quickly identify which items, in which quantities, should be returned. The manager can also use this report to determine which items the pharmacy may no longer need to stock.

## OTHER INVENTORY CONTROL TECHNIQUES

A number of other techniques can be used in conjunction with EOQs and reorder points to help control inventory.

### Manual Techniques

One of the simplest methods of inventory control is a want book. A want book is simply a list of items that the pharmacy needs to order. Before most pharmacies and wholesalers were computerized, a want book typically consisted of a notebook kept in a convenient place. Pharmacists or clerks recorded product names or item numbers and quantities to be ordered in the want book as the items were sold or dispensed. The pharmacist or clerk in charge of inventory then made orders to the wholesaler or manufacturer directly from the information recorded in the want book. Now, the want book is more likely to be a handheld electronic device into which item numbers and quantities are entered. The device records the needed items just as the notebook did, but allows the order to be placed electronically.

Colored or dated price stickers are another simple and effective manual technique. Colored price stickers can be used to indicate the time period during which a product was received. For example, a pharmacy might use blue stickers for products received during the first 6 months of a year, red stickers for products received during the next 6 months, yellow stickers for the first 6 months of the next year, and so on. Because the colors change every 6 months, the manager can readily estimate how long an item has been in inventory by simply glancing at the sticker. The length of time an item has been in inventory gives a rough indication of the quantity of the item needed and of whether the item should be discontinued. Dated stickers are simply a refinement. Rather than depending on color, the date of receipt is placed on the sticker.

## Gross Margin Return on Investment

Managers of pharmacies constantly face choices as to what merchandise they should stock. The manager of a community pharmacy might be faced with a choice among an expanded line of cosmetics, a new line of sports medicine products, or an expanded line of baby products. Once he or she has decided which line of products to carry, he or she must decide which of the competing products to carry within each line. For example, if the manager decided to carry a line of sports medicine products, which particular sports medicine products should he or she stock? In making these decisions, managers focus primarily on gross margin and turnover. That is, they would like to stock those lines and those products that would sell rapidly (high turnover) and at a high markup (gross margin). The manager's choice is complicated by the reality that products with high turnover frequently must be priced competitively—which means a low gross margin— and that products that will yield a high gross margin usually have low turnover.

The gross margin return on investment (GMROI) can help the manager make these decisions because it incorporates both profit and turnover criteria into a single measure of inventory performance. Profit is measured as gross margin. Turnover is measured as the ratio of net sales to average inventory at cost. (This measure is different from the traditional measure of turnover that is calculated as the ratio of cost of goods sold to average inventory at cost.) So, GMROI is calculated as:

$$\text{GMROI} = (\text{Gross margin dollars/Net sales}) \times (\text{Net sales/Average inventory at cost})$$
$$= \text{Gross margin dollars/Average inventory at cost}$$

Because it considers both turnover and profit, GMROI can be used to measure and compare the performance of lines or products that have different turnovers and gross margins. An example will demonstrate how this is done.

The manager of the Friendly Apothecary must decide whether to add a line of sick room supplies—such as crutches, bed pans, sitz baths—or a line of sports medicine products—such as elastic knee and ankle braces. The sick room supplies line carries an average gross margin of 50% and a turnover (as measured by the net sales–to–inventory ratio) of 4. The sports medicine line has a lower gross margin— only 40%—but a turnover of 8. Which line should the manager stock? For sick room supplies, the GMROI is 200% (50% × 4); for sports medicine products, the GMROI is 320% (40% × 8). Based on this, the manager would find it more profitable—in terms of numbers of dollars of profit made over the course of the year—to stock the sports medicine line. In this example, the higher turnover of the sports medicine line more than compensated for the lower margin. Similar calculations can be made to compare products within categories.

One caution must be kept in mind whenever the GMROI is used. Gross margin is a measure of profitability before expenses are considered. If the expenses needed to sell the products or categories being compared are not the same, the use of GMROI will be misleading. For example, it would be incorrect to use GMROI to compare the performance of the prescription department with that of the stationery department of a chain pharmacy. The stationery department is a self-service department; therefore, only minimal expenses are generated in selling stationery. The prescription department requires the services of a pharmacist; thus, selling prescriptions generates high expenses. The GMROI would not take into account the differences in expenses and would not, consequently, give a valid comparison of the profitability of the two departments.

## INVENTORY CONTROL THROUGH PRODUCT SELECTION AND PURCHASING

Pharmacies can make substantial reductions in the number of items in inventory and the total investment in inventory through careful selection of products dispensed and through prudent purchasing practices. The techniques used to implement these practices include generic and therapeutic interchange and purchasing through buying groups and prime vendors. These practices were first used in institutional pharmacies (i.e., those in hospitals, long-term care facilities, clinics, and health maintenance organizations [HMOs] with in-house pharmacies). Over time, they have become more common in community pharmacies.

### Formulary Management

A formulary is a list of drugs that are recommended for use in a health care system or institution. The formulary is compiled by a committee of physicians and pharmacists. Safety, effectiveness, and cost are the primary criteria used in determining which drugs are listed on the formulary.

In many institutional settings physicians agree to prescribe only those drugs listed on the formulary. In such settings, the pharmacy can reduce the number of items and the total dollar investment in inventory by limiting the number and type of drugs on the formulary. *Generic* and *therapeutic interchange* are the most common methods by which formularies are used to reduce inventory investment.

### Generic and Therapeutic Interchange

Products with the same active ingredient, in the same strength and dosage form, are *generic equivalents.* For example, AstraZeneca's Prilosec 20-mg capsules and Mylan's omeprazole 20-mg capsules are generic equivalents because both contain 20 mg of the drug omeprazole in a capsule form. Many brand-name products, such as Prilosec and Percodan, have cheaper, unbranded generic equivalents. Pharmacies can drastically reduce total inventory investment by stocking and dispensing the less expensive, unbranded generic rather than the brand-name product.

Most states have enacted laws that give pharmacists—both community and institutional—the authority to dispense generic substitutes for prescriptions written for branded products. This has allowed both hospital and institutional pharmacies to practice generic interchange.

*Therapeutic equivalents* are "drug products differing in composition or in their basic drug entity that are considered to have very similar pharmacologic and therapeutic activities."[5] For example, there are many different drugs that can be classified as third-generation cephalosporins. The therapeutic differences among them are not significant even though the agents differ chemically. As another example, all multivitamin products produce similar therapeutic effects. Consequently, a hospital pharmacy may choose to carry only one brand of multivitamin. By stocking only one or two, rather than all, of the therapeutic equivalents, a pharmacy can dramatically reduce inventory size and investment. Institutional pharmacies are able to engage in therapeutic interchange because the institutions gain physicians' approval to do so through the formulary system.

## Formularies and Therapeutic Interchange in Community Pharmacies

Formularies and therapeutic interchange have become more common in community pharmacies, but their use and impact are different than in institutional health care settings. Third-party payers, such as insurance companies and HMOs, have formularies that list the products for which they will provide reimbursement. If the community pharmacy dispenses a product that is on the formulary, then part or all of the product's cost is covered by the third-party payer. If a nonformulary drug is dispensed, the patient must pay for the product. As a service to their patients, community pharmacists frequently contact physicians to persuade them to switch the patient to a formulary drug. Thus, community pharmacists have begun to practice a form of therapeutic interchange.

Unfortunately, third-party formularies and therapeutic interchange have not allowed community pharmacies to reduce inventory investments. A community pharmacy typically deals with dozens of different third-party payers, each of which has its own formulary. The community pharmacy must carry a sufficient number and quantity of products to serve the formularies of all the payers with which it deals. Because of this, third-party payers' formularies have not allowed community pharmacies to reduce the number of items that they stock or to reduce the total amount invested in inventory.

## Bid Purchasing

Pharmacies can realize substantial savings on acquisition costs of drugs through bid purchasing. In this process, the pharmacy solicits bids from manufacturers on specific products. It indicates that it will purchase only from those manufacturers submitting the lowest bids, assuming product quality and service are acceptable. The bid process provides manufacturers with a strong incentive to reduce their normal prices. If they do not, they stand the chance of losing all sales to the pharmacy.

Manufacturers usually submit lower bid prices to pharmacies that use more of their products. To take advantage of this, most pharmacies have joined *buying groups* or *group purchasing organizations* (GPOs). The purpose of a buying group is to pool the purchasing power of individual pharmacies to extract better prices from suppliers. Because of their ability to obtain lower prices from manufacturers, buying groups have become prevalent. The Health Industry Group Purchasing Association, the trade association for GPOs, estimates that 96% to 98% of hospitals use a GPO.[6] Buying groups for independent pharmacies have also become common.

The bid process is most widely used for products available from multiple sources—such as generic drugs. Products available from only one source—such as patented, brand-name products—are less frequently purchased on bids. The reason for this is competition. If a pharmacy must stock a patented, brand-name product, as is usually true, then it must buy it from the one manufacturer that makes it. That manufacturer has no incentive to reduce the price because the pharmacy cannot buy the product anywhere else.

If, however, the pharmacy has a limited formulary and practices therapeutic interchange, the situation changes. If there are therapeutic equivalents, the pharmacy may choose among them in deciding which product to place on the formulary. Thus, the brand-name manufacturer of one of the therapeutic equivalents has the choice of submitting a lower price bid in hopes of having its product placed on the formulary, or not submitting the bid and therefore not selling the product to the pharmacy. Thus, therapeutic interchange induces competition, and lower prices, in bidding for products without generic equivalents. This is an example of how bid purchasing, formulary management, and interchange can work together to reduce the pharmacy's inventory investment.

## Prime Vendors

In a prime vendor system, a group of pharmacies, such as a GPO, agrees to make the majority of its purchases through a single wholesaler. This wholesaler is designated as the group's prime vendor. In return for the assured business, the wholesaler will discount its normal price.

Most prime vendor arrangements include products for which bid prices have been negotiated. The pharmacy buying group puts out bids for products as discussed previously. Contracts are awarded to the manufacturers with the lowest acceptable bids. In a prime vendor system, the member pharmacies then purchase the product through the wholesaler. The wholesaler charges the pharmacies the bid price plus a negotiated service fee for handling the merchandise.

### References

1. Ukens C. McKesson on-line tool tames pharmacy ordering monster. Drug Topics 2004;148(21):54.
2. Anon., Drug chains adopt technology that "supports mission." Chain Drug Rev 2004;26(8):75–76.
3. Anon., McKesson's asset management program empowers SWMC with total inventory control. McKesson Health Systems. Available at: http://healthsystems.mckesson. http://www.mckesson.com/static.files/mckesson.com/MckPharma/documents/pt_im_assetmanagement_casestudy.11.02.pdf accessed August 28, 2006.
4. Levin RI, Rubin DS, Stinson JP. Quantitative Approaches to Management. 6th Ed. New York: McGraw-Hill Book Company, 1986.
5. Anon., ASHP statement on the formulary system. Am J Hosp Pharm 1986;43:2839.
6. Anon., About HIGPA. Available at: https://www.higpa.org/about/about_faqs.asp. Accessed February 23, 2006.

### Suggested Readings

Abramowitz PW. Controlling financial variables changing prescribing patterns. Am J Hosp Pharm 1984;41:503.

Burns LR. The Health Care Value Chain. San Francisco: Jossey-Bass, 2002.

Ozcan YA. Supply chain and inventory management. In: Ozcan YA, ed. Quantitative Methods in Health Care Management: Techniques and Applications. San Francisco: Jossey-Bass, 2005.

Sweeney DJ. Improving the profitability of retail merchandising decisions. J Mktg 1973;37:60.

## QUESTIONS

1. Costs of obsolescence, deterioration, storage, and having capital invested in inventory are known as:
   a. carrying costs
   b. procurement costs
   c. stockout costs
2. Costs of placing, processing, and receiving an order are known as:
   a. carrying costs
   b. procurement costs
   c. stockout costs
3. Making fewer and larger orders per year would minimize:
   a. carrying costs
   b. procurement costs
   c. stockout costs
4. High inventory turnover minimizes:
   a. carrying costs
   b. procurement costs
   c. stockout costs
5. The EOQ formula seeks to minimize:
   a. carrying costs
   b. procurement costs
   c. stockout costs
   d. All of the above
   e. a and b only
6. Lead time includes the period of time required:
   a. for the pharmacy to process an order
   b. for the pharmacy to recognize that an order should be placed
   c. for the supplier to process and deliver an order
   d. All of the above
7. If demand and lead time are both known and constant, does a pharmacy need to maintain a safety stock?
   a. Yes
   b. No
8. The reorder point, under real-world conditions, is based on which of the following?
   a. Pharmacy's lead time
   b. Demand for the item
   c. Required safety stock of the item
   d. All of the above
   e. Only a and b

9. Items with more erratic demand require:
   a. larger safety stocks
   b. smaller safety stocks
   c. pattern of demand has no effect on safety stock
10. Which items should the manager control most closely and carefully?
   a. "A" items
   b. "B" items
   c. "C" items
11. The reorder point in a *fixed review period* system is based on:
   a. demand for the item
   b. size of the safety stock
   c. lead time
   d. length of the review period
   e. All of the above
   f. a, b, and c only
12. The GMROI consists of which of the following?
   a. Measure of inventory turnover
   b. Measure of net profitability
   c. Measure of gross profitability
   d. a and b
   e. a and c
13. The GMROI can be used to compare the performance of:
   a. individual products
   b. lines of products
   c. departments within the pharmacy
   d. individual pharmacies
   e. All of the above
14. Home intravenous antibiotics require specialized expertise and equipment and a good deal of pharmacist time to prepare and dispense. Convenience foods are a self-service category of goods. Should a manager use GMROI analysis to compare the inventory performance of home intravenous antibiotics and convenience foods?
   a. Yes
   b. No
15. Convenience foods have a very high turnover. Small appliances have a low turnover. The expenses required to sell both lines are similar. Should a manager use GMROI analysis to compare the inventory performance of convenience foods and small appliances?
   a. Yes
   b. No
16. When hospitals order direct from manufacturers, they typically receive lower prices but must order in larger quantities. When they order from local wholesalers, they receive higher prices but can order in smaller quantities. Could the hospital use GMROI to decide from where it would be best to order?
   a. Yes
   b. No
17. Drug products that have similar effects and actions but different chemical compositions are known as:
   a. generic equivalents
   b. therapeutic equivalents
   c. pharmaceutical equivalents

18. Therapeutic interchange is most likely to occur in:
    a. community pharmacies
    b. hospital pharmacies without a formulary
    c. hospital pharmacies with a formulary
19. The bid purchasing process is most likely to result in savings on acquisition costs for products:
    a. that have generic equivalents
    b. that have therapeutic equivalents
    c. that are available from only one manufacturer
20. A prime vendor is a type of:
    a. pharmacy
    b. wholesaler
    c. manufacturer
    d. Either b or c

## PROBLEMS

1. Calvin's Corner Drugs uses 1,000 bottles of Tanzac per year. Tanzac costs $60 per bottle. Calvin's procurement costs are $10 per order, carrying costs are 25%, and lead time is 5 days.
    a. How much Tanzac should Calvin's order at a time? How many orders per year would Calvin's place at this quantity? Assuming this quantity is ordered, what would total inventory costs associated with Tanzac be for the year?
    b. How much Tanzac should Calvin's order at a time if ordering costs were $25 per order? How many orders per year would Calvin's place?
    c. How much Tanzac should Calvin's order at a time if carrying costs were 35% and procurement costs were $10 per order? How many orders per year would Calvin's place?
    d. What is the reorder point for Tanzac assuming constant and known lead time and demand?
    e. What is the reorder point if a safety stock equal to 5 days supply is kept?
2. The Wahoo Hospital Pharmacy uses 20,000 bottles of Thiozene, a potent antipsychotic, per year. Thiozene costs $50 per bottle. Wahoo Hospital Pharmacy's procurement costs are $50 per order, carrying costs are 30%, and lead time is 3 days.
    a. How much Thiozene should the Wahoo Pharmacy order at a time? What are the total inventory costs associated with Thiozene for a year?
    b. The manufacturer of Thiozene offers the pharmacy a special deal. Thiozene will be sold for $45 per bottle if the quantity ordered is 1,000 bottles or more. Should Wahoo take the deal? Why?
    c. What is the reorder point for Thiozene assuming constant and known lead time and demand?
    d. What is the reorder point if a safety stock equal to 10 days supply is kept?
3. Goodbuy Pharmacy is considering adding a new line of products. It has two choices. The first line (Line A) has expected sales of $40,000 per year and a 25% gross margin, and will require an average inventory of $5,000. Line B has expected sales of $25,000 per year and a 40% gross margin, and will require an average inventory of $6,000. Use GMROI analysis to determine which line to stock. Why is this line preferable?

4. The Higho Hospital Pharmacy has annual generic drug sales of $150,000. Currently, it purchases generics directly from the manufacturer. Purchasing from the manufacturer yielded cost of goods sold of $90,000 and average inventory of $30,000. Purchasing from a local wholesaler would allow the pharmacy to cut its inventory of generics to $20,000 but would increase cost of goods sold to $100,000. Use GMROI analysis to determine the source from which Higho Hospital Pharmacy should purchase generics.

5. It's bonus time at Riteway Chain Drugstores. Managers are given bonuses based on their inventory control and profitability performance. Manager Jones's pharmacy realized a gross profit of $215,000 on sales of $680,000 and an average inventory of $93,000. Manager Smythe's store had a gross profit of $196,000 on sales of $614,000 and an average inventory of $93,000. Who gets the bigger bonus? Why? (Hint: analyze both profitability and turnover using the GMROI formula.)

CHAPTER 15

# Pharmacoeconomics

After reading this chapter the student should be able to:

1. Define and state the goal of pharmacoeconomics,
2. Explain the concepts of costs and consequences in pharmacoeconomics,
3. Define and differentiate between direct and indirect medical costs,
4. Explain the importance of perspective in a pharmacoeconomic analysis,
5. Define and differentiate cost-minimization analysis, cost-effectiveness analysis, cost-utility analysis, and cost-benefit analysis,
6. Differentiate between average and incremental cost-effectiveness ratios and identify which is typically used in pharmacoeconomic analyses,
7. Explain and discuss the concept of quality-adjusted life years and explain how they are calculated,
8. Interpret cost-effectiveness and cost-utility ratios, and
9. Compare and contrast the population perspective taken by pharmacoeconomic analyses and the individual patient perspective used by most clinicians.

Contemporary pharmacy managers face a health care environment that is very concerned with the costs of health care. This results from the high and rising costs of providing care. Several statistics show the magnitude of the problem. National health expenditures in the United States in 2004 were $1.9 trillion.[1] The percentage of the gross national product devoted to health care has risen from 5.2% in 1960[2] to 16.0% in 2004.[1] Annual expenditures on prescription drugs have increased from $51 billion in 1993 to $189 billion in 2004.[1] Further, for the same time period, increases in expenditures on prescription drugs have averaged over 10% per year.[1]

Concerns about the costs of health care have resulted in a number of programs that have a direct impact on pharmacists practicing in all settings. Hospital reimbursement from the federal government and from many private insurers is now based on a set and predetermined payment for a given diagnosis. If the hospital's costs of treating a patient exceed the set amount, the hospital must absorb the loss. This system puts pressure on hospital pharmacy managers to closely control the costs of products and services. State Medicaid agencies have been faced with constant or decreasing budgets and increased demand for pharmaceutical products and services. To cope with this situation, they have cut pharmacy dispensing fees and established prior approval programs that limit patient access to selected drug products. Prescription drug programs offered by managed-care organizations (MCOs) typically feature such cost containment measures as restricted formularies, discounted pharmacy dispensing fees and ingredient cost reimbursement, and prior approval programs. MCOs also demand large discounts from hospitals. The result of these practices is a high level of concern with controlling costs in all pharmacy practice settings.

In the cost-conscious environment, pharmacists are no longer able to simply develop and offer new services and products and assume that consumers and third parties will pay for them. Reimbursement is increasingly dependent on demonstration that new products and services provide value to purchasers. This does not simply mean that they are low cost. It means that their benefits are greater than their costs. Because of the new emphasis on value, pharmacists need to become familiar with the concept and techniques of pharmacoeconomics.

## DEFINITION AND GOALS OF PHARMACOECONOMICS

Pharmacoeconomics is the means by which pharmacists can demonstrate the value of their products and services. It can be defined as "the description and analysis of the costs of drug therapy to healthcare systems and society."[3] "Pharmacoeconomic research identifies, measures, and compares the costs (i.e., resources consumed) and consequences (clinical, economic, and humanistic) of pharmaceutical products and services."[4] The goal of pharmacoeconomics is to help decision makers allocate a fixed amount of resources across competing products and services so as to maximize health benefits to the population of patients they serve.[5,6] Pharmacoeconomics, unlike the decisions made by most clinicians, focuses on *populations* of patients rather than on individual patients. While an individual clinician is concerned with selecting the best drug for an individual patient, pharmacoeconomics focuses on selecting the most cost-effective drug for a population of patients.

Because of cost containment pressures, most pharmacy managers are expected to operate within a fixed budget (a fixed amount of resources). Unlimited funds are not available. This requires the manager to make choices; new products and services can only be purchased if they are cost saving or cost neutral or if purchases of other products and services are reduced. Because the budget is fixed, the pharmacy manager cannot provide all the products and services that are available or that patients may want. To provide the best possible care within the limited budget, the manager must identify and purchase those products and services that provide the best value. This requires the manager to compare the costs and consequences of products and services to determine which provide the most health benefits for the funds available to the pharmacy. Only by comparing products and services, and by choosing those that provide the best value, can the manager provide the best care to the most patients with the limited funds available to the pharmacy.

## COSTS AND CONSEQUENCES

The essence of pharmacoeconomics is balancing the costs and consequences of pharmaceutical products and services. Pharmacoeconomic studies take a broad view of costs and consequences. Pharmacoeconomic studies examine the product's or service's impact on the total cost of therapy, not just its price. In terms of consequences, pharmacoeconomic studies measure the product's or service's effects on clinical outcomes such as cure, disease progression, and symptoms as well as on humanistic measures like patients' quality of life and satisfaction with care.

### Definition of Costs

Three basic elements determine the total cost of therapy:

*Production costs* are the costs of producing or providing the treatment. The production costs of treating hypertension, for example, include the costs of physician office visits to initiate and monitor therapy, the costs of any testing required to diagnose and monitor the disease, and the costs of pharmaceutical products and services used to treat the disease.

*Induced resource losses* are the costs of treating and managing adverse effects of treatment. Patients treated with antihypertensive medications frequently experience side effects such as dizziness, impotence, and nasal congestion. Occasionally these patients may experience drug interactions. The costs of treating or managing these adverse effects are considered part of the cost of treating the disease. These costs are frequently substantial. Johnson and Bootman have estimated that the total cost attributable to preventable drug-related adverse events in ambulatory settings exceeded $76 billion in 1994.[7]

*Induced resource savings* are costs that are prevented as a result of successful treatment. Untreated hypertension results in strokes and heart attacks. Appropriate drug therapy can prevent these problems and save the costs that would be incurred in treating them. These savings must be accounted for in determining the total costs of antihypertensive treatment.

### An Example

A study published by McCombs and Nichol illustrates how focusing on the total costs of treatment, rather than considering only drug costs, can lead to a more accurate estimation of the value of a pharmaceutical product.[8] Several years ago, Medi-Cal (the California Medicaid program) added cefaclor to its formulary. Cefaclor was restricted to use in patients 50 years and older who had lower respiratory tract infections (LRTIs). If Medi-Cal had considered only drug costs, it would not have added cefaclor to its formulary. Cefaclor was much more expensive than other products—such as penicillin VK, erythromycin, and ampicillin—which were commonly used for treatment of LRTIs. However, when total treatment costs were considered, Medi-Cal saved money by using cefaclor. Total treatment costs were $388 per episode lower for this patient group when cefaclor was used than when one of the less expensive antibiotics was used. Drug costs were $56 higher per episode when cefaclor was used. However, hospital costs were $366 lower, physician costs were $28 lower, and lab costs were $3 lower. Cefaclor was more effective in this patient group, and, as a result, using it led to more initial cures and fewer follow-up office visits and hospitalizations. Consequently, cefaclor was a valuable, and cost-saving, addition to the Medi-Cal formulary in spite of its higher cost.

## Direct and Indirect Costs

The costs that we have discussed to this point are direct costs of treatment. They are costs that arise directly from treating or managing the disease. There are *direct medical costs* and *direct nonmedical costs*. Direct medical costs are the costs of health care resources—such as physician visits, hospitalizations, and pharmaceuticals—used to prevent or treat disease. Direct nonmedical costs include costs such as transportation to and from health care facilities, informal caregivers' time, and housekeeping and meal preparation expenses that result from the patient being unable to perform the services for himself or herself. Patients who are unable to care for themselves as a result of disease or disability, such as patients with advanced AIDS or Alzheimer's disease, incur substantial direct nonmedical costs.

Treatments also have *indirect costs*. These result from productivity losses that patients incur as a result of disease or disability. Returning to our antihypertensive example, we know that patients who have strokes and heart attacks suffer a great deal of disability and dysfunction. As a result, they become much less productive. They are not able to work, or work as productively, as they did when they were healthy. They are also less productive in their non–work-related roles as homemakers, parents, and citizens. Thus, the patient, his or her employer, and society all suffer economic loss as a result of the patient's ill health.

The economic losses from reduced productivity are sometimes larger than the direct medical costs of treating the disease or disability. Consequently, from the point of view of patients and society, these losses should be included in pharmacoeconomic analyses. Bootman et al. conducted a classic pharmacoeconomic study that illustrates the importance and magnitude of indirect costs.[9] The study examined the value of using pharmacists to monitor patient blood levels when dosing gentamicin for severely burned patients. The researchers found that pharmacists' interventions increased direct costs. The patients for whom pharmacists provided pharmacokinetic dosing services had higher survival rates and, as a result, stayed longer and received more treatment in the hospital. This resulted in higher treatment costs for these patients. However, surviving patients were eventually able to return to work and to their other roles (such as parents and homemakers). The indirect cost savings—the economic value these patients generated by being able to return to work and home—far exceeded the increase in the direct costs of providing treatment to them.

## Consequences

The other variable that must be considered in a pharmacoeconomic study is the consequences of using the product or service. Consequences are the outcomes of using a product or service. Pharmacoeconomic studies use two types of outcome measures. The first is the *final outcome*. Final outcomes are consequences that measure direct effects on patients' health, well-being, or productivity. Numbers of lives saved and years of life saved are commonly used as final outcome measures. Final outcomes also include more subjective measures such as improvements in quality of life and changes in patient satisfaction. A study of the effects of pharmacist counseling and monitoring of asthma patients might include final outcome measures like symptom-free days and decreases in days of employment lost.

The final outcome of treatment with many pharmaceutical products or services may not occur until many years after treatment has been initiated. For example, pharmacist monitoring, counseling, and education of patients with high serum cholesterol should decrease cardiovascular-related death and disability. However, these decreases may not be apparent until 10, 20, or 30 years after pharmacy services are initiated. In these situations, where use of final outcome measures is impractical, pharmacoeconomic studies use measures of *intermediate outcomes*. Examples of these include reductions in blood pressure and serum cholesterol. These are termed intermediate outcomes because they are outcomes that are necessary steps in achieving the desired final outcomes. For example, serum cholesterol (an intermediate outcome) is measured not because it is an inherently important outcome, but because elevated cholesterol will result in death and disability (final outcomes) later in life. Thus, intermediate outcomes serve as practical substitutes for final outcome measures.

## Perspective

Many different groups use pharmacoeconomic studies. These groups include society, pharmaceutical manufacturers, managed-care organizations, patients, and pharmacies. Different costs and consequences accrue to different groups. Consequently, the cost and consequences that should be included in a pharmacoeconomic study depend on the perspective the study takes.

Society has the broadest perspective. An analysis conducted from society's perspective would include all costs and consequences of using a given pharmaceutical, regardless of which group experiences them. Other groups have more limited perspectives and, as a result, consider a narrower range of costs and consequences.

Payers—such as insurance companies and managed-care organizations—are one such group. Payers are responsible for the direct medical costs of the patients for whom they provide coverage. They are not responsible for indirect costs due to changes in patient productivity or for direct nonmedical costs. Thus, pharmacoeconomic analyses done from the payer's perspective typically include only direct medical costs. An example of a pharmacoeconomic analysis done from a payer's perspective is Johnson and Bootman's study of the costs of drug-related adverse events in ambulatory settings.[7] This study included estimates of "health care costs that were directly associated with the treatment of preventable drug-related mortality and morbidity." It did not include estimates of the economic losses resulting from decreased patient productivity or disease-related costs incurred for transportation or personal care. Had the study been done from society's perspective, it would have included all three types of costs.

Pharmacoeconomic analyses of clinical pharmacy services provided in hospitals typically take the perspective of the hospital. From this perspective, only costs and consequences that affect the hospital's budget—such as decreased drug costs or nursing administration time—are considered. Costs and consequences that do not affect the hospital's budget—such as savings to the health care system as a whole or improved quality of life for patients—are not included. These studies take the hospital's perspective because they are usually done to provide an economic justification for the service to hospital administration.

## PHARMACOECONOMIC TECHNIQUES

Four basic economic techniques are used in pharmacoeconomic studies. They are cost-minimization analysis, cost-effectiveness analysis, cost-utility analysis, and cost-benefit analysis. All consider both the costs and the consequences of the products or services being compared. The identification and measurement of costs is the same for all of the techniques. The major difference among them lies in how they measure effectiveness.

## Cost-Minimization Analysis

The simplest of the pharmacoeconomic tools is cost-minimization analysis (CMA). CMA compares the costs of therapies that achieve the same outcome and that are equally effective. It could be used, for example, to compare the costs of drugs that reduce hypertension, drugs that reduce cholesterol, or drugs that prevent postoperative nausea and vomiting. Only costs are compared because CMA should be used only when the therapies compared are equally effective. For example, ondansetron and granisetron are both used for the prevention of chemotherapy-induced nausea and vomiting. If they are equally effective, then the choice between them could be made using a CMA. That is, since both are equally effective, the least expensive would be preferred. In CMA, as in all pharmacoeconomic studies, the relevant cost is the total cost of therapy, not just the acquisition cost of the drug.

## Cost-Effectiveness Analysis

Frequently, the products or services being compared are not equally effective. Typically, a newer, more expensive, and more effective agent is compared with an older, less expensive, and less effective product, which is the standard of therapy. A cost-effectiveness analysis (CEA) is the appropriate technique for this situation. A CEA seeks to find the least costly means of achieving some particular health outcome. For example, a CEA could be used to determine the least costly product for reducing blood pressure by a certain amount or the least costly method of decreasing smoking in a population of patients by a given amount. CEA meets this goal by simultaneously comparing the costs and effectiveness of treatments that achieve the same type of health outcome—such as prolonging life, reducing blood pressure, or helping patients stop smoking—but that differ in their effectiveness at achieving this outcome.

The effectiveness measure in a CEA is expressed in natural or physical units. For example, a cost-effectiveness study of antihypertensives might use effectiveness measures such as millimeters by which blood pressure was lowered or, over the longer term, additional years of life gained. A study of antiarthritis drugs might use such measures as improvements in grip strength, increases in mobility, or changes in ability to climb stairs.

Costs and consequences are compared in a CEA by means of an *incremental* cost-effectiveness ratio. The ratio is incremental because it measures the additional costs and effectiveness of the product or service being studied as compared with the current standard of therapy. The ratio is calculated as:

$$\text{CER} = (\text{Cost}_{nt} - \text{Cost}_{cst})/(\text{Effectiveness}_{nt} - \text{Effectiveness}_{cst}),$$

where $\quad$ CER = cost-effectiveness ratio,
$\text{Cost}_{nt}$ = cost of the new treatment,
$\text{Cost}_{cst}$ = cost of the current standard of treatment,
$\text{Effectiveness}_{nt}$ = effectiveness of the new treatment, and
$\text{Effectiveness}_{cst}$ = effectiveness of the current standard of treatment.

As with all pharmacoeconomic analyses, the relevant costs are the total costs of treatment.

## An Example of a CEA Study

Smith et al. compared the costs and patient outcomes of two treatments for colon cancer: surgery alone, which was the current standard of treatment, and surgery followed by 52 weeks of chemotherapy.[10] They estimated the direct medical costs of surgery to be $6,000 per patient and the direct medical costs of surgery and chemotherapy to be $13,000. The average life expectancy for a patient receiving surgery alone was estimated to be 13.25 years as compared with 15.65 years for a patient treated with both surgery and chemotherapy. Thus, the incremental cost-effectiveness ratio for surgery plus was chemotherapy was:

$$CER = \text{Additional costs of surgery plus chemotherapy/Additional effectiveness}$$
$$\text{of surgery plus chemotherapy}$$
$$= (\$13,000 - \$6,000)/(15.65 - 13.25)$$
$$= \$2,917$$

The cost-effectiveness ratio is $2,917 per life year saved. This indicates that use of both surgery and chemotherapy will result in longer life for patients, but at an additional cost of $2,917 for each year of life saved.

## Limitations of CEA

CEA has some significant limitations. First of all, CEA can only compare products or services that produce the same type of health outcome; it cannot be used if they produce different outcomes. For example, CEA can be used to compare different drugs that lower blood pressure or to compare different drugs that treat arthritis. CEA cannot, however, be used to compare an antihypertensive product—whose primary effect is on length of life—with an antiarthritic drug—whose primary effect is on quality of life.

Second, CEA cannot readily compare treatments that differ on more than one important outcome. As an example, in the study by Smith et al., the addition of chemotherapy to surgery was more effective than surgery alone, but also more toxic. Patients lived longer when treated with chemotherapy, but the quality of life was diminished by the toxic effects of the chemotherapy. So, the treatments differed on two critical measures of outcome— life expectancy and toxicity. A CEA can include only one measure of outcome. Consequently, it cannot be used to simultaneously deal with the difference in effectiveness and the difference in toxicity.

## Cost-Utility Analysis

A third, and more sophisticated, pharmacoeconomic technique is cost-utility analysis (CUA). CUA differs from CEA in that the health outcome measure used considers changes in both quantity and quality of life. The effectiveness measure most frequently used in CUA is the quality-adjusted life year (QALY). The QALY considers changes in both the length of life and the quality of life resulting from treatment.

The QALY concept is based on the assumption that different health states provide different qualities of life and that, as a result, patients would be willing to trade length of life for quality of life. The QALY concept assumes that patients would be willing to give up some number of years of life in a less preferred health state to live the remaining years in a more preferred state. For example, patients might be willing to trade 15 years of life on dialysis for 13 years of life in good health. That is, they would give up 2 years of length of life on dialysis to live the remaining 13 years in good health.

Life years are converted to QALYs using utility values. Utility values are mathematical estimates of the tradeoffs patients would be willing to make between length of life and quality of life. Figure 15-1 shows utility values estimated for various disease states.[11] On this scale, 1 represents perfect health and 0 represents death. Most other health states fall somewhere between these two extremes. Hospital dialysis for a period of 8 years, for example, has a utility value of 0.56. This indicates that a patient would trade 8 years of life on dialysis for $8 \times 0.56 = 4.5$ years of life in good health. To put it another way, 8 years of life on hospital dialysis are equivalent to 4.5 quality-adjusted life years.

## An Example of a CUA Study

The study of colon cancer treatment by Smith et al., which was discussed earlier, also presented cost-utility estimates to account for both the extension of lifespan and the diminished quality of life accompanying chemotherapy.[10] Subjects in the study were asked to compare a year of life after colon surgery with no chemotherapy with a year of life after colon surgery with chemotherapy. They indicated that a year of life after surgery and on chemotherapy was equivalent to 0.87 years after surgery with no chemotherapy. (The utility value for the surgery plus chemotherapy treatment was 0.87.) The average lifespan for patients treated with both chemotherapy and surgery

| Health State | Utility Value |
|---|---|
| Reference state: perfect health | 1.00 |
| Angina with no chest pain | 0.87 |
| Symptomatic HIV infection | 0.77 |
| Type 1 diabetes requiring insulin therapy alone | 0.75 |
| Depression | 0.70 |
| Severe to profound deafness | 0.58 |
| Type 1 diabetes with blindness | 0.48 |
| Advanced breast cancer | 0.45 |
| Major stroke | 0.40 |
| Severe Alzheimer's—living in nursing home | 0.31 |
| Hepatocellular carcinoma | 0.25 |
| Reference state: dead | 0.00 |

*Source:* The CEA Registry. Catalog of Preference Weights 1998–2001, Tufts-New England Medical Center Institute for Clinical Research and Health Policy Studies. Available at: http://www.tufts-nemc.org/cearegistry/index.html. Accessed May 5, 2006.

**FIGURE 15-1**    Utility values estimated from various studies of patients and the community.

was 15.65 years. Each of these years was equivalent to 0.87 years in good health (defined in this study as the kind of health experienced after colon surgery). So, the chemotherapy plus surgery treatment extended average patient lifespan by 15.65 × 0.87 = 13.62 quality-adjusted life years.[1] The cost-utility ratio (CUR) is calculated as:

CUR = Additional costs of surgery plus chemotherapy/Additional effectiveness
    of surgery plus chemotherapy
  = ($13,000 − $6,000)/(13.62 − 13.25)
  = $18,920

The ratio indicates that treatment with surgery and chemotherapy will extend life, but at an additional cost of $18,920 per quality-adjusted life year saved. In this case, the CUA, which adjusts for the diminished quality of life experienced by patients on chemotherapy, has a substantially higher cost per year of life saved than does the CEA (which does not adjust for quality of life).

## Interpretation of Cost-Effectiveness and Cost-Utility Ratios

One of the major issues in pharmacoeconomics is properly using and interpreting the results of cost-effectiveness and cost-utility analyses. Sometimes the interpretation is simple and straightforward. Oftentimes, it is not. Figure 15-2 shows the four possible results of a CEA study. The figure compares the costs and effectiveness of a new pharmaceutical with the costs and effectiveness of the current standard of therapy. Results that are represented by the upper left and lower right quadrants of the figure have straightforward interpretations. If the new drug or service is both more effective and less costly than the current standard, then obviously it should be used. Doing so would both decrease costs and increase health benefits. Similarly, if the drug or service is both more expensive and less effective than the alternative, it should not be used.

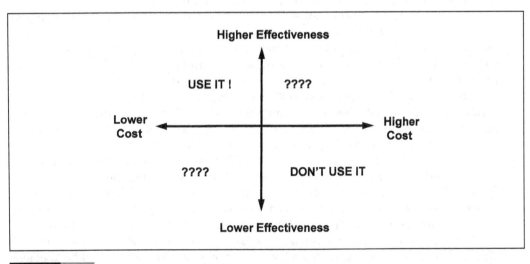

**FIGURE 15-2**  Outcomes of a cost-effectiveness or cost-utility analysis comparing a new treatment with the current standard of therapy.

Results represented by the other two quadrants of the figure are more difficult to interpret. The most common situation occurs when the new drug or service is both more effective and more expensive than the current standard of therapy. In this situation, the question of interest is whether the additional effectiveness is worth the extra cost. To return to our colon cancer example, is one additional quality-adjusted year of life worth an additional $18,920?

Answering this question requires making a value judgment. The judgment can be based either on a specified amount that an organization (such as the Medicaid program or the company paying for an employee's health insurance) is willing to pay for each QALY or on a comparison with the cost per QALY of other commonly used medical procedures.[12]

The provincial government of Ontario provides an example of the first approach. Ontario provides insurance for prescription drugs to all its citizens. To determine which drugs are eligible for reimbursement under the provincial insurance program, Ontario had (at one time but not currently) suggested ranges of acceptable and unacceptable CU ratios.[13] The ranges indicated how much Ontario was willing to pay for a QALY. According to Ontario's guidelines, therapies having CU ratios of less than $20,000 per QALY when compared with current standards of therapy are "almost universally accepted as appropriate uses of society's and the health-care system's resources."[13] That is, Ontario would provide reimbursement for all products with CU ratios of $20,000 or less per QALY.

Therapies with CU ratios between $20,000 and $100,000 per QALY are "provided routinely but the availability of some of these may be limited."[13] The government would provide reimbursement for these products but might limit their availability through such means as restricting their use to specialists or through prior approval programs.

Therapies with CU ratios of greater than $100,000 per QALY would probably not be reimbursable.

Given these guidelines, we would expect Ontario to provide reimbursement for chemotherapy after colon cancer.

The other approach to determining whether the benefits of a new product or service are worth the additional costs is to compare the product's CU ratio with those of commonly used medical procedures. The rationale is that society should be willing to pay as much for new procedures as it does for procedures that are currently in common use. This process is facilitated by the use of "league tables." These tables provide CU (or CE) ratios for a range of different products and procedures. By doing so, they provide decision makers with a comparison for new products.

An example of a league table is shown in Figure 15-3. The league table can be used to interpret the CU ratio for chemotherapy after colon cancer surgery. The information in the table indicates that estrogen therapy for postmenopausal women, a commonly provided medical treatment, has a CU ratio of $27,000. The CU ratio for chemotherapy after colon cancer surgery is $18,920. One could argue that because society (and most insurance companies and health maintenance organizations [HMOs]) commonly pays for estrogen therapy at a cost of $27,000 per QALY gained, society (and insurance companies and HMOs) should also be willing to pay for chemotherapy after colon cancer surgery at the lower $18,920 per QALY saved.

Unfortunately, neither technique addresses the problem of limited resources.[14] Both assume that if a new drug has a low cost-utility ratio, then money will be available to buy it. This will not be true for pharmacies and other health care providers that operate under a fixed budget. For example, a new drug with a cost-utility ratio of $15,000 per

| Treatment | Cost/QALY gained 1983 U.S. dollars |
|---|---|
| Coronary artery bypass surgery for left main coronary artery disease[17] | $4,200 |
| Neonatal intensive care for babies with birthweight of 1000–1499 g[18] | 4,500 |
| Treatment of severe hypertension in males age 40[19] | 9,400 |
| Treatment of mild hypertension in males age 40[19] | 19,100 |
| Estrogen therapy for postmenopausal symptoms in women without a prior hysterectomy[17] | 27,000 |
| Neonatal intensive care for babies with birthweight of 500–999 g[18] | 31,800 |
| Continuous ambulatory peritoneal dialysis[20] | 47,100 |
| Hospital dialysis[20] | 54,000 |

**FIGURE 15–3**   An example of a league table.[16–20]

QALY would be eligible for reimbursement under Ontario's drug program. However, the ratio indicates that the drug would increase expenditures as compared with the current standard of therapy. If a pharmacy really has a fixed budget for drugs, it may not be able to afford the extra expenditure, even if the product is more effective.

League tables and published ranges also require that health effectiveness be measured in life years or quality-adjusted life years saved. The use of these measures is frequently impractical and sometimes not meaningful. As discussed earlier, many studies use intermediate measures—such as decreases in blood pressure or serum cholesterol—because of the long time horizon required to measure final outcomes such as years of life saved. For other types of products, such as those used for mild to moderate pain or other self-limiting conditions, life years may not be appropriate measures because neither the condition being treated nor the drug being tested has a large or lasting effect on either length or quality of life. However, use of quality-adjusted life years in pharmacoeconomic studies has become more common.

## Cost-Benefit Analysis

Cost-benefit analysis (CBA) differs from the other techniques used in pharmacoeconomic analyses in that effectiveness is valued in dollars. Bootman et al.'s evaluation of pharmacist-provided pharmacokinetic dosing services for severely burned patients is an example of a CBA.[9] One of the major outcomes of the service was a decrease in patient mortality. For the CBA, the decrease in mortality had to be valued in dollars. This was done by setting the value of each life saved equal to the earnings that the patient was expected to receive during the remainder of his or her life.

Because both costs and effectiveness (or benefits) are expressed in dollar terms, interpretation of the results of a CBA is simple. Two methods are commonly used to present the results of the CBA: computing the ratio of benefits to costs and computing net benefits. Benefit-to-cost ratios are calculated by dividing the sum of a product's or service's benefits by the sum of its costs. A ratio greater than 1 indicates that benefits exceed costs and, consequently, that there is an economic justification for using the product or service. The net benefit of a product or service is calculated by subtracting the sum of its costs from the sum of its benefits. A positive net benefit indicates that use of the product or service is economically justified. In Bootmanet al.'s study, the total benefits of pharmacokinetic dosing services amounted to $331,068 for the population of patients studied. The costs of providing services were $37,850. Thus, the benefit-to-cost ratio was 8.7 and the net benefit was $293,218.[9]

A major problem in CBA is that of valuing decreases in mortality and morbidity in dollar terms. Two methods have been used. The first, and most widely used, approach is called the *human capital* approach. This method bases the value of a saved life or a shortened incidence of illness on the monetary value of patients' expected future earnings. Using this approach, the benefits of a program that saved lives would be calculated as a function of the number of years of life saved and patients' expected wage rates for these years. The wage rates are usually estimated as the average wages of the age, sex, and racial group to which the patient belongs.

The human capital approach biases CBAs in favor of groups that earn higher wages, such as white males. As a result, a CBA using the human capital approach would favor a program that saved the lives of white males over one that saved an equivalent number of lives of blacks or females. Another problem is that the approach considers only savings from work-related productivity. Other benefits of reducing mortality and morbidity, such as alleviation of pain and grief, are ignored. Because of this limitation, estimates provided by the human capital method should be considered as minimum estimates of the cost of human life.

A second approach to valuing mortality and morbidity savings is the *willingness to pay* approach. This approach asks individuals how much they would be willing to pay to decrease the probability of mortality or morbidity by some set percentage. For example, if a given drug is believed to decrease the probability of stroke by 20%, then potential users might be asked how much they would pay for a 20% reduction in the probability of experiencing a stroke. A major problem with this approach is that of developing reliable estimates. Individuals' estimates of the amounts they would be willing to pay to avoid morbidity and mortality have not been stable from study to study.

## ETHICAL CONSIDERATIONS IN PHARMACOECONOMICS

Pharmacoeconomics takes a societal point of view for allocating resources. It focuses on spending limited resources in a way that provides the most benefit for the most people. Individual practitioners, such as physicians and pharmacists, typically take the point of view of the individual patient. That is, practitioners seek to do all they can for individual patients; they believe that any treatment that could improve a patient's condition should be used. Inevitably, this leads to a conflict about how resources should be used. A real-life example illustrates the conflict.[15]

In 1987, the Oregon legislature decided that the state Medicaid program would no longer pay for transplants. The state faced this decision because it did not have enough money to meet all its needs; as a result, it had to cut some programs. One of the choices that the Medicaid program had to make was whether to pay for transplants. The amount of funding available was sufficient to cover either 30 transplants or basic medical services for 5,700 women and children. The legislature chose the latter option. They believed that the benefits of providing basic medical services to 5,700 women and children would far outweigh the benefits of providing 30 transplants. This was an example of taking the societal perspective. The legislature chose to use its money to do the most good for the most people.

Shortly after the decision was made, a 7-year-old Medicaid patient was diagnosed with acute lymphocytic leukemia. He needed a bone marrow transplant to live. Because Medicaid no longer paid for transplants, the boy's family was unable to afford the transplant, and the boy died. Individual practitioners would argue that the boy should have been given the transplant; not doing so led to his death. On the other hand, if the state's resources had been used to fund the transplant, a large number of women and children would have been denied basic medical services such as prenatal care, immunizations, and hypertensive therapy. The state's best estimate was that number of years of life lost as a result of denying care to these women and children would have substantially exceeded the number lost as a result of not funding transplants.

This story illustrates the basic conflict between pharmacoeconomics, with its emphasis on the group, and the individual practitioner, with his or her emphasis on the individual. This is a conflict that society, individual practitioners, and citizens will increasingly face as the resources available for health care become more limited.

## References

1. Borger C, Smith S, Truffer C, et al. Health spending projections through 2015: changes on the horizon. Health Aff 2006;25:w61–w73.
2. Levit KR, Sensenig AL, Cowan CA, et al. National Health Expenditures, 1993. Health Care Financ Rev 1994;16:247–293.
3. Townsend RJ. Post-marketing drug research and development. Drug Intell Clin Pharm 1987;21:134–136.
4. Bootman JL, Townsend RJ, McGhan WF. Principles of Pharmacoeconomics. Cincinnati: Harvey Whitney Books Company, 2005.
5. Robinson R. Economic evaluation and health care: what does it mean? Br Med J 1993;307:670–673.
6. Detsky AS, Naglie IG. A clinician's guide to cost-effectiveness analysis. Ann Intern Med 1990;113:147–154.
7. Johnson JA, Bootman JL. Drug-related morbidity and mortality: a cost-of-illness study. Arch Intern Med 1995;155:1949–1956.
8. McCombs JS, Nichol MB. Pharmacy-enforced outpatient drug treatment protocols: a case study of Medical restrictions for cefaclor. Ann Pharmacother 1993;27:155–160.
9. Bootman JL, Wertheimer AI, Zaske D, et al. Individualizing gentamicin dosage regimens in burn patients with gram-negative septicemia: a cost-benefit analysis. J Pharm Sci 1979;68:267–272.
10. Smith RD, Hall J, Gurney H, et al. A cost-utility approach to the use of 5-fluorouacil and levamisole as adjuvant chemotherapy for Dukes' colonic carcinoma. Med J Aust 1993;158:319–322.
11. The CEA Registry. Catalog of Preference Weights 1998–2001, Tufts-New England Medical Center Institute for Clinical Research and Health Policy Studies. Available at: http://www.tufts-nemc.org/cearegistry/index.html. Accessed May 5, 2006.
12. Doubilet P, Weinstein MC, McNeil BJ. Use and misuse of the term "cost effective" in medicine. N Engl J Med 1986;314:253–255.
13. Ontario Ministry of Health. Guidelines for Preparation of Economic Analyses to Be Included in Submissions to Drug Programs Branch for Listing in the Ontario Drug Benefit Formulary/Comparative Drug Index. Toronto: Ministry of Health: Drug Programs Branch, 1991.
14. Gafni A, Birch S. Guidelines for the adoption of new technologies: a prescription fro uncontrolled growth in expenditures and how to avoid the problem. Can Med Assoc J 1993;148:913–917.

15. Eddy DM. What's going on in Oregon? JAMA 1991;266:417–420.
16. Torrance GW, Zipursky A. Cost-effectiveness of antepartum prevention of Rh immunization. Clin Perinatol 1984;11:267.
17. Weinstein MC. Tutorial: economic assessments of medical practices and technologies. Med Decis Making 1981;1:309–330.
18. Boyle MH, Torrance GW, Sinclair JC. Economic evaluation of neonatal intensive care of very-low-birth-weight infants. N Engl J Med 1983;425.
19. Stason WB, Weinstein MC. Allocation of resources to manage hypertension. N Engl J Med 1977;296:732–739.
20. Churchill DN, Lemon B, Torrance GW. Cost-effectiveness analysis comparing continuous ambulatory peritoneal dialysis to hospital dialysis. Med Decis Making 1983;3:355.

### Suggested Reading

Bootman JL, Townsend RJ, McGhan WF, eds. Principles of Pharmacoeconomics. 3rd Ed. Cincinnati: Harvey Whitney Books Company, 2005.
Drummond MF, O'Brien B, Stoddart GL, et al. Methods for the Economic Evaluation of Health Care Programmes. Oxford: Oxford University Press, 1997.
Laupacis A, Feeny D, Detsky AS, et al. How attractive does a new technology have to be to warrant adoption and utilization? Tentative guidelines for using clinical and economic evaluations. Can Med Assoc J 1992;146:473–481.

## QUESTIONS

1. Pharmacoeconomics is concerned with:
   a. costs of drug therapy
   b. clinical outcomes of drug therapy
   c. outcomes of drug therapy such as quality of life and patient satisfaction
   d. All of the above
   e. a and b only
2. The goal of pharmacoeconomics is to:
   a. minimize the amount spent on drug therapy
   b. maximize the benefits of drug therapy
   c. maximize the benefits of drug therapy for a set and limited budget
3. A pharmacoeconomic study of a new anticholesterol agent should include which of the following costs if done from society's perspective?
   a. Drug costs
   b. Physicians' fees for initial diagnosis and periodic monitoring
   c. Cost savings that occur as a result of preventing strokes and heart attacks
   d. Costs of treating drug side effects
   e. All of the above
   f. a and b only
4. The indirect costs of treating depression include:
   a. costs of antidepressant drugs
   b. costs of treating side effects of antidepressant drugs
   c. wages lost by patients as a result of being too depressed to work
   d. All of the above

5. Intermediate outcome measures include:
   a. patient satisfaction
   b. health-related quality of life
   c. blood pressure
   d. life years saved
   e. All of the above
   f. a, b, and c
6. Pharmacoeconomic studies done from which of the following perspectives would include patient productivity losses?
   a. Insurer's perspective
   b. Patient's perspective
   c. Society's perspective
   d. All of the above
   e. b and c only
7. CMA differs from CEA in that:
   a. CMA considers changes in both length and quality of life
   b. CMA can only be used when the treatments being compared produce the same type of outcome
   c. CMA can only be used when the treatments being compared produce the same type of outcome and are equally effective in doing so
8. Cost-effectiveness ratios are calculated as the:
   a. effectiveness of the treatment divided by its acquisition cost
   b. effectiveness of the treatment divided by total costs
   c. difference between the total cost of the treatment and the current standard divided by the difference in the effectiveness of the treatment and the current standard
9. CUA differs from CEA in that:
   a. CUA considers changes in both length and quality of life
   b. CUA can only be used when the treatments being compared produce the same type of outcome
   c. CUA can only be used when the treatments being compared produce the same type of outcome and are equally effective in doing so
   d. CUA measures effectiveness in natural or physical units
10. A QALY is:
    a. a quality-adjusted life year
    b. based on the tradeoffs patients make between length of life and quality of life
    c. a measure of effectiveness
    d. All of the above
    e. a and b only
11. It is estimated that the average patient will live for 10 years after a heart attack. Assume that patients would trade 1 year of life in the kind of health experienced after a heart attack for 0.75 years of good health. How many quality-adjusted life years can a patient expect to experience after a heart attack?
    a. 10
    b. 7.5
    c. 2.5
    d. 9.25
12. Livsumore, a new antiarrhythmic drug, has a cost utility ratio of $5,000 per QALY saved as compared with the current standard of therapy for arrhythmias. The cost-utility ratio can be interpreted to mean:

    **a.** Livsumore is more effective and less expensive than the current standard of therapy

    **b.** Livsumore is more effective and more expensive than the current standard of therapy

    **c.** Livsumore is less effective and less expensive than the current standard of therapy

13. Would Livsumore be covered under Ontario's drug reimbursement program?
    
    **a.** Yes
    
    **b.** Yes—but with some restrictions placed on its availability
    
    **c.** No

14. The Good Life HMO is considering adding Livsumore to its formulary. If it added Livsumore, and all of its patients were switched from the current standard of therapy to Livsumore, what would happen to Good Life's drug budget?
    
    **a.** It would increase
    
    **b.** It would decrease
    
    **c.** It would not change

15. Should the Good Life HMO add Livsumore to its formulary?
    
    **a.** Yes
    
    **b.** No
    
    **c.** It depends—if the HMO believes that a year of quality-adjusted life is worth $5,000 or more and if it has sufficient budget, then Livsumore should be added

16. Cost-benefit analysis compares:
    
    **a.** the dollar value of the costs of a program with its effectiveness as measured in natural units
    
    **b.** the dollar value of the costs of a program with its effectiveness as measured in quality-adjusted life years
    
    **c.** the dollar value of the costs of a program with the dollar value of its effectiveness

17. A major problem in cost-benefit analysis is:
    
    **a.** determining the most appropriate measure of effectiveness
    
    **b.** placing a dollar value on human morbidity and mortality
    
    **c.** estimating utility values
    
    **d.** the technique's inability to consider more than one measure of effectiveness

18. Which of the following best describes the view of resource allocation taken by pharmacoeconomics?
    
    **a.** Do the most good for the most people
    
    **b.** Do all the good possible for each individual patient

19. Which of the following best describes the view of resource allocation taken by most health care providers?
    
    **a.** Do the most good for the most people
    
    **b.** Do all the good possible for each individual patient

20. Pharmacoeconomics focuses on:
    
    **a.** cost
    
    **b.** effectiveness
    
    **c.** value

## CHAPTER 16

# Decision Analysis

After reading this chapter, the student should be able to:

1. Use decision analysis to inform and assist in clinical, business, and pharmacoeconomic decision making,
2. Discuss the importance of perspective in a decision analysis,
3. Use sensitivity analysis to examine the effects of uncertainty of estimates used in decision and financial analyses,
4. Discuss the reasons that cost-effectiveness analyses are not appropriate for estimating the budgetary and clinical impact of adding a new drug to a formulary,
5. Use the systems approach to estimate the budgetary and clinical impact of adding a new drug to a formulary,
6. List and discuss the advantages and disadvantages of randomized, controlled, clinical trials and observational studies as sources of probability and outcome information used in pharmacoeconomic decision analysis, and
7. List and discuss ways that decision analysis may improve the quality of decision making.

The pharmacy director for a large health maintenance organization (HMO) must decide which of a new class of anti-influenza agents to add to the formulary. The HMO's current treatment options for influenza include rimantadine, which is an older antiviral agent, and symptomatic treatment. The new agents are also antivirals, but they are more effective than rimantadine in reducing the severity and duration of influenza symptoms and have fewer side effects. They also have much higher acquisition costs.

The new agents—Flu-wonder and Flu-begone—are similar in chemical structure, mechanism of action, and side effect profiles. Flu-wonder is somewhat more effective and more expensive. The pharmacy manager's task is to decide which agent to add to the formulary.

Decision analysis is a technique that the pharmacy manager could use to help make this decision. Decision analysis is defined as "a systematic approach to decision making under conditions of uncertainty."[1] Uncertainty means that we do not know, with a high degree of certainty, what the outcome of the decision will be. Decision analysis is a useful technique because most decisions in life are made under uncertain conditions. The best we can do is gather information, assess probabilities, and make the best decision possible with the information we have. Decision analysis systematizes this process.

Many important decisions that pharmacists face are made under uncertain conditions. Clinical pharmacists select drug therapy for particular patients. Because there is no way to know beforehand how a drug will work in a particular patient, these decisions have to be made under uncertain conditions. Pharmacy managers employed by insurance companies, major employers, and pharmacy benefit managers (PBMs) decide which drugs to include on the formulary. Since there is no sure way of knowing how effective and economical a particular drug will be for a particular population of patients, this decision has to be made under uncertain conditions. Pharmacy managers in community and health system settings make pricing and personnel decisions. Again, there is no way to know with certainty how these decisions will turn out. Decision analysis is a technique that managers can use to assist them in gathering the information needed to make a decision, organizing that information, and logically evaluating it.

Detsky et al.[2] stated that decision analyses are appropriate when two conditions are present. First, there should be some uncertainty about the decision. Some decisions are clear-cut. In treating patients with high cholesterol, for example, the first line of drug treatment is almost always a statin. Since there is no uncertainty about this decision, there is no need for a decision analysis. However, the choice of *which* statin to use is less clear-cut and could benefit from a decision analysis. Second, the alternatives being compared should have tradeoffs among them. If one is clearly better than the others, there is no need for a formal decision analysis. If the most effective statin is also the least expensive and the most convenient for patients to take, there is no need for a decision analysis. But if the cheapest product is less effective or less convenient, then a decision analysis may be needed.

Decision analysis requires that the decision maker explicitly structure the decision, then use quantitative techniques to identify the decision option with the *greatest expected benefit*. Calculation of the greatest expected benefit considers both the probability that a benefit will be attained and the value of the benefit if it is attained. As an example, assume that a clinical pharmacist must select between two life-saving drugs. Drug A has a 75% chance of working, and, if it does work, will extend the patient's life by 5 years. Drug B has a 50% chance of working, but if it works, the patient will live 10 more years. To make a rational decision, the pharmacist should consider both the probability that the drug will work and the benefit the patient will receive if it does work. In other words, he or she must consider and compare the expected benefits of the drugs. Expected benefit is calculated as the product of the probability and magnitude of the benefit. Expected benefits of Drugs A and B are:

Drug A: 0.75 × 5 years = 3.75 years
Drug B: 0.50 × 10 years = 5.00 years

In this case Drug B would be the choice with the highest expected benefit and, consequently, would be the logical choice.

Because it deals with decision making in uncertain conditions, decision analyses are based on the *probabilities* or likelihood of outcomes. Because it is a predictive technique, decision analysis cannot determine what the best choice will be; it can only determine which of a number of options is most likely to be the best choice. This is the choice with the greatest expected benefit.

While decision analysis can be applied to many decisions that pharmacists have to make, it is most commonly used for pharmacoeconomic decision making. It is particularly useful in pharmacoeconomics because it can be used to estimate both expected costs and expected effectiveness of treatment. For example, decision analysis could be used to predict the least costly drug to use to treat a particular disease or condition. In this context, cost refers to total cost of treatment, not just the acquisition cost of the drug product. Decision analysis could also be used to predict the most effective treatment for a particular disease or condition. Effectiveness could be defined as cure of disease, decrease in symptoms, improvement in physiologic measures (such as blood pressure or cholesterol levels), improvement in quality of life, increase in length of life, or increase in patient satisfaction.

## AN EXAMPLE ILLUSTRATING THE USE OF DECISION ANALYSIS

We will continue with the example given at the beginning of the chapter to illustrate the use of decision analysis. In that example, the pharmacy manager must decide which of two new influenza drugs—Flu-wonder or Flu-begone—to add to the formulary.

Influenza is an acute respiratory illness caused by a viral infection. Symptoms include headache, fever, myalgia, malaise, and sore throat. Complete resolution of symptoms typically takes about 5 days in an otherwise healthy patient. Resolution of symptoms usually takes about 3 days for patients treated with Flu-wonder and about 4 days for patients treated with Flu-begone. Secondary bacterial infections, such as pneumonia, can complicate the illness. Secondary infections are more likely in elderly or immunocompromised patients and can lead to hospitalization and death. In general, patients who receive only symptomatic treatment have about a 20% chance of acquiring a secondary bacterial infection. The probability goes down to 15% for those treated both symptomatically and with rimantadine. (All patients, regardless of other treatment, will receive symptomatic treatment. Consequently, when we refer to a patient being treated with another agent—such as Flu-wonder—it is assumed that the patient is also receiving symptomatic treatment.) The probabilities of secondary bacterial infection are 5% for those treated with Flu-wonder and 7% for those treated with Flu-begone. Secondary bacterial infections require treatment with antibiotics. Influenza patients who are successfully treated with antibiotics for secondary infections typically take about 7 days to see complete resolution of influenza symptoms. However, about 0.5% of patients with secondary infections do not respond to antibiotics and have to be hospitalized for further treatment. These patients usually take about 15 days to see complete symptom resolution.

Decision analysis can be used to determine which of the new antivirals—Flu-wonder or Flu-begone—has lower total treatment costs and which has greater effectiveness.

## CONDUCTING THE DECISION ANALYSIS

A decision analysis consists of five steps. These will be described and illustrated with the influenza example.

### Identify and Bound the Decision

The first step in a decision analysis involves identifying and bounding the decision. Identifying the decision consists of concisely stating what decision needs to be made. Bounding the decision consists of setting the ground rules for the analysis. Bounding the decision includes:

- determining the perspective from which the decision will be made,
- stating the criteria that will be used to evaluate the alternatives, and
- deciding on the time frame of the analysis.

The decision to be made in our example is which of the new antivirals to add to the formulary. The alternatives are Flu-wonder and Flu-begone.

The analysis will be conducted from the HMO's perspective (rather than the perspective of the patient or of society). As a result, only costs and benefits that accrue to the HMO will be considered in the analysis. The criteria for judging the alternatives will be total cost of treatment (cost) and decrease in days of symptoms (effectiveness). In this example, the time frame for the analysis is straightforward. It is simply the 3 to 15 days that it takes for patients to become symptom free. In cases where the decision analysis deals with chronic diseases—such as hypertension, high cholesterol, or diabetes—the appropriate time frame is more difficult to determine.

### Structure the Decision

The second step in a decision analysis is structuring the decision. This consists of systematically identifying and stating the consequences of each decision alternative. Typically, a decision tree is used to structure the decision. A decision tree is a graphical representation of the decision alternatives and outcomes. For decisions that involve disease or injury, the decision tree depicts the course of treatment and natural history of the disease. An example of a decision tree for influenza treatment is shown in Figure 16-1.

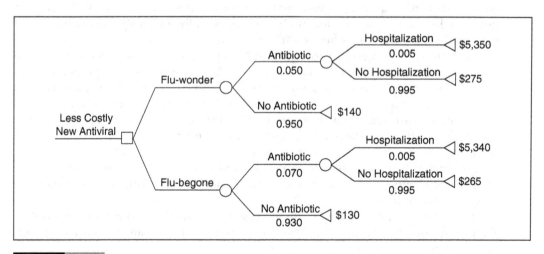

**FIGURE 16—1a**    Decision tree for treatment of influenza (outcomes are costs).

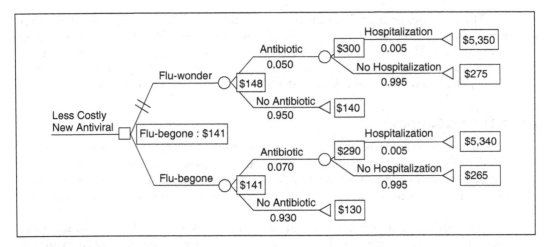

**FIGURE 16–1b**  Decision tree for treatment of influenza (outcomes are costs)—rolled back and averaged out.

By convention, the flow of events in a decision tree goes from left to right. Events that happen earlier are shown to the left and those that occur later to the right. The decision to be made and the decision alternatives are shown on the left side of the tree. The outcomes of each branch, or path, of the tree are shown on the far right.

Figure 16-1a shows a small square from which the three decision alternatives branch off. The small square is called a *choice node* because it indicates that the choice of alternatives is under the decision maker's control. The decision maker can choose to treat with either Flu-wonder or Flu-begone.

As shown in Figure 16-1a, the qualitative consequences are the same for each of the new antivirals. If treatment is successful, the patient will require no further treatment. If treatment is not successful, the patient will develop a secondary bacterial infection. This will require treatment with an antibiotic. If the antibiotic cures the infection, no further treatment is necessary. If not, the patient will require hospitalization. Note the small circles in the figure from which consequences branch. These are called *chance nodes*. Chance nodes indicate that the events to follow are probabilistic events that are not under the control of the decision maker. For example, whether or not a patient initially treated with Flu-wonder requires an antibiotic is not under the decision maker's control. It is a probabilistic event. There is an X% chance it will happen and $(1 - X)\%$ chance it will not.

## Assess the Probabilities

The third step in the decision analysis is to assess the *probabilities* of each consequence. In Figure 16-1, the probability of each consequence is shown under the branch for that consequence. Each decision alternative in the example has the same qualitative consequences, but the probability of each consequence occurring differs among alternatives. As shown in Figure 16-1a, patients are somewhat less likely to develop secondary bacterial infections if they are treated with Flu-wonder than if they are treated with Flu-begone.

The branches coming from a chance node must be mutually exhaustive and exclusive. That is, each must represent a distinct and independent outcome and the sum of the probabilities of all consequences must sum to one (100%) at the chance node.

The branches coming from the first Flu-wonder chance node indicate that either the patient will need an antibiotic or he will not. There is a 5% chance of needing an antibiotic and 100 − 5% = 95% chance of not needing an antibiotic. Similarly, the first Flu-begone node indicates that there is a 7% chance that a patient treated with Flu-begone will need an antibiotic and a 93% chance he or she will not.

## Value the Outcomes

The next step in the decision analysis is to value the outcomes of each branch, or path, of the decision tree. The value of each outcome is expressed in terms of the outcome criteria. In our example, we have both cost and effectiveness outcomes. We will first look at cost outcomes. Cost outcomes indicate the total cost of treatment for each branch.

The cost outcomes are shown at the end of each branch, on the far right (in Figure 16-1a). To calculate the cost outcomes, we determine the cost of treating a patient for each path in the decision tree. Costs of each treatment item are shown in Figure 16-2. We assume that all patients receive symptomatic treatment—a nasal decongestant and cough suppressant—even if they also receive an antiviral. The first path in the tree is for a patient who is treated with Flu-wonder, develops a secondary bacterial infection and requires an antibiotic, does not respond to the antibiotic, and then requires hospitalization. The value of the cost outcome of this path is the cost of treating a patient who follows this path. For this branch, this would include:

- the cost of the initial physician visit ($75) and treatment with Flu-wonder ($45) and symptomatic treatment ($20),
- the cost of a follow-up visit to the physician ($75) and an antibiotic ($60), and
- the cost of another follow-up visit after the antibiotic failed ($75) and a hospitalization ($5,000).

The total costs of treating a patient who followed this path would be $5,350, as shown in Figure 16-1a.

| Cost item | Cost ($) |
|---|---|
| Hospitalization | 5,000 |
| Physician visit | 75 |
| Symptomatic treatment*: | |
| Cough suppressant | 15 |
| Nasal decongestant | 5 |
| Total | 20 |
| Antibiotic | 60 |
| Flu-wonder | 45 |
| Flu-begone | 35 |
| Rimantadine | 2 |

*All patients receive symptomatic treatment, even if they also get an antiviral.

**FIGURE 16-2**   Cost data.

By comparison, the costs of treating a patient who was initially treated with Flu-wonder and required no further treatment would include only the cost of the initial physician visit ($75) and treatment with Flu-wonder ($45) and symptomatic treatment ($20). This amounts to $140.

To complete this step, we would calculate the cost of treatment for each path in the tree.

## Choose the Preferred Course of Action

The final step in the decision analysis is to choose the preferred decision option. The preferred alternative is the one with the best *expected value*. In our case, this would be the alternative with the lowest expected cost and the fewest expected days with symptoms.

The expected value of each decision option is found by a process known as *averaging out and folding back*. This involves starting at the end of each branch (the farthest point on the right side of the decision tree), then calculating the weighted average outcome at each chance node. The weighted average is calculated by multiplying the value of each branch by its probability. The expected values of cost for each agent are shown in Figure 16-1b.

The expected cost of treatment with Flu-wonder would be calculated as follows: patients who are treated with Flu-wonder and who require an antibiotic have a 0.5% chance of requiring hospitalization at a cost of $5,350 and a 99.5% chance of not requiring hospitalization with an associated cost of $275. The expected cost for a patient treated with Flu-wonder and requiring an antibiotic is:

$$0.005 \times \$5,350 + 0.995 \times \$275 = \$300$$

A patient treated with Flu-wonder has a 5% chance of requiring an antibiotic, with an associated expected cost of $300, and a 95% chance of not requiring an antibiotic, with an associated cost of $140. So, the expected cost of treatment for a patient receiving Flu-wonder is:

$$0.050 \times \$300 + 0.950 \times \$140 = \$148$$

The expected cost of treating a patient with Flu-wonder is $148. Averaging out and folding back indicates that the expected cost of treating a patient with Flu-begone is $141. Thus, Flu-begone is the less expensive choice. The hash marks in Figure 16-1b on the branches from Flu-wonder indicate that Flu-begone is the preferred alternative when the cost is the criterion.

The expected days with symptoms for each treatment are also calculated by rolling back and averaging out. Figures 16-3a and 16-3b show the decision tree used to calculate the expected effectiveness (days with symptoms) for each of the new antivirals. A patient treated with Flu-begone and requiring an antibiotic would have a 0.5% chance of being hospitalized and having 15 days of symptoms, and a 99.5% chance of not being hospitalized and having only 7 days of symptoms. So the expected number of days of symptoms for a patient treated with Flu-begone and requiring an antibiotic would be:

$$0.005 \times 15 \text{ days} + 0.995 \times 7 \text{ days} = 7.0 \text{ days}$$

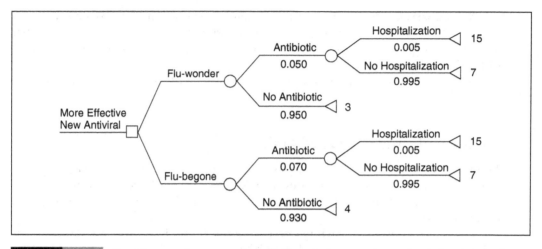

**FIGURE 16–3a**    Decision tree for treatment of influenza (outcomes are days of symptoms).

A patient treated with Flu-begone has a 7% chance of needing an antibiotic and suffering 7 days of symptoms, and a 93% chance of not needing an antibiotic and suffering only 4 days of symptoms. Thus, the expected effectiveness—in days of symptoms—for Flu-begone is:

$$0.07 \times 7 \text{ days} + 0.93 \times 4 \text{ days} = 4.2 \text{ days}$$

The expected effectiveness of Flu-begone is 4.2 days of symptoms. The expected effectiveness of Flu-wonder is 3.2 days of symptoms. The hash marks on the branch from Flu-begone indicate that Flu-wonder is the preferred alternative when effectiveness is the criterion.

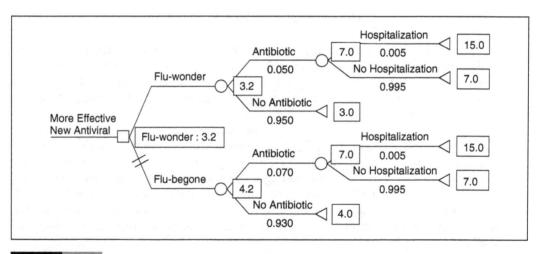

**FIGURE 16–3b**    Decision tree for treatment of influenza (outcomes are days of symptoms)— rolled back and averaged out.

## COST-EFFECTIVENESS ANALYSIS

The preceding discussion has demonstrated how to use decision analysis to determine the less expensive and the more effective antiviral. However, the decision analysis did not answer the question of which should be added to the formulary. Because Flu-wonder was the more effective, but also the more expensive, product, a cost-effectiveness analysis is needed to address this question.

The results of the two decision analyses provide the input for a cost-effectiveness analysis of the two influenza treatments. The cost-effectiveness calculations for use of Flu-wonder compared with Flu-begone are:

$$\text{Cost-effectiveness ratio} = \frac{\text{Cost of Flu-wonder}}{\text{Effectiveness of Flu-wonder}} - \frac{\text{Cost of Flu-begone}}{\text{Effectiveness of Flu-begone}}$$

$$= \frac{\$148}{3.2} - \frac{\$141}{4.2}$$

= $7 per additional day of symptoms avoided (a negative number of days with symptoms would be a positive number of days of symptoms avoided)

The question of whether Flu-wonder is cost effective, and consequently whether it should be added to the formulary, is a value judgment. It depends on whether the HMO believes that saving a patient from a day of symptoms is worth $7. It would certainly be easy to make the case to the employers who paid for their employees' membership in the HMO that it was worth $7 to save a day of influenza symptoms if doing so would eliminate a missed day of work. For any employer that provided paid sick leave to its employees, paying an additional $7 to prevent a lost day from work would be a good deal. This suggests that Flu-wonder probably would be considered cost effective and added to the formulary.

## SENSITIVITY ANALYSIS

Most of the probabilities and outcome measures used in a decision analysis are estimates. Because they are estimates, we are usually not certain of their exact value. This affects the degree of confidence we can have in the results of the decision analysis—the less certain we are of the values of the probability and outcome data, the less confidence we have in the results of the decision analysis. Sensitivity analysis is commonly used to deal with uncertain estimates. Sensitivity analysis does so by indicating the extent to which the uncertainty of estimates of probabilities and outcomes affects the results of the decision analysis or, more importantly, the decision that is made from the decision analysis results.

A sensitivity analysis is conducted by varying the uncertain estimate across some reasonable range to see how the changes affect the result, or outcome, of the decision analysis. If the result stays the same, or varies little, across the full range of reasonable estimates, then we can have greater confidence in the result. If the result changes substantially across the range of the estimate, our confidence in the result is reduced.

In the influenza example, the probability that a patient on Flu-wonder would require an antibiotic was estimated to be 5%. Assume that this estimate was obtained by averaging the results of several clinical trials. Further, assume that the clinical trial estimates ranged from 3% to 7%. In this situation, we cannot be completely sure that the correct probability was 5%. It might be as high as 7% or as low as 3%. This variability would lead us to question whether probability estimates higher or lower than our *baseline* estimate would affect the results of our analysis. (The baseline value is the value of the estimate used in the original decision analysis. It is the best estimate of the value.) This is the issue that sensitivity analysis addresses. To continue our example, assume that the estimate of the probability of needing an antibiotic when treated with Flu-begone is also an average. On average, a patient treated with Flu-begone has a 7% chance of requiring an antibiotic, but it could range as low as 5.0% or as high as 10%.

The simplest type of sensitivity analysis is a *one-way sensitivity analysis*. This is done by varying the values of one estimate across its reasonable range while holding the values of all other estimates constant at their baseline values. The decision tree is used to estimate expected costs and expected effectiveness across all levels at which the uncertain variable is varied. Two-way sensitivity analyses are done by varying the values of two estimates while holding the values of all other estimates constant. It is also possible to do three-way and higher-way analyses.

The first panel of Figure 16-4 shows the results of a one-way sensitivity analysis for the uncertainty of the probability of requiring an antibiotic when treated with Flu-wonder. The analysis shows the effects of varying the probability on days of influenza symptoms. At either end of the range of reasonable estimates (0.03 and 0.07), Flu-wonder is the more effective treatment. Further, days of symptoms vary very little. This indicates that the effectiveness measure (days of symptoms) is not sensitive to the probability of needing an antibiotic (across the range tested). This increases our confidence in the results of the decision analysis because any reasonable estimate of the

| Probability of needing an antibiotic after treatment with Flu-wonder | Days of symptoms if treated with: | |
| --- | --- | --- |
| | Flu-wonder | Flu-begone |
| 0.03 | 3.1 | 4.2 |
| 0.04 | 3.2 | 4.2 |
| 0.05 | 3.2 | 4.2 |
| 0.06 | 3.2 | 4.2 |
| 0.07 | 3.3 | 4.2 |
| Probability of needing an antibiotic after treatment with Flu-begone | Days of symptoms if treated with: | |
| | Flu-wonder | Flu-begone |
| 0.050 | 3.2 | 4.2 |
| 0.063 | 3.2 | 4.2 |
| 0.075 | 3.2 | 4.2 |
| 0.088 | 3.2 | 4.3 |
| 0.100 | 3.2 | 4.3 |

**FIGURE 16-4**    One-way sensitivity analysis: days of symptoms by probability of needing an antibiotic.

| Probability of needing an antibiotic after treatment with Flu-wonder | Total treatment costs ($) if treated with: | |
| --- | --- | --- |
| | Flu-wonder | Flu-begone |
| 0.03 | 145 | 141 |
| 0.04 | 146 | 141 |
| 0.05 | 148 | 141 |
| 0.06 | 150 | 141 |
| 0.07 | 151 | 141 |

| Probability of needing an antibiotic after treatment with Flu-begone | Total treatment costs ($) if treated with: | |
| --- | --- | --- |
| | Flu-wonder | Flu-begone |
| 0.050 | 148 | 138 |
| 0.063 | 148 | 140 |
| 0.075 | 148 | 142 |
| 0.088 | 148 | 144 |
| 0.100 | 148 | 146 |

**FIGURE 16–5**  One-way sensitivity analysis: total treatment costs by probability of needing an antibiotic.

probability of requiring an antibiotic after treatment with Flu-wonder will show Flu-wonder to be the more effective treatment.

The second panel of Figure 16-4 shows a one-way sensitivity analyses for the uncertainty in the probability of needing an antibiotic after Flu-begone treatment. This analysis shows that the results of the original analysis—which indicated that Flu-wonder is more effective—are not sensitive to the probabilities that patients treated with Flu-begone will need antibiotics. At all reasonable levels, Flu-wonder is the more effective agent.

The sensitivity analyses increase our confidence in the results of the decision analysis by indicating that any reasonable values of the probability of needing an antibiotic for either of the new antivirals will lead to the same results. Thus, any uncertainty we have about these estimates is not likely to affect the results. A similar analysis could be done to assess the effects of uncertainty of the probability of hospitalization on days of symptoms.

Sensitivity analysis can also be used for the cost estimates (Fig. 16-5). The analysis indicates that across all reasonable ranges of the estimates of needing an antibiotic, Flu-wonder is the more expensive agent. This, again, increases our confidence in the results.

Sensitivity analyses can also be used for cost-effectiveness analysis. In this case, the analysis shows the effects of variability in an estimate on the incremental cost-effectiveness ratio (ICER). The ICER incorporates both cost and effectiveness. Doing a cost-effectiveness sensitivity analysis by hand is very tedious. It requires calculating the expected costs and expected effectiveness values across the range of estimates, then calculating ICERs for each. Decision analysis software, such as DATA by Treeage,[3] automates and substantially simplifies the process.

| PAntFW | Antiviral | Cost | Incr Cost | Effectiveness | Incr Eff | ICER |
|---|---|---|---|---|---|---|
| 0.03 | Flu-begone | $141 | | 4.2 | | |
| | Flu-wonder | $145 | $4 | 3.1 | 1.1 | $3.64 |
| 0.04 | Flu-begone | $141 | | 4.2 | | |
| | Flu-wonder | $146 | $5 | 3.2 | 1.0 | $5.00 |
| 0.05 | Flu-begone | $141 | | 4.2 | | |
| | Flu-wonder | $148 | $7 | 3.2 | 1.0 | $7.00 |
| 0.06 | Flu-begone | $141 | | 4.2 | | |
| | Flu-wonder | $150 | $9 | 3.2 | 1.0 | $9.00 |
| 0.07 | Flu-begone | $141 | | 4.2 | | |
| | Flu-wonder | $151 | $10 | 3.3 | 0.9 | $11.11 |

PAntFW, probability of needing an antibiotic when treated with Flu-wonder; Incr Cost, incremental cost; Incr Eff, incremental effectiveness; ICER, incremental cost-effectiveness ratio.

**FIGURE 16–6** One-way sensitivity analysis: cost-effectiveness by probability of needing an antibiotic when using Flu-wonder.

A sensitivity analysis for the cost effectiveness of anti-influenza agents is shown in Figure 16-6. The estimate that is varied is the probability of needing an antibiotic when treated with Flu-wonder. Across the range of estimates, Flu-begone is less expensive and Flu-wonder is more effective in every case. The ICERs range from $4.00 to $11.11 per day of symptoms avoided. This suggests that the analysis is relatively insensitive to the probability of needing an antibiotic when treated with Flu-wonder.

Some experts recommend doing one-way sensitivity analyses for all probabilities and outcomes in the decision analysis.[4,5] At minimum, one-way sensitivity analysis should be done for the estimates with the greatest variability and for those likely to have the greatest impact on the results. For two-way and higher-way analyses, it may not be feasible to use all sets of variables. In this case, the analyst must determine which are the most important to test. These are frequently the ones with the greatest levels of uncertainty (the widest range of reasonable values) or the ones that the one-way analysis showed to have the greatest impact on the final results.

## Estimating the Effect of a Formulary Addition on a Health Care Organization's Budget and the Health of Its Population

Pharmacoeconomic analyses, such as cost-effectiveness and cost-utility analysis, are useful for selecting the most cost-effective alternative from a number of mutually exclusive choices. For example, cost-effectiveness analysis was useful for selecting which of two new antivirals should be added to the formulary because the antivirals were very similar to each other. Because of their similarity, the HMO viewed the antivirals as mutually exclusive choices. Once the formulary decision was made, the pharmacy manager needed to estimate the effect that adding the new drug to the formulary would have on the HMO's budget and on the health of the population it serves. The typical pharmacoeconomic analyses—cost-minimization, cost-effectiveness, and cost-utility analyses—are not appropriate for this purpose.

They are not appropriate for estimating budget or health outcomes impact because they assume that the alternatives being tested are mutually exclusive. That is, *all* patients will be treated with the one best drug. This is modeled in the decision tree by estimating the costs and effectiveness of all patients being treated with the first treatment alternative, then estimating the costs and effectiveness of all patients being treated with the second treatment alternative, and so on, until the costs and effectiveness of treating all patients with each of the alternatives have been estimated. In our example, the pharmacoeconomic analysis assumed that patients would be treated with Flu-wonder or Flu-begone.

However, in actual medical practice different patients would be treated with different agents because of differences in disease severity. In our example, physicians would use Flu-wonder to treat the patients most likely to experience influenza-related complications, rimantadine for healthier patients, and symptomatic-only treatment for the healthiest patients. Consequently, an analysis that estimates the impact of the addition of a new agent to a formulary on budget and health outcomes should reflect the fact that different types of patients receive different influenza treatments.

In this section, we will discuss how a manager could use a decision analysis–type approach to estimate the budget and health impact of adding a drug to the formulary. Paul Langley has referred to this as "a systems based approach" to pharmacoeconomics.[6] The Academy of Managed Care Pharmacy (AMCP) has included this approach in its "Format for Formulary Submissions."[7] The AMCP Format describes the information that a health care organization should obtain when considering a product for formulary inclusion.

In using the systems-based approach, the manager would first estimate the effect that adding a new drug would have on patterns of drug use in the population served by the HMO. In our example, adding Flu-wonder would obviously result in increased use of Flu-wonder, but it would also result in changes in the use of complementary or substitute drugs. Specifically, the addition of Flu-wonder to the formulary would decrease the use of rimantadine and symptomatic-only treatment. Based on the projected changes in patterns of drug use, the manager then estimates the effects that adding the new drug will have on medical costs and outcomes. The addition of Flu-wonder would increase drug costs, because Flu-wonder is substantially more expensive than the rimantadine or symptomatic-only treatment. However, because it is more effective, it should also decrease influenza-related physician and hospital costs. We will continue our example to more fully illustrate the systems-based approach.

After selecting Flu-wonder as the antiviral to add to the formulary, the pharmacy manager needs to estimate the effect the addition would have on the HMO's budget and health outcomes. The first step in this process is to examine how influenza is currently treated within the HMO. Assume that the HMO expects to treat 1,000 patients for influenza in the coming year. The manager estimates that, if Flu-wonder were *not* added to the formulary, 100 patients would receive rimantadine and 900 would receive symptomatic-only treatment (Fig. 16-7). The manager estimates that treatment patterns for influenza would change fairly dramatically with the introduction of

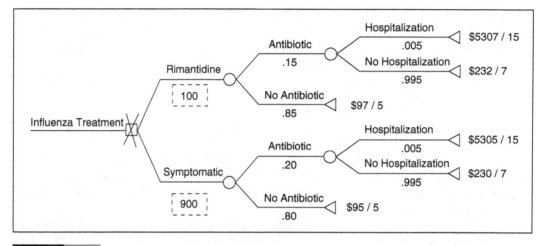

**FIGURE 16-7** Drug use for treating influenza before addition of Flu-wonder to formulary (outcomes are costs and days of symptoms).

Flu-wonder. Specifically, the manager estimates that of the 1,000 patients the HMO expects to treat, 250 will be treated with Flu-wonder, 700 with symptomatic-only treatment, and 50 with rimantadine (Fig. 16-8).

Note that while Figures 16-7 and 16-8 *resemble* decision trees, they are *not* decision trees. Decision trees assume that all patients will be treated with the one best drug.

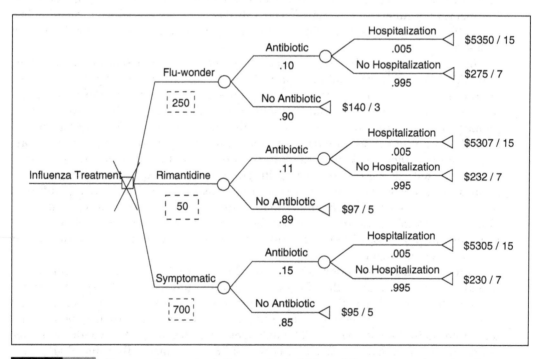

**FIGURE 16-8** Drug use for treating influenza after addition of Flu-wonder to formulary (outcomes are costs and workdays lost).

For our example, if we were using decision trees, this would mean that all 1,000 patients would be treated with Flu-wonder, or all 1,000 would be treated with rimantadine, or all 1,000 would be treated symptomatically only. The purpose of a decision tree analysis is to determine the one best treatment from a group of mutually exclusive alternatives. We are not using Figures 16-7 and 16-8 to identify the one best alternative. That is why the choice node is crossed out. Instead, we are assuming that some patients are treated with one alternative and the remaining patients with other alternatives. Specifically, as shown in Figure 16-8, 250 patients will be treated with Flu-wonder, 50 with rimantadine, and 700 with symptomatic-only treatment. We will use the decision tree *structure* so we can "average out and fold back" to estimate the expected costs and outcomes of each treatment.

The next step in the process is to estimate how changes in drug treatment patterns resulting from the addition of Flu-wonder to the formulary will affect the HMO's cost of treating influenza. This is known as *budget impact analysis*.

Before the manager can estimate the changes in costs due to the addition of Flu-wonder, he or she must first estimate how much the HMO would spend if Flu-wonder were not on the formulary. Figure 16-7 shows the projected patterns of drug use if Flu-wonder were not on the formulary. Rolling back and averaging out indicates that the expected cost of treating a patient with rimantadine is $121 and the expected cost of treating a patient symptomatically is $127. (These estimates are not shown in Figure 16-7, but can be calculated by rolling back and averaging out the tree.) The HMO's total cost of treating patients for influenza, if Flu-wonder is not added to the formulary, is:

$121 per patient × 100 patients treated with rimantadine = $ 12,100
$127 per patient × 900 patients treated symptomatically = 114,300
Total cost of treating patients = $126,400

Next, the manager estimates how much the HMO will spend to treat influenza if it adds Flu-wonder to the formulary. The use of Flu-wonder will increase pharmaceutical costs because Flu-wonder is more expensive than rimantadine or symptomatic-only treatment. However, if Flu-wonder is more effective, it should decrease the number of influenza-related pulmonary infections and hospitalizations. This will decrease the amount the HMO spends on antibiotics, physician visits, and hospitalizations.

These changes are modeled in Figure 16-8. Notice that the proportions of patients getting bacterial infections are different than previously stated. This is because the rates previously quoted assumed that the same population of patients was treated with each agent. For example, the 5% rate of secondary infections for Flu-wonder assumed that all 1,000 patients were treated with Flu-wonder and the 15% rate for rimantadine assumed that all 1,000 patients were treated with rimantadine. However, in Figures 16-7 and 16-8 we are not assuming this. Instead, we are estimating how the drugs would be used in actual medical practice. In practice, physicians will reserve Flu-wonder for older or immunocompromised patients who are most likely to experience complications of influenza. Therefore, the rate of secondary infection will be higher than the 5% rate, which applied to a population including both sicker and healthier patients. They will use rimantadine for patients less likely to experience complications and symptomatic-only treatment for younger, otherwise healthy patients who are least likely to experience complications. Thus, since they apply to a healthier population, the rates of secondary infection would be lower than previously quoted.

Averaging out and rolling back the information in Figure 16.8 indicates expected costs of $156 for each patient treated with Flu-wonder, $115 for each patient treated with rimantadine, and $119 for each patient treated symptomatically. The total cost to the health system is estimated as:

$156 per patient × 250 patients treated with Flu-wonder  = $ 39,000
$115 per patient × 50 patients treated with rimantadine   =   5,750
$119 per patient × 700 patients treated symptomatically   =  83,300
Total cost to health system for 1,000 patients treated      = $128,050

Comparing the cost estimates for adding and not adding Flu-wonder to the formulary indicates that adding Flu-wonder will have a positive impact on the HMO's budget. The total amount spent on treatment of influenza is estimated to be $128,050 − $126,400 = $1,650 higher as a result of adding Flu-wonder to the formulary.

Finally, the manager must estimate how changes in drug treatment patterns will affect the health of the population. As mentioned previously, if Flu-wonder is more effective, there should be a decrease in influenza-related bacterial infections and hospitalizations. This would decrease the number of days with symptoms among patients treated for influenza.

Rolling back and averaging out the information in Figure 16-7 provides an estimate of the total number of days with symptoms that the HMO population would experience if Flu-wonder were not on the formulary. The estimates indicate that the expected number of days with symptoms is 5.3 for patients treated with rimantadine and 5.4 for patients treated symptomatically. The total number of days with symptoms for the HMO's population if Flu-wonder is not on the formulary is:

5.3 days with symptoms per patient × 100 patients treated with rimantadine  =   530
5.4 days with symptoms per patient × 900 patients treated symptomatically    = 4,860
Total days with symptoms                                                     = 5,390

Averaging out and rolling back the health outcomes information in Figure 16-8 estimates the total number of days with symptoms if Flu-wonder is on the formulary. The expected number of days with symptoms for a patient treated with Flu-wonder is 3.4. The expected values for rimantadine and symptomatic treatment are 5.2 and 5.3, respectively. So, the total number of days with symptoms from influenza if Flu-wonder is on the formulary is:

3.4 days with symptoms per patient × 250 patients treated with Flu-wonder   =   850
5.2 days with symptoms per patient × 50 patients treated with rimantadine   =   260
5.3 days with symptoms per patient × 700 patients treated symptomatically   = 3,710
Total days with symptoms                                                     = 4,820

The total number of days with influenza symptoms will be 5,390 workdays −4,820 workdays = 570 days lower if Flu-wonder is added to the formulary. As a result of these analyses, the manager has good reason to believe that adding Flu-wonder to the formulary will result in a healthier population with only a small increase in cost.

## PROBLEMS AND ISSUES IN DECISION ANALYSIS

## How Realistic are Decision Models?

Decision models must make a tradeoff between comprehensively and completely representing all elements of a decision and being simple enough to use. Decision models get very large and complicated when they incorporate all aspects of the decision. Consequently, most models have to be simplified. In this regard, Detsky et al.[2] argued that a decision model does not need to be a complete representation of a decision situation, but only a model that includes the most important elements of the decision. They argued that the decision model, to be useful, only needs to "capture the key issues necessary to fully describe the risk-benefit tradeoff." Thus, good decision models are simplified by concentrating on the most critical elements of the decision and ignoring minor or lesser concerns. The most critical elements are usually those that represent the tradeoffs among the decision options. For the Flu-wonder example, these included the costs of the treatments, their relative effectiveness, and the probability and cost of hospitalization. The lesser concerns included those that will not have a major impact on the decision either because they are extremely rare, are easily and inexpensively handled, or have no lasting effects. For the Flu-wonder example, the cost of antipyretic drugs, such as aspirin or acetaminophen, were ignored because of their low cost.

Detsky et al.[2] also pointed out that the complexity of a model is frequently limited by availability of data. However, they also stated that in their experience, "the insights derived from a simple model are similar to those derived from a complex formulation."

## Where Can Probability Values and Outcome Values Be Found?

The validity of a decision analysis depends on the validity of the data used in it. Thus, it is critical to have valid measures of the probability of events and of the value of their outcomes. These measures can be taken from randomized, controlled clinical trials; observational studies; published literature reviews; or expert opinion.

### Randomized Controlled Clinical Trials

The ISPOR Lexicon[8] defines a randomized, controlled, clinical trial (RCCT) as "an experimental study designed to test the efficacy, safety, or effectiveness of a health care intervention, in which people are randomly allocated to experimental or control groups, and the outcomes are compared. The experimental group or groups receive the intervention of interest, while the control group receives a placebo or usual care." RCCTs are conducted under conditions that are carefully controlled to ensure that the only difference between the experimental and control groups is the intervention of interest. In addition to randomly assigning patients to groups, the determination of which group will receive the intervention and which will be the control group is also randomly determined. Random assignment means that patients and treatments are assigned in such a way that the investigator cannot bias, intentionally or unintentionally, which is assigned to a particular group. For example, assignment of treatments to groups could be made by flipping a coin or assignment of individuals to groups could be made using a table of random numbers.

If a sufficiently large group of patients is involved, random assignment will result in equivalent groups. That is, the groups will be the same in terms of their severity of disease, number and type of comorbidities, age, gender, etc. Because randomization minimizes both differences between groups and investigator bias, any differences found between the groups' outcomes can be attributed to the intervention. If one group were substantially older, or more female, or less ill than the other, then we could not be confident that differences in outcome were due to differences in treatments.

In addition to randomization, RCCTs carefully control other factors in the study. Patients are treated according to strict written protocols so that all get the same level of care. Study monitors are employed to ensure that physicians treat patients according to the protocol. This ensures that differences in outcomes are not due to differences in physician practice patterns. Study nurses are employed to ensure that patients are compliant with their medicines and that they show up for scheduled appointments.

The strength of RCCTs is that any differences found between group outcomes can reliably be attributed to differences in the treatments administered to the groups and not to extraneous factors such as differences in demographics, underlying illness, or physician practice style. Because of this, RCCTs are said to have high *internal validity*.

However, because RCCTs are conducted under highly controlled conditions, they may not accurately reflect real-world medical practice. Thus, the extent to which the results of RCCTs can be applied to populations other than the one in the trial is limited. This is referred to as low *external validity*. As an example of this problem, assume that a certain drug is shown to be very effective in an RCCT. Also assume that the drug nauseates most patients who take it. In the RCCT, the drug may have been effective because patients took it as they were instructed. This would have occurred because study nurses constantly reminded and persuaded patients to take the medicines. In the real world, however, compliance would be much lower due to the side effect. If effectiveness were related to compliance, then this would lead to lower effectiveness in the real world than in the RCCT. The term *efficacy* is frequently used to describe how well a treatment works under ideal conditions (such as an RCCT), while *effectiveness* is used to describe how well the treatment works under real-world conditions.

RCCTs are generally regarded as the best source of medical information—including probability and outcome estimates. They are considered to be the best source of information because of their high internal validity. However, one must keep in mind that the results of RCCTs may not be strictly applicable to the real world. Because of this, estimates from RCCTs should be considered as best-case estimates. In addition, because RCCTs are conducted under strict medical protocols, they are not the best sources of cost information. Because the protocols used in RCCTs do not accurately reflect real-world care, they also fail to accurately reflect real-world costs.

Pharmacists usually get RCCT data from the published literature. They may also be able to get results of unpublished trials from the pharmaceutical company that is marketing the product.

## Observational Studies

The ISPOR Lexicon[8] defines an observational study as "a study in which the actual experiences of the groups being compared are simply observed, often retrospectively (e.g., after the event of interest, such as receipt of a drug or surgical procedure) but also sometimes prospectively." The strength of observational studies is that they reflect real-world practice patterns. Their weakness is lack of internal validity. In observational studies, there is no assurance that the groups being compared are equivalent. They could, and frequently do, differ on important variables such as disease severity, level of education, and age.

An example may clarify this. Several years ago, the federal government published statistics describing mortality rates of hospitals. These data were published to provide information that patients and insurers could use in selecting the highest-quality hospitals. This was an observational study. The results indicated that mortality rates at many teaching hospitals were substantially higher than those at rural and community hospitals. Did this mean that the quality of care was substantially lower at teaching hospitals? This would not be a reasonable conclusion, because patients treated at teaching hospitals are much sicker. Typically, patients are referred to teaching hospitals because they cannot be adequately treated at rural and community hospitals. So, the differences in mortality rates were more a reflection of teaching hospitals treating sicker patients than of teaching hospitals providing lower-quality care.

Well-conducted observational studies measure, and attempt to adjust for, differences between groups. This is frequently done as part of the statistical analysis. Even with these adjustments, observational studies' internal validity is not as high as RCCTs'. Consequently, they may not be as useful as RCCTs for estimates of probabilities and outcomes. As with RCCTs, pharmacists obtain information from observational studies from the published literature and from pharmaceutical companies.

## Literature Reviews

If the treatments being considered are not new, there is a chance that literature reviews evaluating their safety and effectiveness have been published. These are good sources of probability and outcome data because they incorporate the results of numerous studies.

## Expert Opinion

A common problem with pharmacoeconomic analyses for formulary decisions is that there is little published data on the drug of interest because it is a new product. When published data are not available, costs, probabilities, and outcome information for a decision analysis may have to come from expert opinion.

Expert opinion involves gathering information from experts to answer questions in the areas of their expertise. For a decision analysis of a cancer drug, experts would include physicians, pharmacists, and nurses who had substantial experience in treating cancer patients. These professionals would be asked to give their opinions about the potential effectiveness of the drug, the probabilities of different side effects, and the type of care that would normally be provided to patients with this type of cancer.

Expert opinion is believed to be less valid than results from research studies. Consequently, estimates generated from expert opinion should be subjected to rigorous sensitivity analyses.

## Additional Information

Additional information about finding and selecting probabilities and outcomes for decision analyses can be found in Naglie et al.[9] Petitti,[5] and Gold.[10]

## ADVANTAGES OF USING DECISION ANALYSIS

Using decision analysis offers decision makers two advantages over less formal techniques. First, decision analysis requires a systematic approach to making decisions. It requires the decision maker to carefully and logically think through the decision and to define the decision that must be made, the various decision alternatives, the outcomes of those alternatives, and the probabilities associated with each outcome. Structuring the decision in this way aids logical thinking. Having to think through the decision and explicitly list alternatives and their consequences helps the decision maker consider all aspects of the decision.

Second, decision analysis makes the reasoning behind the decision explicit. A well-done decision analysis explicitly states what the decision is and what the decision maker assumed in selecting a particular course of action. In addition, decision analysis makes it easier to communicate the decision and the process of arriving at the decision to others. This allows for more productive discussion of the merits of a particular decision. Rather than simply disagree with the decision, interested parties can examine the process and discuss particular estimates, assumptions, or values with which they disagree. Focusing on particular points of disagreement is likely to lead to a more focused and useful discussion.

## SUMMARY

Decision analysis is a systematic, quantitative means of making decisions in uncertain conditions. It requires the decision maker to explicitly and clearly state the decision to be made, the various decision alternatives, and the probable consequences of each option. Decision analysis is used frequently in pharmacoeconomics because of its utility in helping decision makers determine the expected values of both cost and effectiveness outcomes.

### References

1. Weinstein MC, Fineberg H V. Clinical Decision Analysis. Philadelphia: W.B. Saunders Company, 1980.
2. Detsky AS, Naglie G, Krahn MD, et al. Primer on medical decision analysis: part 1—getting started. Med Decis Making 1997;17:123–125.
3. DATA 4.0. Williamstown, MA: Treeage Software, Inc., 2001.
4. Krahn MD, Naglie G, Naimark D, et al. Primer on medical decision analysis: part 4—analyzing the model and interpreting the results. Med Decis Making 1997;17:142–151.
5. Petitti DB. Meta-analysis, Decision Analysis, and Cost-effectiveness Analysis: Methods for Quantitative Synthesis in Medicine. New York: Oxford University Press, 2000.
6. Langley PC. Meeting the information needs of drug purchasers: the evolution of formulary submission guidelines. Clin Ther 1999;21:768–787.
7. Anon., The AMCP Format for Formulary Submissions, version 2.1. J Manage Care Pharm 2005;11(Suppl):1–21.
8. Anon., ISPOR Lexicon. Princeton, NJ: International Society for Pharmacoeconomics and Outcomes Research, 1998.

9. Naglie G, Krahn MD, Naimark D, et al. Primer on medical decision analysis: part 3—estimating probabilities and utilities. Med Decis Making 1997;17: 136–141.

10. Gold MR, ed. Cost-Effectiveness in Health and Medicine. New York: Oxford University Press, 1996.

## QUESTIONS

1. Decision analysis is most useful for making decisions:
   a. under conditions of uncertainty
   b. when there is not a clearly superior course of action
   c. when tradeoffs must be made among alternate courses of action
   d. All at the above
2. The expected benefit of a decision alternative is based on:
   a. the probability that the alternative will be successful
   b. the benefit the alternative will provide if it is successful
   c. Both of the above
3. Decision analysis involves which of the following?
   a. Probabilities
   b. Use of qualitative techniques
   c. Calculation of expected costs and benefits
   d. All of the above
   e. a and c only
4. On the decision tree, which of the following indicates that the selection of alternatives is under the decision maker's control?
   a. Choice node
   b. Chance node
5. Which type of study has the highest internal validity?
   a. Randomized, controlled, clinical trial
   b. Observational study
6. The extent to which the differences in outcomes between treatment and control groups in a study can be attributed to differences in treatments given to the groups is known as:
   a. internal validity
   b. external validity
7. The results of a randomized, controlled, clinical trial provide an estimate of the treatment's:
   a. efficacy
   b. effectiveness
8. The major weakness of observational studies is:
   a. they poorly reflect real-world practice patterns
   b. differences in outcomes between treatment and control groups may be due to factors other than different treatments
   c. they are conducted in strictly controlled environments
9. Sensitivity analysis is used to:
   a. determine the effects of variations in estimated values on the final result of the decision analysis
   b. deal with uncertainty of estimates

    c.  assess the degree of confidence one should place in the results of the decision analysis

    d.  All of the above

10.  A clinical pharmacist must recommend the best drug for a rheumatoid arthritis patient. Drug A has been shown to be effective in 90% of patients and to result in a 50% decrease in symptoms in those patients in whom it is effective. Drug B is effective in 30% of patients and results in a 90% decrease in symptoms in those patients in whom it is effective. Which drug should the pharmacist recommend? Why?

    a.  Drug A, because it is effective in more patients

    b.  Drug A, because it has the highest expected benefit

    c.  Drug B, because it results in the greatest reduction in symptoms

11.  Which of the following should be used to determine which agent from a new class of pain medications should be added to the formulary?

    a.  Cost-effectiveness analysis

    b.  Systems-based approach

12.  Which of the following should be used to estimate the change in an HMO's budget that will result from the addition of a new pain reliever to the formulary?

    a.  Cost-effectiveness analysis

    b.  Systems-based approach

13.  Which of the following explicitly considers patterns of drug use in the population to be treated?

    a.  Cost-effectiveness analysis

    b.  Systems-based approach

## PROBLEMS

Bleedless is a drug used to reduce the need for blood transfusions in patients undergoing cardiac artery bypass graft (CABG) surgery. CABG patients frequently need blood transfusions. Bleedless decreases bleeding, and consequently the need for transfusions, during CABG surgery. Use the following decision tree to answer the following questions. The outcomes of the paths are cost (e.g., $40,000 in the Yes—Need transfusion path) and probabilities of surviving surgery (1.0 or 100% for the Yes—Need transfusion path).

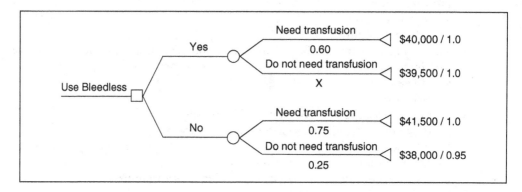

1.  What is the correct value of "X" in the figure?

2.  What is the expected cost of using Bleedless?

3.  What is the expected effectiveness of not using Bleedless?

4.  What is the cost-effectiveness ratio for using Bleedless?

# Answers to Questions and Problems

## CHAPTER 2

## Answers to Questions

1. **a.** Expense
   **b.** Expense
   **c.** Liability
   **d.** Asset
   **e.** Asset
   **f.** Expense
   **g.** Liability
   **h.** Owner equity
   **i.** Revenue

2. **a.** Balance sheet
   **b.** Balance sheet
   **c.** Balance sheet or capital statement
   **d.** Capital statement or statement of retained earnings
   **e.** Income statement, capital statement, or statement of retained earnings
   **f.** Balance sheet, capital statement, or statement of retained earnings

3. **a.** Decrease
   **b.** Decrease
   **c.** Decrease
   **d.** No effect

4. **a.** $5,000
   **b.** $250,000
   **c.** $20,000

      d. ($10,000)—by convention, accountants denote negative values using parentheses
      e. $55,000
      f. $3,000

5. c.

6. c.

7. c.

8. c.

## Answers to Problems

**1.**

| Method | Year | Depreciation Expense | Accumulated Depreciation |
|---|---|---|---|
| Straight line | 1 | 3,000 | 3,000 |
| | 2 | 3,000 | 6,000 |
| | 3 | 3,000 | 9,000 |
| Double declining balance | | | |
| | 1 | 6,667 | 6,667 |
| | 2 | 2,222 | 8,889 |
| | 3 | 111 | 9,000 |

**2.**

| Method | Year | Depreciation Expense | Accumulated Depreciation |
|---|---|---|---|
| Sum of years digits | 1 | 1,667 | 1,667 |
| | 2 | 1,333 | 3,000 |
| | 3 | 1,000 | 4,000 |
| | 4 | 667 | 4,667 |
| | 5 | 333 | 5,000 |
| Double declining balance | | | |
| | 1 | 2,000 | 2,000 |
| | 2 | 1,200 | 3,200 |
| | 3 | 720 | 3,920 |
| | 4 | 432 | 4,352 |
| | 5 | 648 | 5,000 |

**3.**

| Method | Year | Depreciation Expense | Accumulated Depreciation |
|---|---|---|---|
| Sum of years digits | 1 | 8,000 | 8,000 |
| | 2 | 6,000 | 14,000 |
| | 3 | 4,000 | 18,000 |
| | 4 | 2,000 | 20,000 |

Straight line

| | | | |
|---|---|---|---|
| | 1 | 5,000 | 5,000 |
| | 2 | 5,000 | 10,000 |
| | 3 | 5,000 | 15,000 |
| | 4 | 5,000 | 20,000 |

# CHAPTER 3

## Answers to Questions and Problems

1. **a.** Debit
   **b.** Credit
   **c.** Credit
   **d.** Debit
   **e.** Credit
   **f.** Credit
   **g.** Credit
   **h.** Debit
   **i.** Debit
   **j.** Debit

2.

### Journal

| Date | Account Title and Explanation | Dr. | Cr. |
|---|---|---|---|
| 1-1-X1 | Cash | 5,000 | |
| | Sales | | 5,000 |
| | Record cash sales | | |
| 1-5-X1 | Rent expense | 500 | |
| | Cash | | 500 |
| | Record payment of rent expense | | |
| 3-10-X1 | Computer | 9,000 | |
| | Cash | | 9,000 |
| | Record purchase of computer | | |
| 4-1-X1 | Salary expense | 5,000 | |
| | Cash | | 5,000 |
| | Record salary expense | | |
| 5-30-X1 | Utility expense | 200 | |
| | Cash | | 200 |
| | Record payment of utility bill | | |
| 6-1-X1 | Accounts receivable | 500 | |
| | Sales | | 500 |
| | Record credit sales | | |

| 7-3-X1 | Supplies | 200 | |
| | Accounts payable | | 200 |
| | Record purchase of supplies on credit | | |

| 12-27-X1 | Supplies | 500 | |
| | Cash | | 500 |
| | Record purchase of supplies | | |

3.

## Trial Balance
## Big Bill's Consulting Service
## December 31, 20X1

| Account Name | Debit | Credit |
| --- | --- | --- |
| Cash | 950 | |
| Accounts receivable | 1,100 | |
| Supplies | 500 | |
| Furniture | 250 | |
| Accumulated depreciation: furniture | | 50 |
| Accounts payable | | 225 |
| Accrued salaries payable | | 100 |
| Accrued taxes payable | | 100 |
| B. Bill, capital | | 1,900 |
| B. Bill, withdrawal | 100 | |
| Consulting revenue | | 2,200 |
| Rent expense | 100 | |
| Phone expense | 25 | |
| Salary expense | 1,200 | |
| Depreciation expense | 50 | |
| Property tax expense | 100 | |
| Supplies expense | 200 | |
| Totals | 4,575 | 4,575 |

## Big Bill's Consulting Service
## Income Statement Year Ended
## December 31, 20X1

| | | |
| --- | --- | --- |
| Consulting revenue | | $2,200 |
| Expenses | | |
| Salaries | $1,200 | |
| Supplies | 200 | |
| Rent | 100 | |
| Property tax | 100 | |
| Depreciation | 50 | |
| Phone | 25 | |
| Total expenses | | 1,675 |
| Net income | | $ 525 |

**Big Bill's Consulting Service**
**Statement of Capital**
**For the Year Ended December 31, 20X1**

| | |
|---|---:|
| Capital, B. Bill, January 1 | $1,900 |
| Add net income | 525 |
| Less owner withdrawals | 100 |
| Capital, B. Bill, December 31 | $2,325 |

**Big Bill's Consulting Service**
**Balance Sheet**
**December 31, 20X1**

**Assets**

| | | |
|---|---:|---:|
| Cash | | $ 950 |
| Accounts receivable | | 1,100 |
| Supplies | | 500 |
| Furniture | 250 | |
| Less: accumulated depreciation | 50 | |
| Net furniture | | 200 |
| Total assets | | $2,750 |

**Liabilities**

| | |
|---|---:|
| Accounts payable | 225 |
| Accrued taxes payable | 100 |
| Accrued salaries payable | 100 |
| Total liabilities | $ 425 |

**Owner's equity**

| | |
|---|---:|
| B. Bill, capital | $2,325 |
| Total liabilities plus owner's equity | $2,750 |

**Closing Entries**
**Journal**
**Big Bill's Consulting Service**

| Date | Account Title and Explanation | Dr. | Cr. |
|---|---|---:|---:|
| 12-31-X1 | Consulting revenue | 2,200 | |
| | ISA | | 2,200 |
| | Close revenue to ISA | | |
| 12-31-X1 | ISA | 1,675 | |
| | Rent expense | | 100 |
| | Phone expense | | 25 |
| | Salary expense | | 1,200 |
| | Depreciation expense | | 50 |
| | Property tax expense | | 100 |
| | Supplies expense | | 200 |
| | Close expense accounts to ISA | | |

| 12-31-X1 | ISA | 525 | |
| | B. Bill, capital | | 525 |
| | Close ISA to capital | | |
| 12-31-X1 | B. Bill, Capital | 100 | |
| | B. Bill, Withdrawal | | 100 |
| | Close owner withdrawal to capital | | |

4. **a, c.** No adjustment is needed because the expense was incurred and payment was made during the same accounting period.

   **b, d.** An adjustment is needed because the expense was incurred in one period and payment made in a later period.

   **e.** No adjustment is needed because the revenue is recognized when sales are made, not when payment is received.

   **f.** An adjusting entry will be necessary in each year of the car's useful life to reflect use of the car—an expense.

   **g.** Adjusting entries are needed to reflect use of the computer in each year of its life (depreciation expense) and use of the cash from the loan (interest expense). The adjustment for interest expense is needed because no interest will be paid until the end of the fifth year of the loan.

5. Transaction data are collected in income statement accounts for only one accounting period. At the end of each period, income statement accounts are closed; their balances are transferred and reset to zero. Transaction data are collected in balance sheet accounts over the entire life of the business. These accounts are not closed.

6. Closing entries are needed for c, d, e, and f. The remaining accounts are balance sheet accounts that are never closed.

7.

### New Service Company
### Income Statement
### Year Ended December 31, 20X2

| Consulting revenue | | $60,000 |
|---|---|---|
| Expenses | | |
| Salaries | $46,200 | |
| Supplies | 5,000 | |
| Depreciation | 4,000 | |
| Utilities | 1,800 | |
| Misc. | 1,000 | |
| Interest | 375 | |
| Total expenses | 58,375 | |
| Net income | | $ 1,625 |

## New Service Company
## Statement of Capital
## For the Year Ended December 31, 20X2

| | |
|---|---|
| Capital, J. Smith, January 1, 20X2 | $39,000 |
| Add net income | 1,625 |
| Capital, J. Smith, December 31, 20X2 | $40,625 |

## New Service Company Balance Sheet
## December 31, 20X2

**Assets**

| | | |
|---|---|---|
| Cash | | $ 4,000 |
| Accounts receivable | | 17,000 |
| Supplies | | 3,000 |
| Equipment | $40,000 | |
| Less: accum. depreciation | 4,000 | |
| Net equipment | | 36,000 |
| Total assets | | $60,000 |
| **Liabilities** | | |
| Accounts payable | | 9,000 |
| Note payable | | 10,000 |
| Accrued interest payable | | 375 |
| Total liabilities | | $19,375 |
| **Owner's equity** | | |
| J. Smith, Capital | | $40,625 |
| Total liabilities plus owner's equity | | $60,000 |

## Closing Entries
## Journal
## New Service Company

| Date | Account Title and Explanation | Dr. | Cr. |
|---|---|---|---|
| 12-21-X2 | Consulting revenue | 60,000 | |
| | Income summary account | | 60,000 |
| | Close consulting revenue to income | | |
| | Summary account | | |
| 12-31-X2 | Income summary account | 58,375 | |
| | Salary expense | | 46,200 |
| | Utility expense | | 1,800 |
| | Misc. expense | | 1,000 |
| | Depreciation expense | | 4,000 |
| | Supplies expense | | 5,000 |
| | Interest expense | | 375 |
| | Close expense to income | | |
| | Summary account | | |

| 12-31-X2 | Income summary account | 1,625 | |
| | J. Smith, capital | | 1,625 |
| | Close income summary to capital | | |

8.

## Journal
## Long-Term Care Consultants

| Date | Account Title and Explanation | Dr. | Cr. |
|---|---|---|---|
| 8-1-X5 | Cash | 1,000 | |
| | L. Smith, capital | | 1,000 |
| | Record owner investment in business | | |
| 8-3-X5 | Supplies | 100 | |
| | Cash | | 100 |
| | Record purchase of supplies | | |
| 8-5-X5 | Furniture | 500 | |
| | Accounts payable | | 500 |
| | Record purchase of office furniture on account | | |
| 8-7-X5 | Accounts receivable | 250 | |
| | Consulting fees | | 250 |
| | Record billing to Golden Agers Home for services provided | | |
| 8-10-X5 | Cash | 400 | |
| | Consulting fees | | 400 |
| | Record billing to Old Sailors Home for services provided | | |
| 8-18-X5 | Rent expense | 250 | |
| | Cash | | 250 |
| | Record payment of August rent | | |
| 8-25-X5 | L. Smith, withdrawals | 100 | |
| | Cash | | 100 |
| | Record owner withdrawal | | |
| 8-28-X5 | Utilities expense | 50 | |
| | Cash | | 50 |
| | Record payment of August utilities | | |
| 8-30-X5 | Accounts payable | 100 | |
| | Cash | | 100 |
| | Record payment on account for furniture | | |

### Long-Term Care Consultants
### Trial Balance
### August 31, 20X5

| Account Name | Debit | Credit |
| --- | --- | --- |
| Cash | 800 | |
| Accounts receivable | 250 | |
| Supplies | 100 | |
| Furniture | 500 | |
| Accounts payable | | 400 |
| L. Smith, capital | | 1,000 |
| P. Smith, withdrawal | 100 | |
| Consulting fees | | 650 |
| Rent expense | 250 | |
| Utilities expense | 50 | |
| Salary expense | | |
| Totals | 2,050 | 2,050 |

### Long-Term Care Consultants
### Income Statement
### Month Ended August 31, 20X5

| | | |
| --- | --- | --- |
| Consulting revenue | | $650 |
| Expenses | | |
| Rent | $250 | |
| Phone | 50 | |
| Total | | 300 |
| Net income | | $350 |

### Long-Term Care Consultants
### Statement of Capital
### For the Month Ended August 31, 20X5

| | |
| --- | --- |
| Capital, L. Smith, August 1 | $1,000 |
| Add: net income | 350 |
| Less: L. Smith, withdrawal | 100 |
| Capital, L. Smith, August 31 | $1,250 |

## Long-Term Care Consultants
## Balance Sheet
## August 31, 20X5

**Assets**

| | | |
|---|---|---|
| Cash | $800 | |
| Accounts receivable | 250 | |
| Supplies | 100 | |
| Furniture | 500 | |
| Total assets | | $1,650 |
| **Liabilities** | | |
| Accounts payable | $400 | |
| Total liabilities | | 400 |
| **Owner's equity** | | |
| L. Smith, capital | | $1,250 |
| Total liabilities plus owner's equity | | $1,650 |

## CHAPTER 4

## Answers to Questions

1. **a.**

2. **a.**

3. **a.** Perpetual
   **b.** Periodic
   **c.** Perpetual
   **d.** Perpetual
   **e.** Perpetual
   **f.** Periodic
   **g.** Perpetual

4. **c.**

5. **c.**

6. **c.**

## Answers to Problems

1. Weighted average method: COGS = $616.35; EI = $58.70
   FIFO: COGS = $615.00; EI = $60.00
   LIFO: COGS = $622.50; EI = $52.50

2. The *calculated* values are as follows:
   Weighted average method: COGS = $5,332; EI = $318
   FIFO: COGS = $5,350; EI = $300
   LIFO: COGS = $5,280; EI = $370

However, ending inventory must be valued at the lower of cost or market. Because the cost of amoxicillin has declined over the year, the ending inventory must be valued at the replacement cost. Hence, in all three cases ending inventory must be valued at $300. This is calculated as 20 bottles on hand multiplied by $15—the current market or replacement cost. To recognize that it has suffered a loss on the value of inventory, as calculated in the weighted average or LIFO system, the pharmacy must also record and expense—"Write Down on Inventory Loss." This loss would amount to $18 in the weighted average system and $70 in LIFO.

3. COGS = $325,000; EI = $50,000

# CHAPTER 5

## Answers to Problems

1. Financial statement analysis for Apple Blossom Pharmacy.

|  | Computed Ratios | |
| --- | --- | --- |
|  | Apple Blossom | Typical Pharmacy |
| *Overall performance* | | |
| Return on equity | 24.0 | 41.9 |
| Return on assets | 3.9 | 23.2 |
| *Profitability* | | |
| GM% | 32.1 | 42.8 |
| NI% | 1.4 | 8.9 |
| *Liquidity* | | |
| Current ratio | 1.8 | 3.2 |
| Quick ratio | 1.2 | 2.4 |
| Accounts payable period | 71.4 | 33.5 |
| *Efficiency* | | |
| ARCP | 51.0 | 57.7 |
| Inventory turnover | 7.2 | 7.3 |
| Asset turnover | 2.8 | 2.6 |
| *Solvency* | | |
| CL/OE | 277 | 50 |
| LTD/OE | 247 | 30 |
| TD/OE | 523 | 81 |
| Financial leverage | 6.2 | 1.8 |

Comparing Apple Blossom Pharmacy's computed ratios with those of comparable pharmacies reveals several major problems. Both ROE and ROA are much below average. Both the gross margin and net income percents are below average. The problems with net profitability and overall performance result from the lower than average gross margin. If the gross margin were average or above, the net income percent and overall performance measures would be adequate.

Liquidity is a problem. The current and quick ratios are less than average, and the accounts payables period is more than twice the average. This suggests difficulty paying bills on time. Gross margin may be lower as a result of losing cash discounts or of having to purchase merchandise from higher-priced sources.

Apple Blossom Pharmacy's debt-to-equity ratios are very high. The common size statements indicate that the pharmacy has higher than average accounts payables and long-term debt and much lower than average owner equity.

The DuPont Model reveals a similar picture. ROE is lower than average. This is primarily due to much lower than average net profitability, which is, in turn, a result of a low gross margin. Asset turnover is average and, therefore, not a reason for low ROE. Financial leverage is much higher than average. This leads to higher ROE but also to high financial risk. Apple Blossom needs to reduce its financial leverage. The common size statements indicate that financial leverage is high due to high accounts payables and long-term debt and low owner equity.

In addressing the pharmacy's problems, the manager should concentrate on improving the gross margin percent. This may require examining the pharmacy's purchasing practices and identifying lower-cost sources of merchandise. Finding a way to pay for purchases on time might also improve the gross margin (assuming the pharmacy was losing purchase discounts). Increasing the gross margin percent would increase net income in both percent and dollars. The extra profit could be retained in the business (which would increase owner equity) and used to decrease debt. Both would improve solvency. Finally, the additional cash flow from increased profits would improve liquidity.

2. Financial statement analysis for Tarboro Pharmacy.

| | Computed Ratios | | |
|---|---|---|---|
| | Tarboro Pharmacy | | Comparable Pharmacies |
| | 20X1 | 20X2 | 20X2 |
| *Overall performance* | | | |
| Return on equity | 31.7 | 32.6 | 22.6 |
| Return on assets | 21.6 | 15.6 | 13.6 |
| *Profitability* | | | |
| GM% | 31.3 | 29.9 | 27.3 |
| NI% | 5.5 | 3.9 | 3.6 |
| *Liquidity* | | | |
| Current ratio | 3.2 | 2.6 | 3.2 |
| Quick ratio | 0.9 | 0.7 | 1.5 |
| Accounts payable period | 33.1 | 41.2 | 23.4 |
| *Efficiency* | | | |
| ARCP | 25.0 | 25.4 | 34.3 |
| Inventory turnover | 4.1 | 4.1 | 5.9 |
| Asset turnover | 3.9 | 4.0 | 3.7 |
| *Solvency* | | | |
| CL/OE | 42.1 | 76.0 | 45.8 |
| LTD/OE | 4.7 | 33.5 | 20.3 |
| TD/OE | 46.8 | 109.5 | 66.1 |
| Financial leverage | 1.5 | 2.1 | 1.7 |

For 20X2, Tarboro Pharmacy's ROE and ROA were substantially better than average. The gross margin percent was better than average, and the net income percent was somewhat better than average. Common size statements show that Tarboro's expenses were higher than average.

The current ratio was lower than average, but acceptable. The quick ratio suggested some problem with liquidity. Tarboro's accounts payables period was much longer than normal, which suggested that the pharmacy did not pay its trade creditors on time.

The debt-to-equity ratios were higher than average, which suggests solvency problems. In terms of efficiency, both the accounts receivables collection period and asset turnover were better than average. Inventory turnover, on the other hand, was substantially worse than average.

The DuPont Model shows Tarboro's ROE to be above average. This is due to higher than average net profitability, asset turnover, and financial leverage.

Comparison of changes from 20X1 to 20X2 provided a more negative view of Tarboro Pharmacy's performance. Profitability, both gross and net, declined substantially, as did ROA. ROE increased slightly but only because of the substantial decrease in owner's equity. Solvency and liquidity deteriorated due to major increases in accounts payables and long-term debt. The manager of Tarboro Pharmacy needs to determine why performance deteriorated so much over the year.

A major question for this pharmacy is why owner equity declined during 20X2. If all of a pharmacy's net income is retained in the business, the owner equity will increase by the amount of net income. Thus, Tarboro's owner equity for 20X2 should have increased by $41,100. This would have yielded a year-end owner equity of $238,100. In fact, owner equity was $126,100. This indicates that the owner withdrew $112,000 from the business. Over the same time period, the pharmacy took on additional long-term debt of $33,000. A major question is why these events occurred. They had a detrimental effect on both solvency and liquidity. The manager would also want to investigate the decrease in gross margin percent in 20X2. This was responsible for the decreases in net income percent, ROE, and ROA.

3. Sawbones's hospital pharmacy had an inventory turnover of 8.75, a drug expense per patient day of $120, and a personnel expense per patient day of $11.42. Compared with the typical hospital pharmacy of this type, Sawbones Pharmacy uses inventory less efficiently and personnel much more efficiently than the typical pharmacy.

4. Computed ratios for Rivbo Pharmacy and averages for a comparable group of chain pharmacies:

|  | Chain Averages | Rivbo— 20X4 | Rivbo— 20X3 |
|---|---|---|---|
| ROE | 20.0 | 15.4 | 7.7 |
| ROA | 9.8 | 7.3 | 3.3 |
| GM% | 28.3 | 30.4 | 30.1 |
| NI% | 3.7 | 3.1 | 1.6 |
| CR | 1.9 | 1.7 | 1.7 |
| QR | 0.3 | 0.2 | 0.2 |
| APP | 30.1 | 37.6 | 35.6 |
| CL to OE | 57.6 | 68.2 | 72.7 |
| LTD to OE | 44.1 | 44.0 | 57.5 |

| TD to OE | 101.8 | 112.2 | 130.2 |
|---|---|---|---|
| Fin. leverage | 2.0 | 2.1 | 2.3 |
| ITO | 4.1 | 3.5 | 3.3 |
| ATO | 2.7 | 2.4 | 2.1 |

Comparing Rivbo's ratios with those of similar pharmacies indicates problems in the areas of overall performance, profitability, and efficiency. Rivbo's liquidity and solvency are somewhat worse than average but probably are not major problems. Both ROE and ROA are well below average. The gross profit margin is above average, while net income percent is below average. This suggests that expenses are above average. Examination of common size statements shows this to be true. The lower than average net income is a major reason for lower than average ROE and ROA. Efficiency problems are suggested by lower than average inventory turnover and asset turnover. Examination of common size statements indicates that inventory and fixed assets are higher than normal. A trend analysis indicates that Rivbo has improved its performance in all areas except liquidity since 20X3. Although the accounts payables period was a little longer in 20X4, overall liquidity was about the same as in 20X3.

The DuPont Model results provide little additional insight. They indicate that Rivbo Pharmacy's ROE is less than average because of lower than average net income percent and asset turnover. The results of the analyses indicate that Rivbo's main problems are expense control and inventory turnover. These are the areas managers should focus on to improve Rivbo Pharmacy's financial performance. The improvement in these areas from 20X3 to 20X4 suggests that management is aware of the problems and is successfully addressing them. In addition, the higher than average accounts payables period should be investigated further. This would include determining whether Rivbo Pharmacy was losing discounts as a result of late payment and whether the long payment period was a result of managers' skill in prolonging the payment period or of cash flow problems.

## CHAPTER 6

## Answers to Questions

1. e

2. d

3. f

4. e

5. a

6. b

7. e

8. c

9. e

10. b

11. a

12. e

13. d

14. d

15. c

16. e

17. e

18. c

19. d

## Answers to Problems

1. **a.** Steady-gro Pharmacy had sales increases of 12.0% in 20X2; 12.5% in 20X3; 7.9% in 20X4; and 11.8% in 20X5. The average increase for this period was 11.1%. If the manager assumes stable economic conditions, then estimated sales for 20X6 will be about 11.1% greater in 20X6 than in 20X5. This would yield estimated 20X6 sales of $422,000.

   **b.** An additional 5% increase in inflation would probably result in a 5% increase in sales. Thus, 20X6 sales would be estimated as 20X5 sales, plus the 11.1% increase under stable conditions, plus an additional 5% increase for inflation. This would amount to $422,000 × 1.05 = $443,000.

   **c.** The increase attributable to advertising would be in addition to that normally expected. Thus, estimated sales for 20X6 would consist of the expected 11.1% increase plus the 10% or 15% for advertising. This would amount to $422,000 × 1.10 = $464,000 for a 10% increase or $422,000 × 1.15 = $485,000 for a 15% increase.

2. **a.** Market potential = 50,000 visits per year × 4 days per visit
                         = 200,000 patient days per year.

   **b.** Demand forecast = Market potential × Market share
                         = 200,000 patient days × 0.3
                         = 60,000 patient days

   **c.** Expense budget

   | | |
   |---|---|
   | Purchases | $3,000,000 |
   | Personnel | 1,200,000 |
   | Other direct expenses | 300,000 |
   | Total expenses | $4,500,000 |

   Flexible expense budget

   | | | | |
   |---|---|---|---|
   | Patient days | 40,000 | 60,000 | 80,000 |
   | Fixed expenses | | | |
   | Personnel | $1,200,000 | $1,200,000 | $1,200,000 |
   | Other direct expenses | 300,000 | 300,000 | 300,000 |
   | Total fixed expenses | 1,500,000 | 1,500,000 | 1,500,000 |
   | Variable expenses | | | |
   | Purchases | 2,000,000 | 3,000,000 | 4,000,000 |
   | Total expenses | $3,500,000 | $4,500,000 | $5,500,000 |

3. **a.** The significant variances include sales and gross margin—both of which exceed 10% of the budgeted amounts—and pharmacist salaries, housekeeping, and advertising expenses.

   **b.** A comparison indicates that budgeted and actual gross margin *percents* are the same. Thus, it is unlikely that prices are lower than planned or that the pharmacy sold a different mix of merchandise. Hence, the sales variance is most likely due to a decrease in unit sales.

   **c.** The expense variances are favorable because the actual amount was less than the budgeted amount so net income was increased. However, if these variances occur regularly, they could be contributing to the unfavorable sales variance. The lower than budgeted advertising expense may be responsible for lower sales because customers are not as likely to be attracted to the pharmacy. The lower housekeeping expense may be indicative of a dirty, poorly kept store. The lower pharmacist expense could indicate that pharmacists do not have time to give personal attention to patients. All three factors could lead to a loss of sales.

# CHAPTER 7

## Answers to Problems

1. Cash budget for Urbana Pharmacy

| Sales forecast | June | July | Aug. | Sept. | Oct. | Nov. |
|---|---|---|---|---|---|---|
| Cash sales (30%) | $15,900 | $14,400 | $17,700 | $2,7900 | $24,300 | $37,800 |
| Credit sales (70%) | 37,100 | 33,600 | 41,300 | 65,100 | 56,700 | 88,200 |
| Total | 53,000 | 48,000 | 59,000 | 93,000 | 81,000 | 126,000 |
| Cash receipts | | | | | | |
| Cash sales (this month) | | | 17,700 | 27,900 | 24,300 | 37,800 |
| 75% of last month's credit sales | | | 25,200 | 30,975 | 48,825 | 42,525 |
| 25% of credit sales 2 months ago | | | 9,275 | 8,400 | 10,325 | 16,275 |
| Total monthly cash receipts | | | 52,175 | 67,275 | 83,450 | 96,600 |
| Cash payments | | | | | | |
| Purchases (70% of next month's sales) | | | 65,100 | 56,700 | 88,200 | 108,500 |
| Salaries | | | 11,000 | 12,000 | 12,000 | 15,000 |
| Rent | | | 1,750 | 1,750 | 1,750 | 1,750 |
| Other expenses (5% of monthly sales) | | | 2,950 | 4,650 | 4,050 | 6,300 |
| Total monthly cash payments | | | 80,800 | 75,100 | 106,000 | 131,550 |
| Monthly cash gain (loss) | | | (28,625) | (7,825) | (22,550) | (34,950) |
| Financing | | | | | | |
| Cash balance: beginning of month | | | 10,000 | 5,000 | 5,000 | 5,000 |

| | | | | |
|---|---|---|---|---|
| Monthly cash gain (loss) | (28,625) | (7,825) | (22,550) | (34,950) |
| Cash balance: end of month before financing | (18,625) | (2,825) | (17,550) | (29,950) |
| Borrowing | 23,625 | 7,825 | 22,550 | 34,950 |
| Repayment | 0 | 0 | 0 | 0 |
| Cash balance: end of month after financing | 5,000 | 5,000 | 5,000 | 5,000 |
| Cumulative borrowing | 23,625 | 31,450 | 54,000 | 88,950 |

| Sales forecast | Dec | Jan | Feb |
|---|---|---|---|
| Cash sales (30%) | $46,500 | $21,000 | $19,500 |
| Credit sales (70%) | 108,500 | 49,000 | 45,500 |
| Total | 155,000 | 70,000 | 65,000 |
| Cash receipts | | | |
| Cash sales (this month) | 46,500 | 21,000 | |
| 75% of last month's credit sales | 66,150 | 81,375 | |
| 25% of credit sales 2 months ago | 14,175 | 22,050 | |
| Total monthly cash receipts | 126,825 | 124,425 | |
| Cash payments | | | |
| Purchases (70% of next month's sales) | 49,000 | 45,500 | |
| Salaries | 15,000 | 11,000 | |
| Rent | 1,750 | 1,750 | |
| Other expenses (5% of monthly sales) | 7,750 | 3,500 | |
| Total monthly cash payments | 73,500 | 61,750 | |
| Monthly cash gain (loss) | 53,325 | 62,675 | |
| Financing | | | |
| Cash balance: beginning of month | 5,000 | 5,000 | |
| Monthly cash gain (loss) | 53,325 | 62,675 | |
| Cash balance: end of month before financing | 58,325 | 67,675 | |
| Borrowing | 0 | 0 | |
| Repayment | 53,325 | 35,625 | |
| Cash balance: end of month after financing | 5,000 | 32,050 | |
| Cumulative borrowing | 35,625 | 0 | |

**2. Cash budget for Williams Pharmacy**

| | Jan | Feb | Mar | Apr | May |
|---|---|---|---|---|---|
| Total sales estimate | $50,000 | $45,000 | $50,000 | $40,000 | $35,000 |
| Cash sales (85%) | 42,500 | 38,250 | 42,500 | 34,000 | 29,750 |
| Credit sales (15%) | 7,500 | 6,750 | 7,500 | 6,000 | 5,250 |

|  |  |  |  |  |  |
|---|---|---|---|---|---|
| **Collections** |  |  |  |  |  |
| Cash sales (this month) | 42,500 | 38,250 | 42,500 | 34,000 | 29,750 |
| Credit sales (last month) | 4,800 | 6,000 | 5,400 | 6,000 | 4,800 |
| Credit sales (2 months ago) | 1,080 | 1,200 | 1,500 | 1,350 | 1,500 |
| Total monthly cash | 48,380 | 45,450 | 49,400 | 41,350 | 36,050 |
| **Payments** |  |  |  |  |  |
| Purchases | 25,600 | 32,000 | 28,800 | 32,000 | 25,600 |
| Operating expenses | 13,150 | 13,150 | 13,150 | 13,150 | 13,150 |
| Total payments | 38,750 | 45,150 | 41,950 | 45,150 | 38,750 |
| Net cash gain (loss) | 9,630 | 300 | 7,450 | (3,800) | (2,700) |
| Cash balance (beg. month) | 12,000 | 21,630 | 21,930 | 29,380 | 25,580 |
| Monthly gain (loss) | 9,630 | 300 | 7,450 | (3,800) | (2,700) |
| Cash bal. bef. financing | 21,630 | 21,930 | 29,380 | 25,580 | 22,880 |
| Borrowing to meet minimum | 0 | 0 | 0 | 0 | 0 |
| Cash bal. after financing | 21,630 | 21,930 | 29,380 | 25,580 | 22,880 |
| Cumulative borrowing before repayment | 0 | 0 | 0 | 0 | 0 |
| Repayment | 0 | 0 | 0 | 0 | 0 |
| Net cumulative borrowing | 0 | 0 | 0 | 0 | 0 |
| Cash balance EOM | 21,630 | 21,930 | 29,380 | 25,580 | 22,880 |

| June | July | Aug | Sept | Oct | Nov | Dec |
|---|---|---|---|---|---|---|
| $35,000 | $20,000 | $20,000 | $25,000 | $40,000 | $40,000 | $50,000 |
| $29,750 | 17,000 | 17,000 | 21,250 | 34,000 | 34,000 | 42,500 |
| 5,250 | 3,000 | 3,000 | 3,750 | 6,000 | 6,000 | 7,500 |
| 29,750 | 17,000 | 17,000 | 21,250 | 34,000 | 34,000 | 42,500 |
| 4,200 | 4,200 | 2,400 | 2,400 | 3,000 | 4,800 | 4,800 |
| 1,200 | 1,050 | 1,050 | 600 | 600 | 750 | 1,200 |
| 35,150 | 22,250 | 20,450 | 24,250 | 37,600 | 39,550 | 48,500 |
| 22,400 | 22,400 | 12,800 | 12,800 | 16,000 | 25,600 | 25,600 |
| 13,150 | 13,150 | 13,150 | 13,150 | 13,150 | 13,150 | 13,150 |
| 35,550 | 35,550 | 25,950 | 25,950 | 29,150 | 38,750 | 38,750 |
| (400) | (13,300) | (5,500) | (1,700) | 8,450 | 800 | 9,750 |
| 22,880 | 22,480 | 10,180 | 10,680 | 10,980 | 10,430 | 11,230 |
| (400) | (13,300) | (5,500) | (1,700) | 8,450 | 800 | 9,750 |
| 22,480 | 9,180 | 4,680 | 8,980 | 19,430 | 11,230 | 20,980 |
| 0 | 1,000 | 6,000 | 2,000 | 0 | 0 | 0 |
| 22,480 | 10,180 | 10,680 | 10,980 | 19,430 | 11,230 | 20,980 |
| 0 | 1,000 | 7,000 | 9,000 | 9,000 | 0 | 0 |
| 0 | 0 | 0 | 0 | 9,000 | 0 | 0 |
| 0 | 1,000 | 7,000 | 9,000 | 0 | 0 | 0 |
| 22,480 | 10,180 | 10,680 | 10,980 | 10,430 | 11,230 | 20,980 |

## 3. Cash budget for Cooper-Con

| Sales forecast | Nov | Dec | Jan | Feb | Mar | Apr | May | Jun |
|---|---|---|---|---|---|---|---|---|
| Credit sales (100%) | $15,000 | $12,000 | $15,000 | $12,000 | $8,000 | $8,000 | $10,000 | $12,000 |
| *Cash receipts* | | | | | | | | |
| 60% of last month's credit sales | | | 7,200 | 9,000 | 7,200 | 4,800 | 4,800 | 6,000 |
| 40% of credit sales 2 months ago | | | 6,000 | 4,800 | 6,000 | 4,800 | 3,200 | 3,200 |
| Total monthly cash receipts | | | 13,200 | 13,800 | 13,200 | 9,600 | 8,000 | 9,200 |
| *Cash payments* | | | | | | | | |
| Salaries | | | 6,000 | 6,000 | 6,000 | 6,000 | 6,000 | 6,000 |
| Rent and utilities | | | 4,000 | 4,000 | 4,000 | 4,000 | 4,000 | 4,000 |
| Other expenses  (14% of sales) | | | 2,100 | 1,680 | 1,120 | 1,120 | 1,400 | 1,680 |
| Total monthly cash payments | | | 12,100 | 11,680 | 11,120 | 11,120 | 11,400 | 11,680 |
| Monthly cash gain (loss) | | | 1,100 | 2,120 | 2,080 | (1,520) | (3,400) | (2,480) |
| *Financing* | | | | | | | | |
| Cash balance: beginning of month | | | 2,000 | 3,100 | 5,220 | 7,300 | 5,780 | 2,380 |
| Monthly cash gain (loss) | | | 1,100 | 2,120 | 2,080 | (1,520) | (3,400) | (2,480) |
| Cash balance: end of  month before financing | | | 3,100 | 5,220 | 7,300 | 5,780 | 2,380 | (100) |
| Borrowing | | | 0 | 0 | 0 | 0 | 0 | 3,000 |
| Repayment | | | 0 | 0 | 0 | 0 | 0 | 0 |
| Cash balance: end of month after financing | | | 3,100 | 5,220 | 7,300 | 5,780 | 2,380 | 2,900 |
| Cumulative borrowing | | | 0 | 0 | 0 | 0 | 0 | 3,000 |

285

## CHAPTER 8

### Answers to Questions

1. a
2. c
3. e
4. a
5. a
6. b

### Answers to Problems

1. CM% = 0.280, BEP = $1,258,929

2. SEP = $1,346,429; sales increase = $21,429

3. New sales volume = $1,258,750; new CM% = 0.242; SEP = $1,533,058; sales increase needed to maintain current profit = $274,308

4. CM% = 0.236; BEP = $2,176.91 (million)

5. New CM% = .220; SEP = $2,685.23 (million); sales increase = $231.31 (million)

6. BEP = 9,375 IVs. This is about 26 per day so the service cannot be run profitably.

7. BEP = 7,143 IVs. This is about 20 per day so the service can break even at a $30 per IV charge.

## CHAPTER 9

### Answers to Questions

1. a
2. b
3. b
4. b
5. c
6. b
7. c
8. c
9. a
10. b
11. d

12. c

13. c

14. e

15. a

16. c

17. c

18. a

19. b

20. a

21. c

22. d

23. e

24. e

25. e

26. a

27. a

28. b

29. e

## Answers to Problems

1. CTD = $5.54

2. CTD at 18,000 prescriptions = $6.80; CTD at 30,000 prescriptions = $4.28

3. a. $18.98
   b. $2.35
   c. $10.67
   d. $52.25

4. $17.00 price and 29.4% markup; $17.50 price and 31.4% markup

5. MU-R:
   a. $12.50
   b. $3.63
   c. $40.71
   d. $106.15
   e. $40.32

   MU-C:
   a. $10.50
   b. $2.90
   c. $37.05
   d. $93.15
   e. $34.50

## CHAPTER 10

### Answers to Questions

    1. c

    2. d

    3. e

    4. a

    5. b

    6. b

    7. a

### Answers to Problems

    1. **a.** The pharmacy would find it profitable to participate. Differential revenues =$15,000, differential costs = $7,500, and contribution margin = $7,500.

       **b.** The pharmacy would find it profitable to participate. Differential revenues = $15,000, differential costs = $2,500, and the contribution margin = $12,500.

       **c.** The pharmacy would not find it profitable to participate. Differential revenues = $15,000, differential costs = $17,500, and the contribution margin is ($2,500).

    2. Differential revenues = ($750,000), differential costs = ($725,000), contribution margin = ($25,000). Thus, the chain's profits would *decrease* by $25,000 if it closed the store.

    3. **a.** Differential revenues = $1,200, differential costs = $150, contribution margin = $1,050. Net income increases by $1,050.

       **b.** Differential revenue = ($2,400), differential costs = 0 because the same number of prescriptions are dispensed, contribution margin = ($2,400). Net income decreases by $2,400.

       **c.** Differential revenue = ($3,600), differential costs = ($150), contribution margin = ($3,450). Net income decreases by $3,450.

## CHAPTER 11

### Answers to Questions

    1. f

    2. b

    3. a

    4. b

    5. a

    6. d

7. b

8. a

9. b

10. b

## Answers to Problems

1. **a.** $3,180
   **b.** $15,135
   **c.** $2,580
   **d.** $13,450
   **e.** $965
   **f.** $1,553
   **g.** $9,478
   **h.** $15,363
   **i.** $3,667
   **j.** $1,815

2. PV inflows:

| | | |
|---|---|---|
| Year 1: 5,000 × 0.909 | = | $4,545 |
| Year 2: 25,000 × 0.826 | = | 20,650 |
| Year 3: 50,000 × 0.751 | = | 37,550 |
| Year 4: 50,000 × 0.683 | = | 34,150 |
| Year 5: 50,000 × 0.621 | = | 31,050 |
| Year 6: 50,000 × 0.564 | = | 28,200 |
| Year 7: 50,000 × 0.513 | = | 25,650 |
| Year 8: 50,000 × 0.467 | = | 23,350 |
| Year 9: 50,000 × 0.424 | = | 21,200 |
| Year 10: 50,000 × 0.386 | = | 19,300 |
| Total | | $245,645 |

| | |
|---|---|
| PV inflows | $245,645 |
| PV outflow | 200,000 |
| NPV | 45,645 |

Because the NPV is positive, the investment should be made.

3. NPV at $12,000 annual savings:

| | |
|---|---|
| Cash in: | |
| Pretax cash inflow | $12,000 per year |
| Annual depreciation (50,000/5) = | 10,000 |
| Additional taxable income | 2,000 |
| Tax rate | × .40 |
| Additional tax | $    800 |
| After-tax cash inflow 12,000 − 800 = | 11,200 |
| PV at 10% for 5 years = 11,200 × 3.791 = | 42,460 |

PV of cash inflows     $42,460
PV of cash outflows      50,000
NPV                              (7,540)

NPV at $15,000 annual savings:

Cash in:

| | |
|---|---|
| Pretax cash inflow | $15,000 per year |
| Annual depreciation (50,000/5) | 10,000 |
| Additional taxable income | 5,000 |
| Tax rate | × .40 |
| Additional tax | $2,000 |
| After-tax cash inflow 12,000 − 2,000 = | 13,000 |
| PV at 10% for 5 years = 13,000 × 3.791 = | 49,283 |

PV of cash inflows     $49,283
PV of cash outflows      50,000
NPV                              (717)

The investment should not be made because even at the higher savings estimate, the NPV is negative.

4. Cash in:

| | |
|---|---|
| Pretax cash inflow | $25,000 per year |
| Annual depreciation (80,000/5) | 16,000 |
| Additional taxable income | 9,000 |
| Tax rate | × .30 |
| Additional tax | $2,700 |
| After-tax cash inflow 25,000 − 2,700 = | 22,300 |
| PV at 12% for 5 years = 22,300 × 3.605 = | 80,392 |

PV of cash inflows     $80,392
PV of cash outflows      80,000
NPV                              392

Because the NPV is positive, the investment should be made.

## CHAPTER 12

## Answers to Questions

1. b

2. e

3. a

4. e

5. e

6. a

7. e

# Answers to Problems

1.

## Sources and Uses Statement

### Rose Pharmacy
### 20X5

| | |
|---|---:|
| Sources of cash | |
| Net income | $17,375 |
| Depreciation | 1,000 |
| Increase in accounts payable | 6,500 |
| Increase in note payable—current | 400 |
| Total sources | $25,275 |
| | |
| Uses of cash | |
| Owner withdrawal | $6,375 |
| Increase in cash account | 2,400 |
| Increase in accounts receivable | 1,000 |
| Increase in inventory | 12,500 |
| Decrease in long-term debt | 3,000 |
| Total uses | $25,275 |

Rose Pharmacy's major sources of cash were net income plus depreciation and, to a lesser extent, the increase in accounts payable. Major uses were an increase in inventory and an owner withdrawal. Because the major source is net income plus depreciation, Rose Pharmacy is able to generate sufficient cash through operations to meet its cash needs.

Long-term sources of cash consisted of net income plus depreciation and totaled $18,375. Long-term uses were repayment of long-term debt and an owner withdrawal. These totaled $9,375. Thus, long-term sources exceeded long-term uses by a large amount. Technically, this suggests potential cash flow problems. However, because the source was primarily cash from operations (net income plus depreciation), a cash flow problem should not be likely.

2.

## Sources and Uses Statement
### King's Pharmacy
### Year Ended 12/31/20X1

| | |
|---|---:|
| Sources of cash | |
| Net income | $48,251 |
| Add depreciation | 1,825 |
| Net cash from sale of property and equipment | 34,093 |
| Increase in accounts payable | 4,180 |
| Total sources | $88,349 |

| Uses of cash | |
|---|---|
| Owner withdrawal | $41,324 |
| Increase in cash account | 19,339 |
| Increase in accounts receivable | 3,831 |
| Increase in inventory | 7,992 |
| Decrease in long-term debt | 15,863 |
| Total uses | $88,349 |

King's Pharmacy's major sources of cash were net income plus depreciation and cash generated by sale of property and equipment. Major uses were an owner withdrawal, repayment of long-term debt, and an increase in the cash account. King's Pharmacy appears to be able to meet its cash needs primarily through the profitable operation of the pharmacy. A large source of cash was sale of assets. However, much of this was used to pay off long-term debt.

Long-term sources of cash included net income plus depreciation and cash generated from sale of property and equipment. These totaled $84,169. Long-term uses were repayment of long-term debt and owner withdrawal. These totaled $57,187. Thus, long-term sources exceeded long-term uses by a large amount. This is an unusual situation. King's Pharmacy's manager sold property and equipment and used the proceeds to pay off long-term debt and finance increases in the current accounts. Normally, the fact that long-term sources and uses do not match indicates a potential cash flow problem. However, in this case, where much of the excess of long-term sources end up as an increase in the cash account, the possibility of a problem is small.

3.

### Sources and Uses Statement
### Goodwill Pharmacy
### Year Ended 12/31/20X1

| Sources of cash | |
|---|---|
| Net income | $229,631 |
| Add depreciation | 18,479 |
| Decrease in cash | 25,563 |
| Decrease in prepaid expenses | 19,883 |
| Increase in accounts payable | 18,201 |
| Increase in accrued expenses | 8,362 |
| Total sources | $320,119 |
| | |
| Uses of cash | |
| Owner withdrawal | $172,793 |
| Expenditures on fixed assets | 6,989 |
| Increase in accounts receivable | 116,455 |
| Increase in inventory | 1,540 |
| Decrease in note payable—current | 9,560 |
| Decrease in long-term debt | 12,782 |
| Total uses | $320,119 |

Goodwill Pharmacy's major source of cash was net income plus depreciation. Major uses were an owner withdrawal and an increase in the accounts receivables. Goodwill Pharmacy appears to be able to meet its cash needs primarily through the profitable operation of the pharmacy.

Long-term sources of cash included only net income plus depreciation. These totaled $248,110. Long-term uses were repayment of long-term debt, owner withdrawal, and purchase of fixed assets. These totaled $192,564. Thus, long-term uses were financed with appropriate sources.

The large increase in accounts receivables and the disproportionate increase in accounts payables (as compared with inventory) suggest potential problems with receivables management and liquidity. These should be further investigated with ratio analysis.

## CHAPTER 13

### Answers to Questions

1. **c.** The most appropriate investment for a pharmacy's idle cash would be the savings account. This investment offers low risk and high liquidity. Thus, when the pharmacy needs the cash, it will be readily available. The common stock is probably too risky. The return is high but has been very variable. By investing in this stock, the pharmacy stands the chance of losing cash that it may need to operate the business during the year. The certificate of deposit has a 1-year maturity. If the pharmacy needs the cash during the year, it will not be able to get it without losing any interest that has accumulated.

2. **b.** Pharmacies offer credit with the expectations of increasing sales. Credit programs almost invariably hinder cash flow. The pharmacy hopes that increased profits from increased sales will more than compensate for increased costs and cash flow problems caused by a credit program.

3. The immediate effect of a discount program will be to hinder cash flow. This occurs because a discount program decreases gross margin and, consequently, decreases the amount of cash flowing into the business. The long-run effect would depend on how much the discount increased sales. If the discount program results in a substantial increase in sales, it could increase cash flow in the long run. If the discount did not result in higher sales, it would diminish cash flow.

4. Medicaid programs are a type of credit program. Hence, participation will hinder cash flow in the short run. However, accepting Medicaid reimbursement could increase sales. The long-run effect depends on the extent to which sales are increased.

5. By closing the accounts of habitual late payers, the pharmacy will increase its overall collection rate. This will improve cash flow.

## CHAPTER 14

### Answers to Questions

1. a

2. b

3. b

4. a

5. e

6. d

7. b

8. d

9. a

10. a

11. e

12. e

13. e

14. b

15. a

16. a

17. b

18. c

19. a

20. b

## Answers to Problems

1. **a.** EOQ = 37 bottles; 27 orders per year; TC = $60,548
   **b.** EOQ = 58 bottles; 18 orders per year
   **c.** EOQ = 31 bottles; 33 orders per year
   **d.** ROP = 14 bottles
   **e.** ROP = 28 bottles

2. **a.** EOQ = 365 bottles; TC = $1,005,477
   **b.** Yes, take the deal because it decreases TC to $907,750
   **c.** ROP = 165 bottles
   **d.** ROP = 713 bottles

3. Line A should be stocked because it has the higher GMROI (200% vs. 166%). Although line A has the lower gross margin, its turnover is sufficiently higher than line B's to give the higher GMROI.

4. The hospital pharmacy should purchase from the wholesaler. The wholesaler yields a GMROI of 247% versus 200% for the manufacturer.

5. Both pharmacies realized gross margins of 31%. Jones's had a turnover of 7.31, whereas Smythe's had a turnover of 6.6. Consequently, Jones's Pharmacy's GMROI was higher—231% versus 211%—than Smythe's. Jones should get the bigger bonus.

## CHAPTER 15

### Answers to Questions

1. d
2. c
3. e
4. c
5. c
6. e
7. c
8. c
9. a
10. d
11. b
12. b
13. a
14. a
15. c
16. c
17. b
18. a
19. b
20. c

## CHAPTER 16

### Answers to Questions

1. d
2. c
3. e
4. a
5. a
6. a
7. a
8. b

9. d

10. b

11. a

12. b

13. b

## Answers to Problems

1. 0.40

2. $39,800

3. 99% probability of survival

4. No ratio is calculated because using Bleedless dominates not using Bleedless. That is, Bleedless is more effective and less expensive, so using it (compared with not using it) would result in fewer surgical deaths and would save money.

# Index